New Techniques, Materials and Technologies in Dentistry

New Techniques, Materials and Technologies in Dentistry

Editors

Ricardo Castro Alves
José João Mendes
Ana Cristina Mano Azul

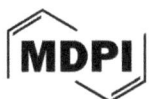

Basel • Beijing • Wuhan • Barcelona • Belgrade • Novi Sad • Cluj • Manchester

Editors

Ricardo Castro Alves
Clinical Research Unit (CRU),
CiiEM, Egas Moniz School of
Health and Science
Almada
Portugal

José João Mendes
Clinical Research Unit (CRU),
CiiEM, Egas Moniz School of
Health and Science
Almada
Portugal

Ana Cristina Mano Azul
Clinical Research Unit (CRU),
CiiEM, Egas Moniz School of
Health and Science
Almada
Portugal

Editorial Office
MDPI
St. Alban-Anlage 66
4052 Basel, Switzerland

This is a reprint of articles from the Special Issue published online in the open access journal *Applied Sciences* (ISSN 2076-3417) (available at: https://www.mdpi.com/journal/applsci/special_issues/dentistry_materials).

For citation purposes, cite each article independently as indicated on the article page online and as indicated below:

Lastname, A.A.; Lastname, B.B. Article Title. *Journal Name* **Year**, *Volume Number*, Page Range.

ISBN 978-3-7258-0097-1 (Hbk)
ISBN 978-3-7258-0098-8 (PDF)
doi.org/10.3390/books978-3-7258-0098-8

© 2024 by the authors. Articles in this book are Open Access and distributed under the Creative Commons Attribution (CC BY) license. The book as a whole is distributed by MDPI under the terms and conditions of the Creative Commons Attribution-NonCommercial-NoDerivs (CC BY-NC-ND) license.

Contents

About the Editors ix

Ricardo Castro Alves, José João Mendes and Ana Cristina Mano Azul
Special Issue on New Techniques, Materials and Technologies in Dentistry
Reprinted from: *Applied Sciences* **2023**, *13*, 11483, doi:10.3390/app132011483 1

José Maria Cardoso, Sofia Duarte, Ana Clara Ribeiro, Paulo Mascarenhas, Susana Noronha and Ricardo Castro Alves
Association between IL-1A, IL-1B and IL-1RN Polymorphisms and Peri-Implantitis: A Systematic Review and Meta-Analysis
Reprinted from: *Applied Sciences* **2022**, *12*, 6958, doi:10.3390/app12146958 5

Ayshe Salim, Sirma Angelova, Bogdan Roussev, Todorka Sokrateva, Yoana Kiselova-Kaneva, Stefan Peev, et al.
Salivary Interleukin-6, Interleukin-1β, and C-Reactive Protein as a Diagnostic Tool for Plaque-Induced Gingivitis in Children
Reprinted from: *Applied Sciences* **2023**, *13*, 5046, doi:10.3390/app13085046 23

Ana-Madalina Raducanu, Sebastian Mihai, Ion Sandu, Andreea Anghel, Cristina Furnica, Raluca Ozana Chistol, et al.
Quantification of Salivary Nitric Oxide in Patients with Fixed Orthodontic Treatment
Reprinted from: *Applied Sciences* **2022**, *12*, 8565, doi:10.3390/app12178565 35

Perrine Saïz, Nuno Taveira and Ricardo Alves
Probiotics in Oral Health and Disease: A Systematic Review
Reprinted from: *Applied Sciences* **2021**, *11*, 8070, doi:10.3390/app11178070 44

Marcela Alcota, Jimena Osorio, Claudia Díaz, Ana Ortega-Pinto, Cristián Peñafiel, Juan C. Rivera, et al.
Effect of the Passive Ultrasonic Irrigation and the Apical Diameter Size on the Debridement Efficacy of Infected Root Canals: A Multivariate Statistical Assessment of Histological Data
Reprinted from: *Applied Sciences* **2021**, *11*, 7495, doi:10.3390/app11167495 63

Kacper Wachol, Tadeusz Morawiec, Agnieszka Szurko, Domenico Baldi, Anna Nowak-Wachol, Joanna Śmieszek-Wilczewska, et al.
Advantages of Dynamic Navigation in Prosthetic Implant Treatment in Terms of the Clinical Evaluation and Salivary Pro-Inflammatory Biomarkers: A Clinical Study
Reprinted from: *Applied Sciences* **2023**, *13*, 9866, doi:10.3390/app13179866 74

Monica Blazquez-Hinarejos, Constanza Saka-Herrán, Victor Diez-Alonso, Raul Ayuso-Montero, Eugenio Velasco-Ortega and Jose Lopez-Lopez
Reliability and Agreement of Three Devices for Measuring Implant Stability Quotient in the Animal Ex Vivo Model
Reprinted from: *Applied Sciences* **2021**, *11*, 3453, doi:10.3390/app11083453 88

Cristiana Gomes Rebelo, Juliana Campos Hasse Fernandes, Nuno Bernardo, Patrícia Couto and Gustavo Vicentis Oliveira Fernandes
Bisphosphonates and Their Influence on the Implant Failure: A Systematic Review
Reprinted from: *Applied Sciences* **2023**, *13*, 3496, doi:10.3390/app13063496 96

Bora Lee, Na-Eun Nam, Seung-Ho Shin, Jung-Hwa Lim, June-Sung Shim and Jong-Eun Kim
Evaluation of the Trueness of Digital Implant Impressions According to the Implant Scan Body Orientation and Scanning Method
Reprinted from: *Applied Sciences* **2021**, *11*, 3027, doi:10.3390/app11073027 111

Hani Tohme, Ghida Lawand, Rita Eid, Khaled E. Ahmed, Ziad Salameh and Joseph Makzoume
Accuracy of Implant Level Intraoral Scanning and Photogrammetry Impression Techniques in a Complete Arch with Angled and Parallel Implants: An In Vitro Study
Reprinted from: *Applied Sciences* 2021, *11*, 9859, doi:10.3390/app11219859 122

Hwa-Jung Lee, June-Sung Shim, Hong-Seok Moon and Jong-Eun Kim
Alteration of the Occlusal Vertical Dimension for Prosthetic Restoration Using a Target Tracking System
Reprinted from: *Applied Sciences* 2021, *11*, 6196, doi:10.3390/app11136196 133

Hwa-Jung Lee, Jeongho Jeon, Hong Seok Moon and Kyung Chul Oh
Digital Workflow to Fabricate Complete Dentures for Edentulous Patients Using a Reversing and Superimposing Technique
Reprinted from: *Applied Sciences* 2021, *11*, 5786, doi:10.3390/app11135786 141

Mariana Manaia, Larissa Rocha, José Saraiva, Ana Coelho, Inês Amaro, Carlos Miguel Marto, et al.
Minimally Invasive Dentistry for Pre-Eruptive Enamel Lesions—A Case Series
Reprinted from: *Applied Sciences* 2021, *11*, 4732, doi:10.3390/app11114732 145

Eva Magni, Wadim Leontiev, Sebastian Soliman, Christian Dettwiler, Christian Klein, Gabriel Krastl, et al.
Accuracy of the Fluorescence-Aided Identification Technique (FIT) for Detecting Residual Composite Remnants after Trauma Splint Removal—A Laboratory Study
Reprinted from: *Applied Sciences* 2022, *12*, 10054, doi:10.3390/app121910054 152

Norberto Quispe-López, Antonio Castaño-Séiquer, Beatriz Pardal-Peláez, Pablo Garrido-Martínez, Cristina Gómez-Polo, Jesús Mena-Álvarez, et al.
Clinical Outcomes of the Double Lateral Sliding Bridge Flap Technique with Simultaneous Connective Tissue Graft in Sextant V Recessions: Three-Year Follow-Up Study
Reprinted from: *Applied Sciences* 2022, *12*, 1038, doi:10.3390/app12031038 162

Joana Santos de Cunha Pereira, José Alexandre Reis, Francisco Martins, Paulo Maurício and M. Victoria Fuentes
The Effect of Feldspathic Thickness on Fluorescence of a Variety of Resin Cements and Flowable Composites
Reprinted from: *Applied Sciences* 2022, *12*, 6535, doi:10.3390/app12136535 175

Cristina Gómez-Polo, Ana María Martín Casado, Norberto Quispe, Eva Rosel Gallardo and Javier Montero
Colour Changes of Acetal Resins (CAD-CAM) In Vivo
Reprinted from: *Applied Sciences* 2023, *13*, 181, doi:10.3390/app13010181 185

Ziaullah Choudhry, Sofia Malik, Zulfiqar A. Mirani, Shujah A. Khan, Syed M. R. Kazmi, Waqas A. Farooqui, et al.
Antifungal Efficacy of Sodium Perborate and Microwave Irradiation for Surface Disinfection of Polymethyl Methacrylate Polymer
Reprinted from: *Applied Sciences* 2022, *12*, 7004, doi:10.3390/app12147004 196

Vitor Anes, Cristina B. Neves, Valeria Bostan, Sérgio B. Gonçalves and Luís Reis
Evaluation of the Retentive Forces from Removable Partial Denture Clasps Manufactured by the Digital Method
Reprinted from: *Applied Sciences* 2023, *13*, 8072, doi:10.3390/app13148072 208

João Cenicante, João Botelho, Vanessa Machado, José João Mendes, Paulo Mascarenhas, Gil Alcoforado, et al.
The Use of Autogenous Teeth for Alveolar Ridge Preservation: A Literature Review
Reprinted from: *Applied Sciences* **2021**, *11*, 1853, doi:10.3390/app11041853 . . . . **223**

Masae Okuno, Sho Aoki, Saki Kawai, Rie Imataki, Yoko Abe, Kyoko Harada, et al.
Effect of Non-Thermal Atmospheric Pressure Plasma on Differentiation Potential of Human Deciduous Dental Pulp Fibroblast-like Cells
Reprinted from: *Applied Sciences* **2021**, *11*, 10119, doi:10.3390/app112110119 . . . . **236**

About the Editors

Ricardo Castro Alves

Ricardo Castro Alves graduated from the Egas Moniz School of Health and Science (Portugal) in 2003, obtained his MSc in Dentistry from Egas Moniz in 2010 and completed his PhD at Granada University (Spain) in 2016. He is a Specialist in Periodontology of the Portuguese Dental Association (OMD) and Secretary of the General Assembly of the Portuguese Society of Periodontology.

Between 2007 and 2016, he was an Assistant Professor of Periodontology. Since 2018, he has been Head of the Periodontology Department at Egas Moniz. He is coordinator of the postgraduate program in Periodontology at Egas Moniz, Head of the Clinical Research Unit of Centro de Investigação Interdisciplinar Egas Moniz and former Secretary and current member of the Egas Moniz Ethics Committee.

José João Mendes

José João Mendes (Prof. Dr.) has served as President of the Egas Moniz School of Health and Science since 2017, and is the elected President of the Egas Moniz Center for Interdisciplinary Research. He completed a DDS at the Egas Moniz School of Health and Science in Portugal in 1995, completed his postgraduate studies in Implantology at the Universitat Bern (Switzerland,1997), obtained an MBA in Health Unit Management from Universidade Católica Portuguesa (2002) and received his PhD in Biomedical Sciences from the ICBAS School of Medicine and Biomedical Sciences (2010). He is Section Editor of the *European Journal of Dentistry* and Associate Editor of *Frontiers in Oral Medicine*. To date, he has authored more than 80 articles and served as the supervisor/co-supervisor of 52 master's and 10 PhD students. Furthermore, he served as Assistant Professor of Conservative Dentistry (MSc in Dentistry of the ISCSEM/IUEM) in 1996, Assistant Professor of Physiology in 1999 (MSc in Dentistry of the ISCSEM/IUEM)—and has been Head of the same Curricular Unit since 2020—Head of the Integrated Dental Clinic Curricular Unit (MSc in Dentistry of the ISCSEM/IUEM) in 2008 and Head of the Curricular Unit on Management and Entrepreneurship in Dental Medicine in 2020. Since 2010, he has held the position of Clinical Director at the Egas Moniz Dental Clinic.

Ana Cristina Mano Azul

Ana Cristina Mano Azul completed her international education at Lycée Français Charles Lepierre (Lisbon). She graduated from the Faculty of Dental Medicine (Lisbon) and obtained a European PhD degree from the Universitat de València (Spain). Ana is an Associate Professor at the Egas Moniz School of Health and Science. Over the last 36 years, she has focused on teaching dental material and conservative dentistry as Head of the school's Conservative Dentistry units. She also serves as Coordinator of the Integrated MSc in Dentistry and the PG Diploma in International Clinical Endodontics. Ana is an integral member of the Egas Moniz Center for Interdisciplinary Research, and her research focuses on materials science and aesthetic dentistry. She has served as President of the Fiscal Council of the Portuguese Dental Association and is currently a member of its General Council. She is currently President of the General Assembly of the Portuguese Society of Stomatology and Dental Medicine.

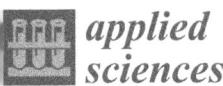

Editorial

Special Issue on New Techniques, Materials and Technologies in Dentistry

Ricardo Castro Alves *, José João Mendes and Ana Cristina Mano Azul

Clinical Research Unit (CRU), CiiEM, Egas Moniz—Cooperativa de Ensino Superior, Caparica, 2829-511 Almada, Portugal; jmendes@egasmoniz.edu.pt (J.J.M.); aazul@egasmoniz.edu.pt (A.C.M.A.)
* Correspondence: ralves@egasmoniz.edu.pt

1. Introduction

Dentistry has seen significant technical and technological advances in recent years. These achievements have made it possible to increase the accuracy of diagnoses and treatment plans, improve the predictability and durability of certain treatments, make procedures safer and faster and improve patient experience and acceptance, among other benefits.

The speed at which these advances are developing justifies the publication of this Special Issue helping clinicians to stay up to date on the latest breakthroughs in this field. This Special Issue covers practically all areas of dentistry: implantology, periodontology, operative dentistry, pediatric dentistry, orthodontics, endodontics and oral rehabilitation. Of the 29 papers submitted to this Special Issue, 21 were accepted. In this Editorial, we highlight some of the main conclusions and impacts of these studies.

2. New Techniques, Materials and Technologies in Dentistry

All patients are different, so the "one size fits all" approach to prevention, diagnosis and treatment is evolving into a more personalized concept of medicine. Better knowledge of patients' genetic profile can help guide clinical decisions. An example of this is peri-implantitis, a growing problem that requires better approaches in terms of prevention and treatment. Cardoso et al. [1] carried out a systematic review via a meta-analysis with the aim of evaluating the association between IL-1A, IL-1B and IL-1RN polymorphisms and peri-implantitis. The results showed that patients who have the polymorphic allele at position +3954 of the IL-1B gene have on average almost twice the risk of developing peri-implantitis.

In the area of disease diagnosis, the use of biomarkers can enable timely diagnosis and better monitoring of disease progression and response to treatment. In an innovative study, Salim et al. [2] evaluated salivary interleukin-6, interleukin-1β and C-reactive protein as a diagnostic tool for plaque-induced gingivitis in children. Based on the results, the authors suggest that salivary IL-1β and CRP can be used as potential diagnostic tools to differentiate between moderate and severe plaque-induced gingivitis.

In another field, Raducanu et al. [3] tested the potential use of salivary nitric oxide as a biomarker of bone response following the application of different types of orthodontic appliances. The results showed that metal brackets lead to a significant temporary increase in oral oxidative stress as an adaptive reaction to the presence of foreign bodies in the oral cavity.

Conventional prevention and treatment strategies of caries, periodontal and peri-implant diseases present some limitations, making it necessary to search for alternatives or adjuvants. Probiotics may play an important role in this context. Saiz et al. [4] carried out a systematic review on the use of probiotics in the prevention and treatment of oral diseases, supporting the existing evidence in this regard. In relation to novel therapeutic approaches, the effect of passive ultrasonic irrigation on the elimination of organic remnant tissue from infected, narrow and curved mandibular root canals during their instrumentation was

---

Citation: Alves, R.C.; Mendes, J.J.; Azul, A.C.M. Special Issue on New Techniques, Materials and Technologies in Dentistry. *Appl. Sci.* **2023**, *13*, 11483. https://doi.org/10.3390/app132011483

Received: 13 October 2023
Accepted: 18 October 2023
Published: 19 October 2023

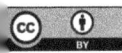

Copyright: © 2023 by the authors. Licensee MDPI, Basel, Switzerland. This article is an open access article distributed under the terms and conditions of the Creative Commons Attribution (CC BY) license (https://creativecommons.org/licenses/by/4.0/).

evaluated in an in vitro study by Alcota et al. [5]. The results suggest that clinicians should incorporate passive ultrasonic irrigation in their regular therapeutic strategy.

Several articles focused on the use of digital technologies in dentistry. This area has seen extremely rapid development in recent years, with a strong impact on clinical practice. For instance, digital technologies bring several advantages, such as reducing errors and complications, faster treatments and faster patient recovery. Wachol et al. [6] evaluated the advantages of dynamic navigation in prosthetic implant treatment in terms of clinical results and salivary pro-inflammatory biomarkers. Dynamic navigation and the application of the flapless technique reduced surgical trauma, leading to a reduced risk of infection, reduced patient discomfort and faster recovery. Implant stability is critical in implant therapy, and there are several devices on the market that allow it to be assessed through resonance frequency analysis and the implant stability coefficient to be calculated. However, there are few studies that have compared the reliability and agreement of different devices. In an in vitro study, Blazquez-Hinarejos et al. [7] compared inter- and intra-rater reliability and the agreement level among three of these devices. Rebelo et al [8] carried out a systematic review on the use of bisphosphonates and implant failure, also identifying other factors such as smoking, poor hygiene, diabetes and hypertension, which increase the risk of failure.

In prosthetic procedures, digital techniques have assumed an increasingly relevant role. Intraoral scanners have gained great clinical acceptance and undergone constant improvements in recent years. Despite this, there are still some relevant issues that need to be investigated. Lee et al. [9] presented a strategy with which operators could acquire more accurate digital impressions in single implant cases in terms of the orientation of the scan body and the scanning method. Until now, stereophotogrammetry has scarcely been investigated in cases of tilted implants. Thome et al. [10] evaluated, in an in vitro study, the accuracy of implant-level intraoral scanning and photogrammetry impression techniques in a complete arch with angled and parallel implants. The alteration of the occlusal vertical dimension for prosthetic restoration using a target-tracking system was evaluated by Lee et al. [11]. This new technique seeks to overcome some of the limitations of conventional methods using mechanical articulators. Also, in oral rehabilitation, concerning removable prosthesis, Lee et al. [12] proposed a digital workflow to fabricate complete dentures for edentulous patients using a reversing and superimposing technique. This four-step, completely digital workflow eliminates the need for conventional impressions and reduces patient discomfort and the number of visits.

Another current trend in dentistry is the use of minimally invasive techniques. Manaia et al. [13] presented a case series of patients with pre-eruptive enamel defects in esthetically compromised tooth regions, which were treated with the microabrasion technique. This technique does not require local anesthesia, is less destructive than restorative interventions and allows good esthetic outcomes with no significant postoperative sensitivity. Distinguishing composite remnants from tooth structure after trauma splint removal can be challenging. Magni et al. [14] compared the fluorescence-aided identification technique with conventional light illumination in terms of accuracy and time required for the detection of composite remnants after trauma splint removal.

In terms of new surgical techniques, [15] evaluated the clinical results of the double lateral sliding bridge flap technique with connective tissue graft in the treatment of isolated and multiple gingival recessions. Treating gingival recessions in the mandibular anterior region is a challenge due to anatomical constraints. This study adds more evidence regarding a technique that is still little addressed in the literature.

Five studies in the field of dental materials were published in this Special Issue. The effect of feldspathic thickness on the fluorescence of a variety of resin cements and flowable composites was evaluated in an in vitro study by Pereira et al. [16]. Color changes in temporary acetal resins manufactured by a fully computerized design and fabrication process were evaluated in vivo by Gómez-Polo et al. [17], with clinically relevant results.

Choudhry et al. [18] tested the antifungal efficacy of sodium perborate and microwave irradiation for the surface disinfection of polymethyl methacrylate polymer, providing a new perspective on the best disinfection strategy for this material.

Also, building a bridge with the digital area, Anes et al. [19] evaluated the retentive forces from removable partial denture clasps manufactured using the digital method. The objective of this study was to evaluate retentive forces and the change in clasps with digitally manufactured different designs over time.

Regarding biomaterials used in bone regeneration and an intersection with the field of new therapeutic approaches, Cenicante et al. [20] carried out a literature review on the use of autogenous dentin in alveolar preservation procedures. In this article, the authors summarize new evidence on the use of autogenous teeth as a biomaterial in ARP, different protocols and future directions.

In terms of translational science, the effect of non-thermal atmospheric pressure plasma on the differentiation potential of human deciduous dental pulp fibroblast-like cells was evaluated by Okuno et al. [21], revealing a potential tool to expand the population of various adult stem cells in vitro for medical applications.

These investigations are united by the common final objective of improving diagnosis accuracy and providing more predictable and long-lasting treatments for patients and with better acceptance. For clinicians, some of these innovative techniques and materials will also make work simpler, faster and more effective.

3. Future Perspectives

Some important topics could not be covered in this Special Issue, and others will require further investigation. Technical and technological advances in dentistry will continue to grow at an incredible speed.

Although this Special Issue is now closed, the success it achieved led us to launch a second edition of "New Techniques, Materials and Technologies in Dentistry". Submissions are now open, so we invite everyone to participate and share their research work.

Acknowledgments: This Special Issue would not be possible without the collaboration of the various talented authors. We would like to take this opportunity to express our sincere gratefulness to all reviewers, who contributed to improving the final quality of the manuscripts. Finally, we would like to thank the editorial team of *Applied Sciences*, and a special thanks goes out to the Section Managing Editor of the MDPI Beijing Office.

Conflicts of Interest: The authors declare no conflict of interest.

References

1. Cardoso, J.; Duarte, S.; Ribeiro, A.; Mascarenhas, P.; Noronha, S.; Alves, R. Association between IL-1A, IL-1B and IL-1RN Polymorphisms and Peri-Implantitis: A Systematic Review and Meta-Analysis. *Appl. Sci.* **2022**, *12*, 6958. [CrossRef]
2. Salim, A.; Angelova, S.; Roussev, B.; Sokrateva, T.; Kiselova-Kaneva, Y.; Peev, S.; Ivanova, D. Salivary Interleukin-6, Interleukin-1β, and C-Reactive Protein as a Diagnostic Tool for Plaque-Induced Gingivitis in Children. *Appl. Sci.* **2023**, *13*, 5046. [CrossRef]
3. Raducanu, A.; Mihai, S.; Sandu, I.; Anghel, A.; Furnica, C.; Chistol, R.; Dinu, C.; Tutunaru, D.; Earar, K. Quantification of Salivary Nitric Oxide in Patients with Fixed Orthodontic Treatment. *Appl. Sci.* **2022**, *12*, 8565. [CrossRef]
4. Saïz, P.; Taveira, N.; Alves, R. Probiotics in Oral Health and Disease: A Systematic Review. *Appl. Sci.* **2021**, *11*, 8070. [CrossRef]
5. Alcota, M.; Osorio, J.; Díaz, C.; Ortega-Pinto, A.; Peñafiel, C.; Rivera, J.; Salazar, D.; Manríquez, G.; González, F. Effect of the Passive Ultrasonic Irrigation and the Apical Diameter Size on the Debridement Efficacy of Infected Root Canals: A Multivariate Statistical Assessment of Histological Data. *Appl. Sci.* **2021**, *11*, 7495. [CrossRef]
6. Wachol, K.; Morawiec, T.; Szurko, A.; Baldi, D.; Nowak-Wachol, A.; Śmieszek-Wilczewska, J.; Mertas, A. Advantages of Dynamic Navigation in Prosthetic Implant Treatment in Terms of the Clinical Evaluation and Salivary Pro-Inflammatory Biomarkers: A Clinical Study. *Appl. Sci.* **2023**, *13*, 9866. [CrossRef]
7. Blazquez-Hinarejos, M.; Saka-Herrán, C.; Diez-Alonso, V.; Ayuso-Montero, R.; Velasco-Ortega, E.; Lopez-Lopez, J. Reliability and Agreement of Three Devices for Measuring Implant Stability Quotient in the Animal Ex Vivo Model. *Appl. Sci.* **2021**, *11*, 3453. [CrossRef]
8. Rebelo, C.; Fernandes, J.; Bernardo, N.; Couto, P.; Fernandes, G. Bisphosphonates and Their Influence on the Implant Failure: A Systematic Review. *Appl. Sci.* **2023**, *13*, 3496. [CrossRef]

9. Lee, B.; Nam, N.; Shin, S.; Lim, J.; Shim, J.; Kim, J. Evaluation of the Trueness of Digital Implant Impressions According to the Implant Scan Body Orientation and Scanning Method. *Appl. Sci.* **2021**, *11*, 3027. [CrossRef]
10. Tohme, H.; Lawand, G.; Eid, R.; Ahmed, K.; Salameh, Z.; Makzoume, J. Accuracy of Implant Level Intraoral Scanning and Photogrammetry Impression Techniques in a Complete Arch with Angled and Parallel Implants: An In Vitro Study. *Appl. Sci.* **2021**, *11*, 9859. [CrossRef]
11. Lee, H.; Shim, J.; Moon, H.; Kim, J. Alteration of the Occlusal Vertical Dimension for Prosthetic Restoration Using a Target Tracking System. *Appl. Sci.* **2021**, *11*, 6196. [CrossRef]
12. Lee, H.; Jeon, J.; Moon, H.; Oh, K. Digital Workflow to Fabricate Complete Dentures for Edentulous Patients Using a Reversing and Superimposing Technique. *Appl. Sci.* **2021**, *11*, 5786. [CrossRef]
13. Manaia, M.; Rocha, L.; Saraiva, J.; Coelho, A.; Amaro, I.; Marto, C.M.; Vale, F.; Ferreira, M.M.; Paula, A.; Carrilho, E. Minimally Invasive Dentistry for Pre-Eruptive Enamel Lesions—A Case Series. *Appl. Sci.* **2021**, *11*, 4732. [CrossRef]
14. Magni, E.; Leontiev, W.; Soliman, S.; Dettwiler, C.; Klein, C.; Krastl, G.; Weiger, R.; Connert, T. Accuracy of the Fluorescence-Aided Identification Technique (FIT) for Detecting Residual Composite Remnants after Trauma Splint Removal—A Laboratory Study. *Appl. Sci.* **2022**, *12*, 10054. [CrossRef]
15. Quispe-López, N.; Castaño-Séiquer, A.; Pardal-Peláez, B.; Garrido-Martínez, P.; Gómez-Polo, C.; Mena-Álvarez, J.; Montero-Martín, J. Clinical Outcomes of the Double Lateral Sliding Bridge Flap Technique with Simultaneous Connective Tissue Graft in Sextant V Recessions: Three-Year Follow-Up Study. *Appl. Sci.* **2022**, *12*, 1038. [CrossRef]
16. Pereira, J.; Reis, J.; Martins, F.; Maurício, P.; Fuentes, M. The Effect of Feldspathic Thickness on Fluorescence of a Variety of Resin Cements and Flowable Composites. *Appl. Sci.* **2022**, *12*, 6535. [CrossRef]
17. Gómez-Polo, C.; Martín Casado, A.; Quispe, N.; Gallardo, E.; Montero, J. Colour Changes of Acetal Resins (CAD-CAM) In Vivo. *Appl. Sci.* **2023**, *13*, 181. [CrossRef]
18. Choudhry, Z.; Malik, S.; Mirani, Z.; Khan, S.; Kazmi, S.; Farooqui, W.; Ahmed, M.; AlAali, K.; Alshahrani, A.; Alrabiah, M.; et al. Antifungal Efficacy of Sodium Perborate and Microwave Irradiation for Surface Disinfection of Polymethyl Methacrylate Polymer. *Appl. Sci.* **2022**, *12*, 7004. [CrossRef]
19. Anes, V.; Neves, C.; Bostan, V.; Gonçalves, S.; Reis, L. Evaluation of the Retentive Forces from Removable Partial Denture Clasps Manufactured by the Digital Method. *Appl. Sci.* **2023**, *13*, 8072. [CrossRef]
20. Cenicante, J.; Botelho, J.; Machado, V.; Mendes, J.; Mascarenhas, P.; Alcoforado, G.; Santos, A. The Use of Autogenous Teeth for Alveolar Ridge Preservation: A Literature Review. *Appl. Sci.* **2021**, *11*, 1853. [CrossRef]
21. Okuno, M.; Aoki, S.; Kawai, S.; Imataki, R.; Abe, Y.; Harada, K.; Arita, K. Effect of Non-Thermal Atmospheric Pressure Plasma on Differentiation Potential of Human Deciduous Dental Pulp Fibroblast-like Cells. *Appl. Sci.* **2021**, *11*, 10119. [CrossRef]

Disclaimer/Publisher's Note: The statements, opinions and data contained in all publications are solely those of the individual author(s) and contributor(s) and not of MDPI and/or the editor(s). MDPI and/or the editor(s) disclaim responsibility for any injury to people or property resulting from any ideas, methods, instructions or products referred to in the content.

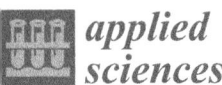

Systematic Review

Association between IL-1A, IL-1B and IL-1RN Polymorphisms and Peri-Implantitis: A Systematic Review and Meta-Analysis

José Maria Cardoso [1,2,*,†], Sofia Duarte [2,†], Ana Clara Ribeiro [1,3], Paulo Mascarenhas [1,3], Susana Noronha [4] and Ricardo Castro Alves [1,2]

1. Centro de Investigação Interdisciplinar Egas Moniz (CiiEM), Instituto Universitário Egas Moniz, Campus Universitário, Quinta da Granja, Monte de Caparica, 2829-511 Almada, Portugal; acribeiro@egasmoniz.edu.pt (A.C.R.); pmascarenhas@egasmoniz.edu.pt (P.M.); ralves@egasmoniz.edu.pt (R.C.A.)
2. Periodontology Department, Instituto Universitário Egas Moniz, Campus Universitário, Quinta da Granja, Monte de Caparica, 2829-511 Almada, Portugal; sofia.alves.duarte@gmail.com
3. Molecular Biology Laboratory, Instituto Universitário Egas Moniz, Campus Universitário, Quinta da Granja, Monte de Caparica, 2829-511 Almada, Portugal
4. Periodontology Department, Faculdade de Medicina Dentária da Universidade de Lisboa, Cidade Universitária, R. Prof. Teresa Ambrósio, 1600-277 Lisboa, Portugal; susanacnoronha@gmail.com
* Correspondence: josencardoso@egasmoniz.edu.pt
† These authors contributed equally to this work.

Featured Application: Feature Application: The evaluation of genetic polymorphisms may have great clinical relevance since they can be measured before the onset of the disease and may be of great benefit for treatment planning and prognosis at an early stage.

Abstract: Recent studies report that individuals with polymorphisms in the genes that encode for interleukin (IL)-1α and IL-1β (IL-1A and IL1B, respectively) and for IL-1 receptor antagonist (IL-1RN) may be more susceptible in developing peri-implantitis. Therefore, the current systematic review evaluates what is reported about the role of genetics, more specifically of single nucleotide polymorphisms (SNP) on IL-1 and variable number of tandem repeats (VNTR) on IL-1RN, in the development of peri-implantitis. This systematic review was carried out by screening PubMed, B-on, Cochrane and Scopus databases, for articles English, Spanish, and Portuguese, with no limit regarding the publication year. Eight articles were selected for systematic review and four for meta-analytic syntheses. Our results show that although there is a lack of consensus in the literature, there seems to be an association between IL-1A, IL-1B, and IL-1RN polymorphisms with peri-implantitis. The results of the meta-analysis showed that patients who have the polymorphic allele at position +3954 of the IL-1B gene have on average almost twice the risk of developing peri-implantitis (*odds ratio* = 1.986, 95% confidence interval).

Keywords: genetics; peri-implantitis; interleukin-1; interleukin-1 receptor antagonist; interleukin-1 genotype; genetic polymorphisms; peri-implant disease

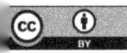

1. Introduction

Dental implants are now considered as an effective and predictable treatment modality for the functional and aesthetic rehabilitation of either partially or completely edentulous patients [1,2]. This rehabilitation method has a success rate of more than 90% for implants in function for more than five years [3]. However, despite the high success rates associated with implant rehabilitation, biological complications may arise in the peri-implant soft tissues, such as peri-implantitis, which can compromise the permanence of the implant [4]. Peri-implantitis is a plaque-associated pathological condition occurring in tissues around dental implants, characterized by inflammation in the peri-implant mucosa and progressive loss of supporting bone [5,6]. This definition is in accordance with the more recent classification of periodontal and peri-implant diseases (American Academy of Periodontology—AAP and European Federation of Periodontology—EFP 2018) [6].

According with the Consensus report of workgroup 4 of the 2017 World Workshop on the Classification of Periodontal and Peri-Implant Diseases and Conditions, there is strong evidence from animal and human experimental studies that plaque is the etiological factor for peri-implant mucositis, which is assumed to precede peri-implantitis [6]. Data indicate that patients diagnosed with peri-implant mucositis may develop peri-implantitis, especially in the absence of regular maintenance care. However, the features or conditions characterizing the progression from peri-implant mucositis to peri-implantitis in susceptible patients have not been identified [6].

With a growing number of dental implants inserted, the potential number of sites for implant-associated diseases increases [7]. But the actual value of the incidence/prevalence of this disease is uncertain since the method of classifying peri-implantitis has varied between authors over the years and, in addition, few studies follow up and evaluate the sample for several years [8]. The characteristics of the populations included also vary between studies, which may influence the results [8]. In a systematic review carried out by Atieh et al., the prevalence of peri-implantitis obtained per patient was 18.8% while the prevalence per implant was 9.6% [9]. Lee et al. conducted a systematic review and meta-analysis, that included forty-seven articles, and concluded that the mean prevalence of peri-implantitis, at implant and subject level was 9.25% and 19.83%, respectively [10].

There are some similar features in the sequence of immunopathological events in peri-implant and periodontal infections [11]. Both are initiated primarily by Gram-negative anaerobic bacteria, while the inflammatory process goes faster and deeper around implants than around natural teeth and thus is a more significant problem for patients with dental implants [12]. However, Becker et al. in a study in which the transcriptome profiling using mRNA from patients suffering from either peri-implantitis or periodontitis was compared, the authors observed that these two pathologies react in a different way [13]. These differences may be explained by the anatomy, which is very different comparing the scar tissue in peri-implantitis with the specialized fibers inserting the surface of the teeth. In peri-implantitis tissue, transcripts associated to innate immune responses, and defense responses were dominating, while in periodontitis tissues, bacterial response systems prevailed [13].

Research evidence indicates that implant complications tend to be clustered in a subset of individuals rather than being randomly distributed in the population implying that patient's host response might play a role for the implant success [14,15].

Interleukin-1 (IL-1) is the pivotal mediator of the immune-inflammatory response that acts both in response to bacterial infection and in bone metabolism [16]. IL-1 family has at least 11 cytokines; clustered on the long arm of chromosome 2q, and the three most studied members are IL-1A, IL-1B, and IL-1RN genes, which encode the agonistic proteins IL-1α and IL-1β, and IL-1 receptor antagonist (IL-1Ra), respectively [17]. The effect of IL-1 is determined by the balance between IL-1α, IL-1β, and IL-1Ra through competitive binding of IL-1Ra to the IL-1 receptor to block the activity of IL-1α or IL-1β. IL1 is strongly induced by lipopolysaccharides from the cell walls of Gram-negative bacteria and acts either directly or indirectly to initiate and amplify inflammatory responses through inducing expression of a substrate of effectors including cytokines/chemokines and matrix metalloproteinases [18].

The variations of IL-1 gene cluster, including IL-1A and IL-1B genes, and the variations of IL-1 RN are the most commonly studied functional polymorphisms for peri-implantitis.

Many studies have investigated different single nucleotide polymorphisms (SNPs) in the IL-1 genes as a risk factor for peri-implantitis. Among them, the IL-1A −889 C/T (rs1800587) and IL-1B +3954 C/T (rs1143634) have been mostly investigated [19]. The IL-1B-511 (rs16944) is also studied in some studies. These polymorphisms are characterized by the substitution of cytosine with thymine in the DNA sequence, which has been demonstrated to be associated with directly changed levels of gene expression and secreted cytokines, respectively [20]. In the IL-1RN gene, there is a genetic polymorphism located in intron 2 which is composed of a variable number of tandem repeats (VNTR) of 86 base pairs length. Several studies have analyzed the relationship between these polymorphisms and peri-implantitis. However, studies have yielded conflicting results on this issue [21–26].

A clarification of the genetic basis associated with peri-implant pathology could be used to predict peri-implantitis occurrence and to improve treatment and monitoring of patients with dental implants [21].

Most of these studies had a relatively small sample size and thus had insufficient statistical power to detect the genetic associations. Some of them do not refer to confounding variables such as periodontal condition, ethnicity and smoking habits. Furthermore, many studies, including published systematic reviews, assess the relationship of these polymorphisms with the peri-implant disease, pooling in the same group patients with bone loss, implant loss, and peri-implantitis [27–29]. However, peri-implant tissue health can exist around implants with variable levels of bone support [6]. In addition, an implant can fail without having an associated chronic inflammatory reaction as occurs in peri-implantitis.

Therefore, we performed a systematic review and meta-analysis, quantitatively synthesizing previous studies, to evaluate the association of common functional polymorphisms in the IL1 and IL-1RN genes with susceptibility to peri-implantitis.

2. Materials and Methods

2.1. Study Design

The guidelines of PRISMA were followed while reporting this systematic review and meta-analysis.

The research question used for this systematic review was: "What is the importance of the interleukin-1 genotype (IL-1A −889 (rs1800587), IL-1B −511 (rs16944), and IL-1B +3954 (rs1143634)) and the IL-1 receptor antagonist genotype (IL-1 RN (rs2234663)) in the development of peri-implantitis, in adults, smokers or not, after at least one year of the implant in function?". In addition, the PECO nomenclature was also used:

P (Population)—Adult patients
E (Exposure)—Genotype including selected polymorphisms of interleukin-1 and its antagonist
C (Control)—Genotype not including selected polymorphisms of interleukin-1 and its antagonist
O (Outcomes/Outcome)—Development of peri-implantitis

A search protocol was specified in advance and registered at PROSPERO (International Prospective Register of Systematic Reviews ID 322662).

2.2. Search Strategy

Two authors (J.M.C.) (S.D.) extracted the specific studies from the databases, and the same authors removed duplicates and irrelevant studies. Discrepancies, if occurred, were resolved by a third researcher (P.M.).

Systematic searches were performed on the PubMed, B-on, Cochrane and Scopus literature databases for studies published until January 2022.

The MESH terms and other keywords were used in combination, and Boolean operators such as AND and/or OR and/or NOT were added to obtain more relevant studies regarding the topic in question [30].

We used a specific search strategy with the following focused key terms:

("dental implants" or "oral implants") and ("polymorphism" or "interleukins" or "interleukin-1"); ("peri-implantitis") and ("interleukin-1" or "interleukins") and ("gene polymorphism" OR "genotype") not animal.

2.3. Inclusion and Exclusion Criteria

The inclusion criteria were: (1) Human case-control studies; (2) peri-implantitis as the outcome of interest in functional implants with at least one year follow up; (3) studies reporting IL-1A −889, IL-1B −511, IL-1B +3954 and IL-1RN (VNTR), and composite genotype of IL-1A −889/IL-1B +3954 polymorphisms; (4) articles written in English, Spanish or Portuguese.

The exclusion criteria were: (1) Studies that included patients with uncontrolled systemic diseases; (2) studies in which patients with peri-implantitis were included in a general category disease group of peri-implant diseases or other conditions (presence of suppuration, development of fistula, radiographic bone loss or implant loss).

The author (S.D.) screened all the titles and abstracts based on the eligibility criteria and included/excluded studies for full-text review. Another author (J.M.C.) rechecked relevant articles. Discrepancies, if occurred, were resolved by a third researcher (P.M.).

2.4. Data Extraction

One author (S.D.) independently extracted the information or data from each study and another author (J.M.C.) rechecked them.

2.5. Risk of Bias Assessment

Two authors (S.D. and P.M.) evaluated the quality of included articles using the Joanna Brigs Institute (JBI) checklist [31]. This tool evaluates "cross-sectional analytical" studies regarding eight domains. These domains evaluate if the criteria in the sample were clearly defined, if the study subjects and the setting were described in detail, if the confounding factors were identified and strategies to deal with, and if the outcomes were measured in a valid and reliable way.

2.6. Statistical Analysis

Statistical analysis was performed using the Open Meta [Analyst] for Windows 8 (built 04/06/2015) software, from Center for Evidence Synthesis in Health (Brown University, Providence, RI, USA), which allowed us to obtain all meta-analysis and meta-regression plots, which are described later [32]. Allele frequencies against peri-implantitis incidence were converted in odds ratios effect size and associated 95% confidence intervals in a binomial model framework. Model parameters were estimated applying the restricted maximum likelihood method.

Heterogeneity was assessed using the I^2 index and it was considered high if it was above 50%. A high I^2 value means that the authors of the different articles analyzed are not in consensus. To counteract this value, covariates can be added [33].

We used 95% confidence intervals and considered the *p*-value test results lower than 0.05 to correspond to a statically significant result.

A subgroup analysis was done in relation of the odds ratio (OR) of the ethnicity in the difference in the frequency of the mutated allele between the disease and control group.

Meta-regressions were carried out for longitude and latitude of the sample's provenance, the mean age, the percentage of males and females, the representative ratio of the mutated allele, sample size and year of publication.

3. Results

3.1. Study Selection

Initially, 324 articles were obtained from all databases. After excluding the duplicates, 218 articles remained, of which the titles and abstracts were read. Since 199 were not included in the theme of this systematic review, they were excluded, leaving only 19. These were read in full and, as eleven articles did not meet the inclusion and exclusion criteria, only eight articles remained, which were included in this systematic review [21–26,34,35]. However, only four of these articles contained eligible quantitative data, and were included in the meta-analysis [21,23,24,26].

A PRISMA flowchart was carried out to systematize the selected information throughout the different research phases (Figure 1).

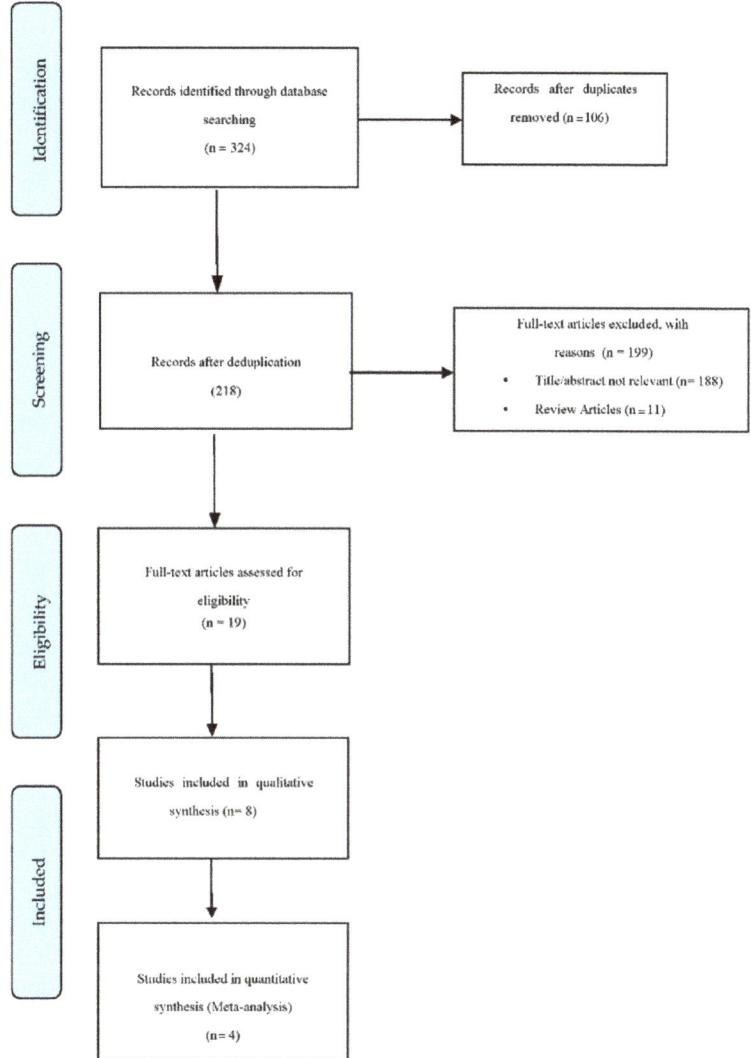

Figure 1. Flow chart of the study selection.

3.2. Results of the Bias Risk Assessment

In order to know the risk of bias in the articles, by completing the JBI checklist, a Traffic Plot-type graph was obtained (Figure A1), where it is possible to clearly observe the risk of bias for each article selected for this systematic review. None of the articles had three or more high risk judgments and they were all included in the review.

3.3. Characteristics of the Studies

The Table 1 provides the characteristics of eight articles [21–26,34,35] included in the systematic review. Four articles included individuals from Europe [21,25,34,35], two from Asia [24,26], one from North Africa [22] and one from South America [23]. Five studies reported IL-1A −889 polymorphism [21,22,24,25,34], two IL-1B −511 [21,23], seven IL-1B +3954 polymorphism [21–26,34], two IL-1RN (VNTR) polymorphism [21,35] and five composite genotype of IL-1A −889 and IL-1B +3954 polymorphisms [21,22,24,25,34].

Table 1. Systematic review table of the eight articles included in the present study.

Year & Author	Type of Study	Polymorphisms Evaluated	Geographic Region	Inclusion Criteria	Exclusion Criteria	Smoking Habits	Time of Implant in Function (Months)	Outcome
Garcia-Delaney, 2015 [34]	Case-control	IL-1A −889 IL-1B +3954 IL-1RN +2018	Spain	Systemically healthy patients; Peri-implantitis group: BOP or SUP (+); BL > 2 mm Control group: BOP (−); SUP (−); BL < 2 mm	- Cases with incomplete data or with dubious diagnosis	All smokers	≥18	IL-1 genotypes do not seem to be good predictors of peri-implantitis in the great majority of smoking patients. Furthermore, no synergic effect was found between IL-1 genotypes and heavy smokers. Patients with a previous history of periodontitis were more prone to peri-implantitis.
Hamdy, 2011 [22]	Case-control	IL-1A −889 IL-1B +3954	Egypt	Systemically healthy patients; Peri-implantitis group: BOP (+); PPD > 4 mm; BL (+)	- Smokers; - History of antibiotic intake or periodontal treatment in previous 6 months	Non-smokers	≥36 (implant placement)	The combination of the polymorphism in IL-1A −889 and IL-1B +3954, in patients with inflamed periodontal or peri-implant tissues, may act as a risk factor that increases tissue destruction. IL-1 gene polymorphism (IL-1A −889 and IL-1B +3954) may have a negative effect on treatment outcomes of peri-implantitis.
He, 2019 [24]	Case-control	IL-1A −889 IL-1B +3954 TNFα −308	China	Peri-implantitis group: PPD ≥ 4 mm; BOP (+); GI (+); BL involving ≥ 2 threads compared to prosthetic placement Control group: Healthy peri-implant tissue: PPD < 3mm; BOP (−); BL (−)	- Smokers; - Pregnant or lactation; - General health problems (diabetes mellitus, HIV infection); - Intake of any antibiotics and anti-inflammatories in the last 3 months.	Non-smokers	≥24	The IL-1A −889 or IL-1B +3954 genetic polymorphisms were associated with the risk of peri-implantitis and periodontal status.
Lachmann, 2007 [25]	Case-control	IL-1A −889 IL-1B +3954	Germany	- Systemic health in general; - Absence of medical conditions that compromise the immune system. Peri-implantitis group—PPD > 4 mm; BOP (+); BL (+)	ND	ND	≥12	The composite IL-1A −889 and IL-1B +3954 genotype investigated exerted only little influence on the peri-implant crevicular immune response, and this influence appeared to be of limited impact in sites with established peri-implantitis lesions.
Laine, 2006 [21]	Case-control	IL-1A −889 IL-1B +3954	Sweden	Peri-implantitis group: BL involving ≥ 3 threads; BOP and/or SUP (+)	ND	Peri-implantitis group—76% smokers Control group—49% smokers	≥24	IL-1RN gene polymorphism is associated with peri-implantitis and may represent a risk factor for this disease.
Melo, 2011 [23]	Case-control	IL-1B +3954 IL-1B −511 IL-6 −174	Brazil	- No medical history of chronic illness; - No history of antibiotic therapy or use of steroidal or AINE medications in the 6 months prior to the study. Control group: no mucosal bleeding, PD ≤ 4 mm, BOP and SUP (−)	- Smokers; - Pregnant or lactation; - Periodontitis	Non-smokers	ND	There was no correlation between the concentration of IL-1β and IL-6 in the crevicular sulcular fluid present in healthy or diseased osseointegrated implants in comparison with healthy teeth. The studied genetic polymorphisms had no influence on peri-implant disease.
Petkovic-Curcin, 2017 [35]	Case-control	IL-6 −174 IL-10 −1082 TNF-α −308 CD14 −159 IL-1RN (VNTR)	Serbia	Peri-implantitis group: PPD ≥ 4 mm, BOP +, GI (+); PI (+) and BL involving ≥ 2 threads compared to prosthetic replacement Control group: Healthy peri-implant tissue, BOP (−), PPD < 4 mm, BL (−)	ND	C—42% smokers PI—71% smoker	≥24	Smoking and the presence of TNFα-308 polymorphism may increase the risk for peri-implantitis, while CD14-159 polymorphism decreases the risk. The results also indicate significant association of CD14-159, TNFα-308, and IL6-174 genotypes and clinical parameters in the Serbian population.

Table 1. *Cont.*

Year & Author	Type of Study	Polymorphisms Evaluated	Geographic Region	Inclusion Criteria	Exclusion Criteria	Smoking Habits	Time of Implant in Function (Months)	Outcome
Saremi, 2021 [26]	Case-control	IL-1B +3954 IL-10 −819 IL-10 −592 TNF-α −308 TNF-α −857	Iran	- No history of periodontitis Peri-implantitis group: PPD > 5 mm; BOP (+) with or without SUP; BL ≥ 2 mm Control group: PPD < 4 mm; BL (−)	- Oral and periodontal diseases (except caries); - Current orthodontic treatment; - History of systemic diseases or any complication that compromises the immune system (diabetes, HIV, hepatitis, chemotherapy); - Pregnant or lactation	ND	≥12	Genetic polymorphisms of IL-10 −819, IL-10 −592 and IL-1B +3954 may play a role in the pathogenesis of peri-implantitis and increase its risk of occurrence.

(+)—presence, (−)—absent, BL—bone loss, BOP—bleeding on probing, SUP—suppuration, GI—gingival index, ND—non-defined, PPD—probing pocket depth, PI—plaque index, VNTR—Variable number of tandem repeats, AINE—non-steroid anti-inflammatory.

The Table A1 provides the percentage of men and women, from which it is possible to conclude that there is a predominance of female individuals in five of the eight articles [21,23,25,26,34]. The mean age varies between 41 and 67 years. The mean age of the sample of each study was considered, since between the group with peri-implantitis and the control group there was no difference in mean age of more than five years.

The mean percentage of the mutated allele in the sample are indicated in four of the eight articles [21,23,24,26]. Some articles only indicated the genotype of the individuals, without referring to whether they were homozygous or heterozygous for the mutated allele, which could influence the results.

3.4. Meta-Analysis

To carry out the meta-analysis, only four articles were used, as explained above [21,23,24,26]. However, due to the lack of information and the different types of polymorphisms analyzed by each article, it was only possible to perform the meta-analytic study for the IL-1B +3954 polymorphism, which was the only common polymorphism in the previously selected articles. In addition, these four articles contained information about the amount of mutated alleles in the sample.

Figure 2 shows the odds ratio (OR) meta-analysis as a forest plot. The OR values extracted from each study are graphically illustrated. This graph performs an analysis of heterogeneity that is expressed in the form of I^2, in %, and presents the mean value of the ORs and the respective uncertainty in the form of a 95% confidence interval. On the left, the authors and the year of the included studies are indicated, followed by the corresponding analytical values obtained.

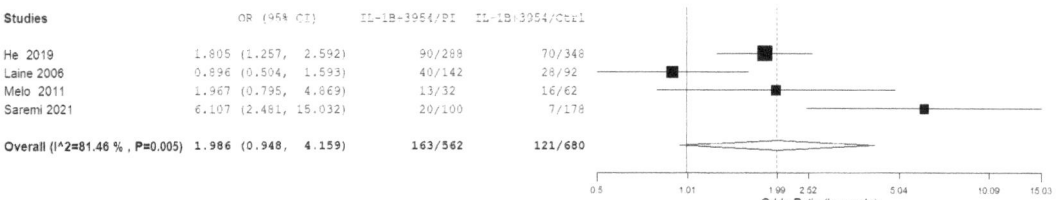

Figure 2. Meta-analysis Forest Plot. (OR—odds ratio, CI—confidence interval, PI—peri-implantitis group, Ctrl—control group). Laine et al., 2006 [21]; Melo et al., 2011 [23]; He et al., 2019 [24]; Saremi et al., 2021 [26].

The odds ratio of these studies is 1.986 (chi square test, $p < 0.001$), which means that this polymorphism increases the risk of carriers of the mutated allele in the IL-1B +3954 to have peri-implantitis, by almost twice, as compared to the control group, patients that do not have this polymorphism.

The I^2 in this case is quite high, which may indicate that the authors are not in agreement with the results they present.

3.5. Subgroup Analysis

The subgroup analyses (based on the ethnicity) of the association between the frequency of the mutated allele in the IL-1B +3954 gene and the risk of peri-implantitis is shown in Figure 3. The results showed that the ethnicity, Asian, is one factor that affects the difference in frequencies of the mutated allele in the IL-1 B3954 gene between the disease and the control groups (OR = 3.088, chi square test, $p < 0.001$). The ethnicity, Caucasian, does not affect the difference in frequencies of the mutated allele in the IL-1 B3954 gene between the disease and the control groups (OR = 0.896, chi square test, $p = 0.709$). Regarding mixed ethnicity, further studies are needed to understand its influence in the difference in frequencies of the mutated allele in the IL-1 B3954 gene between peri-implantitis and control groups (OR = 1.967, chi square test, $p = 0.140$).

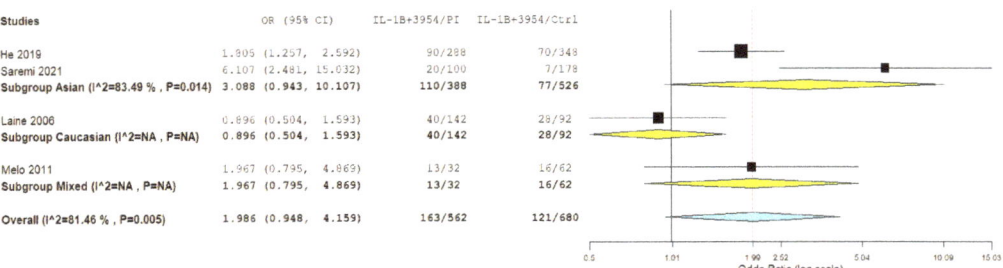

Figure 3. The subgroup analyses (based on the ethnicity) of the association between the frequency of the mutated allele in the IL-1B +3954 gene and the risk of peri-implantitis. (OR—odds ratio, CI—confidence interval, PI—peri-implantitis group, Ctrl—control group). Laine et al., 2006 [21]; Melo et al., 2011 [23]; He et al., 2019 [24]; Saremi et al., 2021 [26].

3.6. Meta-Regression

Regarding meta-regressions, in all there is a limitation, since there are only four points represented in the graphs, only four articles were analyzed. There is, therefore, a limitation to being able to extrapolate this trend to other populations or other geographic regions. Therefore, further studies are recommended in order to confirm this trend.

The size of the circles in all figures represents the weight that this article contributed to the average. Since the OR logarithm is proportional to the OR, with negative coefficient, as the latitude increases, there is a tendency for the OR to decrease, and in this case the trend is statistically supported/significant since the *p*-value obtained was 0.025 (Figure 4). The result of the coefficient statistical test in the longitude-relative meta-regression presents a value of $p = 0.295$, so it is not statistically significant (Figure A2).

Regarding the mean age, the *p*-value in this meta-regression has a value of 0.005, thereby it is statistically significant (Figure 5).

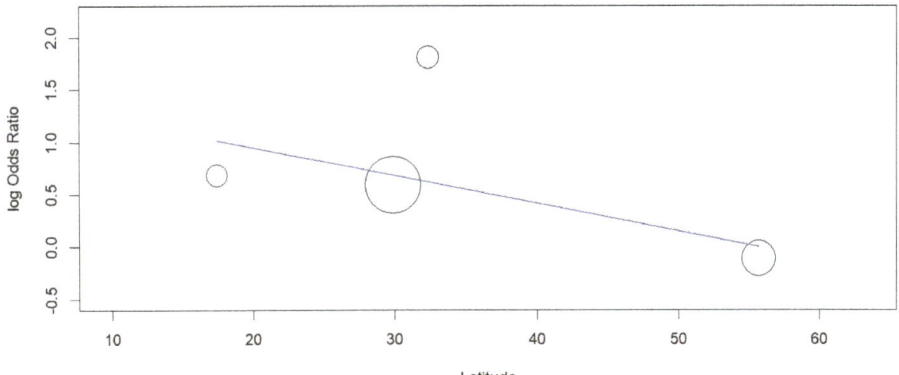

Figure 4. Log OR meta-regression for IL-1B +3954 polymorphism as a function of latitude covariate (*p*-value = 0.025, coefficient = −0.026).

Analyzing the meta-regression analysis regarding the percentage of male subjects, it is possible to conclude that, as the proportion of male individuals increases, there is an increase in the OR, therefore, there is an increase in risk, however, it is not statistically significant (Figure A3).

We can also observe that as the percentage of the mutated allele increases, the OR decreases. It is necessary to consider that the value of the mutated allele corresponds to the entire sample, both for control patients and patients with peri-implantitis. The effect of the lower percentage of the mutated allele on the risk for peri-implantitis is statistically significant (p-value < 0.05) (Figure 6).

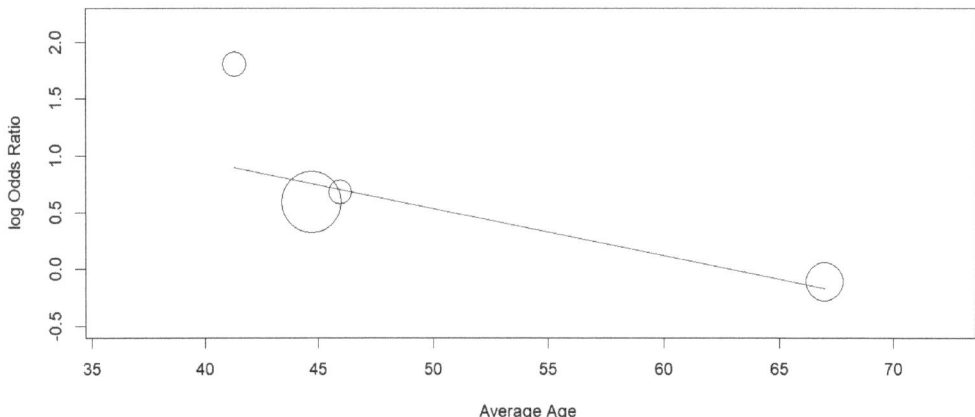

Figure 5. Log OR meta-regression for the IL-1B +3954 polymorphism as a function of the mean age covariate (p-value = 0.005, coefficient = −0.041).

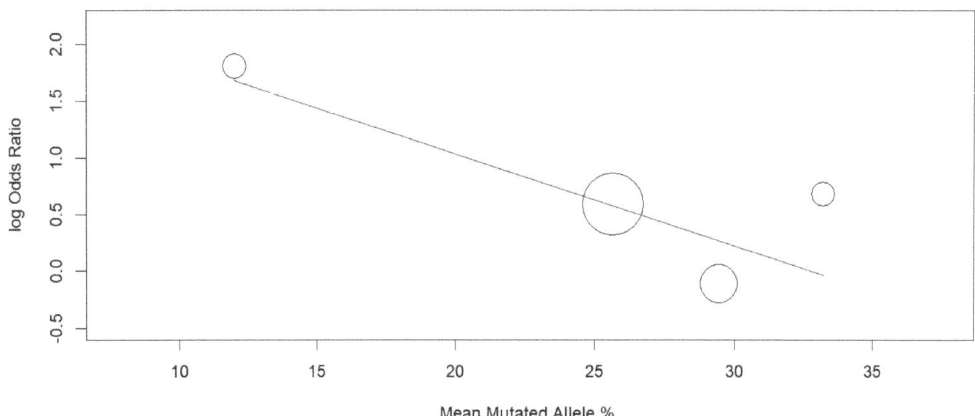

Figure 6. Log OR meta-regression for the IL-1B +3954 polymorphism as a function of the covariate percentage of the mutated allele in the s ample (p-value = 0.003, coefficient = −0.081).

Performing a meta-regression analysis regarding the year of publication (Figure 7) and the sample size (Figure A4) of the included studies, we can conclude that the effect of year of publication is statistically significant while the effect of the sample size is not statistically significant. We can observe that as the year of publication increases, the risk for peri-implantitis also increases.

Through the interpretation of this meta-analysis, we were able to analyze the historical perspective from the oldest to the most recent article. From the Figure 8, we concluded that, with these successive assessments, there is an increased risk of carriers of the IL-1B +3954 polymorphism to have peri-implantitis.

3.7. Sensitivity Analysis

Both "leave-one-out" and "cumulative analysis" were performed within the sensitivity analysis for the IL-1B +3954 polymorphism study effects sizes. Results are illustrated in Figure A5. All studies seem to have had a balanced contribution to the pooled results although recent studies seem to overestimate the effect in comparison with previous ones.

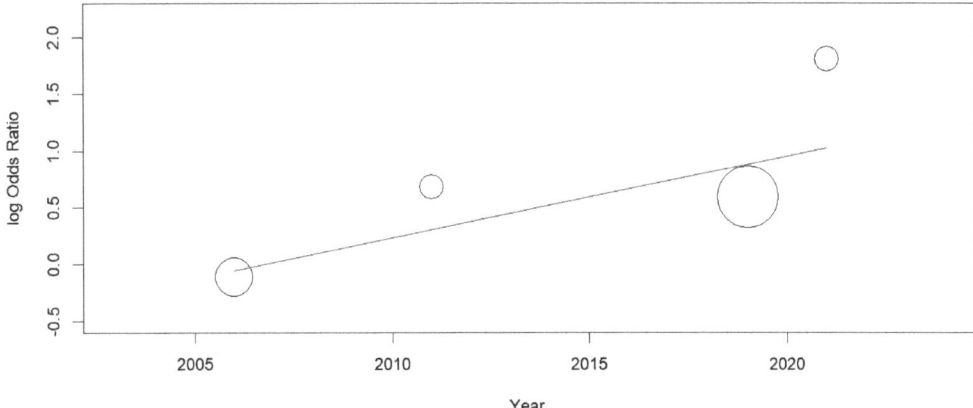

Figure 7. Log OR meta-regression for the IL-1B +3954 polymorphism as a function of the year of publication (*p*-value = 0.014, coefficient = 0.067).

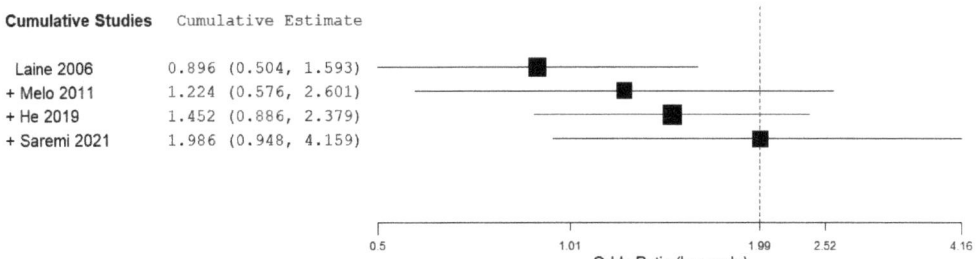

Figure 8. Forest Plot of the cumulative meta-analysis for the IL-1B +3954 polymorphism. Laine et al., 2006 [21]; Melo et al., 2011 [23]; He et al., 2019 [24]; Saremi et al., 2021 [26].

4. Discussion

This study aimed to verify if there is an association between the polymorphisms of the IL-1A, IL-1B, and IL-1RN genes and peri-implantitis. It is a relevant topic since, if this association is confirmed, it is possible to identify patients who have this polymorphism and the physician's approach can be adjusted in order to prevent the onset of this disease, considered a public health problem. Genetic polymorphisms are constant and can be measured before disease onset, thus it could be of great benefit for treatment planning and prognosis in an early stage. Despite the fact that peri-implantitis etiology and pathology are complex, the identification of genetic biomarkers associated with peri-implantitis risk could be a valuable tool in daily clinical practice. They could be used for early identification of individuals predisposed to increased peri-implantitis risk, and this would help practitioners (after estimating dental implants prognosis) in individualizing their treatment plan.

The future of disease diagnosis must involve not only identifying more susceptible patients but also identifying disease-associated biomarkers. Biomarkers are biological indicators with high prognostic and predictive value that can be related to the onset or development of a pathology. Frequently they must be able to predict the presence of a disease or its progression. A recent paper that has focused on five promising host derived biomarkers as candidate for early diagnosis of periodontitis, IL-1 β was one of them [36].

After a systematic search, which is described in the flowchart in Figure 1, eight articles were obtained for the present systematic review [21–26,34,35].

Table 1 shows the general conclusions of each of the eight articles. Four of these articles concluded that individuals with the IL-1 gene polymorphisms had a higher risk for the development of peri-implantitis [21,22,24,26]. These results are in agreement with what is found in the systematic review of Dereka et al. [27]. In this systematic review, the authors observed that in two of the three studies which evaluated peri-implantitis in relation to IL-1 genotype, the findings indicate that IL-1RN, IL-1A −899, IL-1B +3954 gene polymorphisms were correlated to increased peri-implant tissue infection and destruction [27]. In 2008, Huynh-Ba et al. carried out a systematic review [37] where two articles were included [38,39], and they concluded that there is not enough evidence to support or refute an association between the IL-1 genotype status and peri-implantitis. It should be mentioned that the articles included in this review evaluated peri-implantitis based on bone loss [37,38].

The number of studies in the literature evaluating this association is limited and some of these do not refer to confounding variables such as periodontal condition, ethnicity, and smoking status. These factors may explain the differences found between the different studies. The ethnicity of the populations included in the studies varies and there are studies that include patients who smoke and others who do not. On the other hand, the definition of peri-implantitis varies between studies, which makes comparisons between studies difficult. In our systematic review, we only included articles in which peri-implantitis was the evaluated outcome. From 2018, with the new Classification of Periodontal and Peri-implant Diseases and Conditions, it will be easier to standardize the definition of peri-implantitis between studies [6]. This new classification is the product of the World Workshop on the Classification of Periodontal and Peri-implant Diseases and Conditions organized jointly by the American Academy of Periodontology (AAP) and the European Federation of Periodontology (EFP) to create a consensus knowledge base for a new classification to be promoted globally.

Furthermore, some aspects such as the surface and position of the implants (anterior or posterior), the type of prosthetic restoration used (removable or fixed), type of retention (screw or cemented), the need for guided bone regeneration before or at the time of implant placement, general oral cavity health conditions were not referred or varied between studies. The techniques of DNA isolation also differ between studies, with some studies obtaining DNA from oral mucosal cells using swabs [22–25,34] and others using mouthwashes [21]. Other authors obtain DNA from blood [26,35].

Within the limits of this systematic review, it might be concluded that there is no obvious association between specific genetic polymorphism of IL-1 and IL-1RN and peri-implantitis, although a tendency should be underlined showing the potential link between IL-1 genotype and peri-implantitis.

For the meta-analysis, it was only possible to include four articles [21,23,24,26] since, in order to obtain a more real result on the true influence of the polymorphism in the disease, allele frequencies were evaluated. The remaining studies were excluded as they did not mention whether the patients were homozygous or heterozygous for the mutated allele, which may influence the interpretation of the results. The common polymorphism in these four studies was IL-1B +3954, which was evaluated.

In the present study, it was found that individuals who had the polymorphism in the IL-1B +3954 had an almost twice higher risk of developing peri-implantitis (OR 1.986). This result is in agreement with a meta-analysis performed by Jin et al. where the association between IL-1A −889, ILB +3954, IL-1B -511, composite genotype of IL-1A −889 and ILB +3954, and TNF-α −308 and risk of peri-implant disease (PID) was evaluated [29]. The PID included implant failure/loss, marginal bone loss and peri-implantitis. When a subgroup analysis is performed, it is observed that only IL-1B +3954 is associated with a higher risk of peri-implantitis (OR 1.87).

In a meta-analysis carried out by Liao et al., that included four articles regarding the relationship of IL-1 polymorphisms and peri-implantitis, the composite genotype of IL-1 −889 and IL-1B +3954 was associated with increased risk of peri-implantitis (OR 2.34) [19]. The inclusion criteria differed from the present study, which allowed the authors to assess the relationship between the composite genotype and peri-implantitis.

In a recent meta-analysis, which evaluated association between interleukin-1 polymorphisms and susceptibility to PID, the authors observed that there was no association between IL−1A −889, IL−1B −511 and IL−1RN (VNTR) polymorphisms and the risk of PID [28]. In contrast, an association was observed between the composite genotype of IL−1A −889 and IL−1B +3954 and PID. In addition, the T allele and CT genotype of IL−1B +3954 polymorphism were also associated with an elevated risk of PID. In subgroup analysis no association was found between the polymorphisms evaluated and the risk of peri-implantitis [28]. However, the results of the study have to be interpreted with caution because the authors included in the same group of PID, patients with peri-implantitis, patients with marginal bone loss and patients with implant failure. However, bone loss can occur with or without the sign of infection, whereas peri-implantitis is an inflammatory lesion associated with loss of supporting bone around implant [5]. On the other hand, not all implant failures are caused by peri-implantitis and not all peri-implantitis lead to implant loss.

Regarding meta-regressions carried out in our meta-analysis, we observed that as the latitude increases, there is a tendency for the OR to decrease, so with increasing latitude, the risk for peri-implantitis decreases. The result of the coefficient statistical test in the longitude-relative meta-regression is not statistically significant. The influence of ethnic and racial variations in the frequency of gene polymorphisms in terms of the genetic susceptibility to a specific disease has been reported [40,41]. It has been demonstrated that there is low prevalence of the periodontitis-associated IL-1A +4845 and IL-1B +3954 gene polymorphisms in Chinese (2.3%) [41] compared with that reported for Caucasians (36%) [40]. The IL-1A +4845 polymorphism is more than 99% in linkage disequilibrium with the IL-1A −889 polymorphism (if one is present, the other usually is present) [42]. In our study, it was observed that in populations where the allele frequency of the mutated allele is higher, the risk of peri-implantitis is lower. Furthermore, in a subgroup analysis we also found that the Asian population was at a greater risk for the disease than the Mixed or Caucasian subgroup. This is not in agreement with the information that exists regarding certain geographic areas, such as the Asian continent. In these areas, there is a low prevalence of the mutated allele in the population and a lower risk for inflammatory diseases such as periodontitis, compared to other geographic areas. We were only able to evaluate four articles in our meta-analysis so we can´t extrapolate these results.

Through the interpretation of our meta-analysis, we were able to analyze the historical perspective from the oldest to the most recent article. We concluded that with these successive assessments, there is an increased risk of carriers of the IL-1B +3954 polymorphism to have peri-implantitis. This finding may be related to a more adequate definition of peri-implantitis over the years in the various published studies.

In carrying out this work, there were some limitations. Not all articles presented information about the follow-up period, the inclusion and exclusion criteria were not similar between the various articles and there were parameters that some articles evaluated while others did not. In addition, there were also factors, such as age, gender, and ethnicity, which were not analyzed in the same way in all studies. These factors contributed to the heterogeneity obtained in this work.

The definition of peri-implantitis itself was not the same in all studies. Another limitation is the fact that some of the articles referred only to the genotype of the individuals and in this study the allele frequency was studied, since it is more specific.

The number of studies in the literature evaluating this association is limited, had small samples and some of them do not refer to confounding variables such as periodontal condition, ethnicity and smoking status. The inequality of these study designs necessitates the conduction of further studies using proper methodologies and from different ethnic groups. A clarification of the genetic basis associated with peri-implant pathology could be used to predict peri-implantitis occurrence and to improve treatment and monitoring of patients with dental implants.

5. Conclusions

It is possible to conclude that there are still no studies with an adequate sample size or sufficient studies to reach robust conclusions about the influence of interleukin 1 and interleukin 1 receptor antagonist polymorphisms on the development of peri-implantitis. However, the available evidence, while constrained by the above mentioned issues, shows that there seems to be a possible influence of these polymorphisms on the development of the disease. Regarding the meta-analysis performed, it was observed that individuals with the polymorphism in the IL-1B +3954 gene have a higher risk for the development of peri-implantitis.

Nevertheless, there is a need for further studies, with larger samples and in different ethnic groups, to increase scientific evidence about the possible role of these polymorphisms in the development of peri-implantitis.

Author Contributions: Conceptualization, J.M.C. and S.D.; methodology, S.D. and P.M.; software, P.M.; validation, J.M.C., S.D. and P.M.; formal analysis, J.M.C., S.D. and P.M.; investigation, J.M.C. and S.D.; resources, J.M.C. and P.M.; data curation, J.M.C., S.D. and P.M.; writing—original draft preparation, J.M.C. and S.D.; writing—review and editing J.M.C., A.C.R., P.M., S.N. and R.C.A.; funding acquisition, J.M.C. and R.C.A. All authors have read and agreed to the published version of the manuscript.

Funding: This work was supported by national funds through the FCT—Foundation for Science and Technology, I.P., (under the project UIDB/04585/2020).

Institutional Review Board Statement: Not applicable.

Informed Consent Statement: Not applicable.

Data Availability Statement: The data used to support the findings of this study are included in the article.

Conflicts of Interest: The authors declare no conflict of interest.

Appendix A

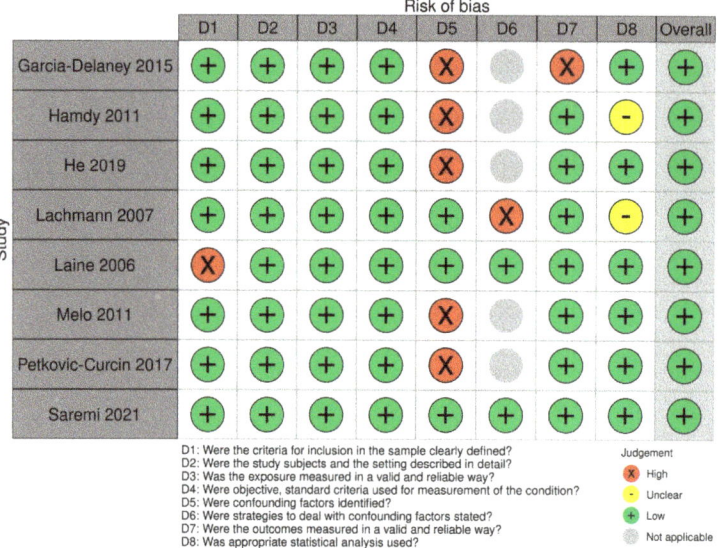

Figure A1. Risk of bias assessment of the included studies. Laine et al., 2006 [21]; Lachmann et al., 2007 [25]; Hamdy et al., 2011 [22]; Melo et al., 2011 [23]; Garcia-Delaney et al., 2015 [33]; Petkovic-Curcin et al., 2017 [34]; He et al., 2019 [24]; Saremi et al., 2021 [26].

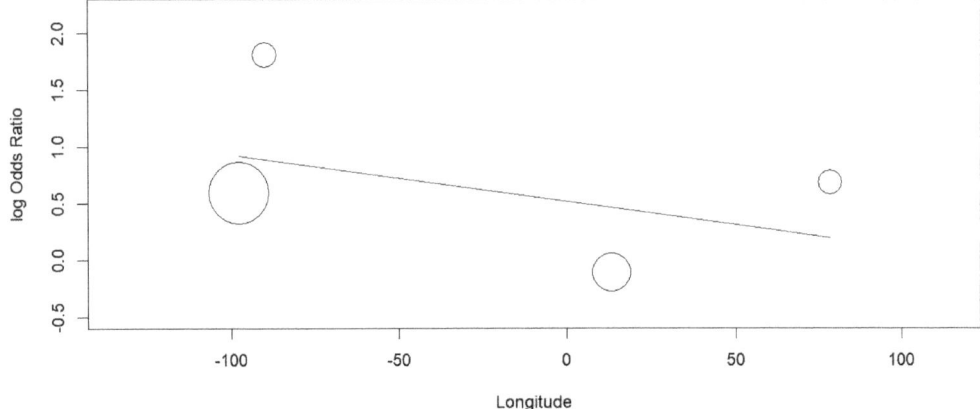

Figure A2. Log OR meta-regression for the IL-1B +3954 polymorphism as a function of the longitude covariate (*p*-value = 0.295, coefficient = −0.004).

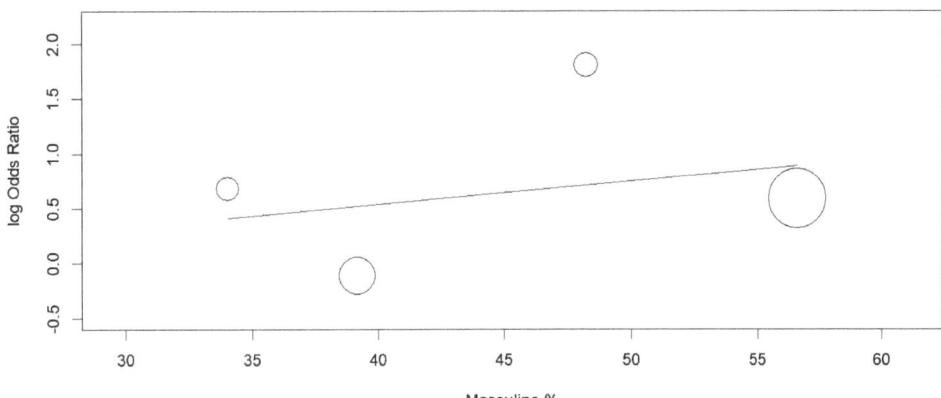

Figure A3. Log OR meta-regression for IL-1B +3954 polymorphism as a function of the covariate percentage of male subjects (*p*-value = 0.531, coefficient = 0.021).

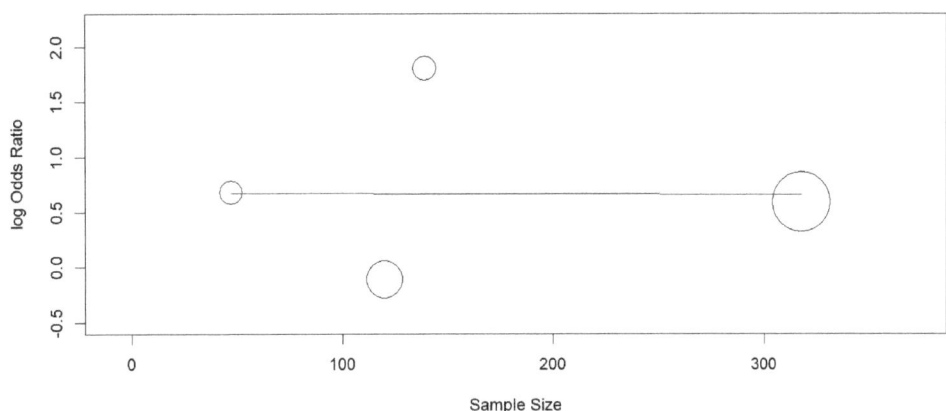

Figure A4. Log OR meta-regression for the IL-1B +3954 polymorphism as a function of sample size (*p*-value = 0.989, coefficient = −0.000).

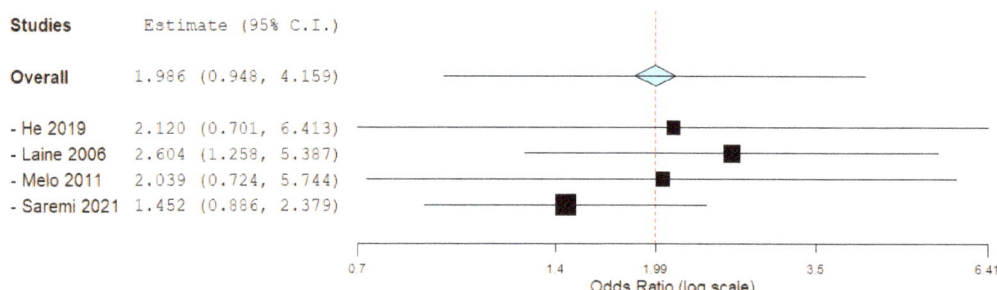

Figure A5. Sensitivity Analysis (CI—confidence interval). Laine et al., 2006 [21]; Melo et al., 2011 [23]; He et al., 2019 [24]; Saremi et al., 2021 [26].

Table A1. Systematic review table relating to the sample characteristics of the different articles.

Year & Author	Latitude; Longitude (Degrees)	Sample Size	M/F (%)	Average Age of the Sample	Mean % of Mutated Allele
Garcia-Delaney, 2015 [33]	32.363890; −86.298190	Total: 54 PI: 27 Control: 27	37/63	53	ND
Hamdy, 2011 [22]	−35.052770; 147.349560	Total: 50 PI: 25 Control: 25	76/24	41	ND
He, 2019 [24]	29.894920; −97.677800	Total: 318 PI: 144 Control: 174	57/43	45	IL-1B +3954: 25.65
Lachmann, 2007 [25]	−13.848923; −171.751145	Total: 29 PI: 11 Control: 18	34/66	66	ND
Laine, 2006 [21]	55.702888; 13.194710	Total: 120 PI: 71 Control: 49	39/61	67	IL-1B +3954: 29.45
Melo, 2011 [23]	17.433660; 78.339010	Total: 47 PI: 16 Control: 31	34/66	46	IL-1B +3954: 33.22
Petkovic-Curcin, 2017 [34]	40.772770; −111.839100	Total: 98 PI: 34 Control: 64	71/29	58 *	ND
Saremi, 2021 [26]	32.331050; −90.170660	Total: 139 PI: 50 Control: 89	49/51	41	IL-1B +3954: 12

ND—non-defined, PI—peri-implantitis group, * In this article, the median age of the sample is exceptionally represented.

References

1. Karoussis, I.K.; Kotsovilis, S.; Fourmousis, I. A comprehensive and critical review of dental implant prognosis in periodontally compromised partially edentulous patients. *Clin. Oral Implant. Res.* **2007**, *18*, 669–679. [CrossRef]
2. Bornstein, M.M.; Halbritter, S.; Harnisch, H.; Weber, H.P.; Buser, D. A retrospective analysis of patients referred for implant placement to a specialty clinic: Indications, surgical procedures, and early failures. *Int. J. Oral Maxillofac. Implants* **2008**, *23*, 1109–1116. [CrossRef] [PubMed]
3. Tey, V.H.S.; Phillips, R.; Tan, K. Five-year retrospective study on success, survival and incidence of complications of single crowns supported by dental implants. *Clin. Oral Implant. Res.* **2017**, *28*, 620–625. [CrossRef] [PubMed]
4. Frizzera, F.; De Oliveira, G.J.P.L.; Shibli, J.A.; De Moraes, K.C.; Marcantonio, E.B.; Junior, E.M. Treatment of peri-implant soft tissue defects: A narrative review. *Braz. Oral Res.* **2019**, *33*, e073. [CrossRef] [PubMed]
5. Lang, N.P.; Berglundh, T.; Working Group 4 of Seventh European Workshop on Periodontology. Periimplant diseases: Where are we now?—Consensus of the Seventh European Workshop on Periodontology. *J. Clin. Periodontol.* **2011**, *38*, 178–181. [CrossRef] [PubMed]
6. Berglundh, T.; Armitage, G.; Araujo, M.G.; Avila-Ortiz, G.; Blanco, J.; Camargo, P.M.; Chen, S.; Cochran, D.; Derks, J.; Figuero, E.; et al. Peri-implant diseases and conditions: Consensus report of workgroup 4 of the 2017 World Workshop on the Classification of Periodontal and Peri-Implant Diseases and Conditions. *J. Clin. Periodontol.* **2018**, *45* (Suppl. S20), S286–S291. [CrossRef]
7. Heitz-Mayfield, L.J.A. Peri-implant diseases: Diagnosis and risk indicators. *J. Clin. Periodontol.* **2008**, *35* (Suppl. 8), 292–304. [CrossRef]

8. Zitzmann, N.U.; Berglundh, T. Definition and prevalence of peri-implant diseases. *J. Clin. Periodontol.* **2008**, *35*, 286–291. [CrossRef]
9. Atieh, M.A.; Alsabeeha, N.H.M.; Faggion, C.M., Jr.; Duncan, W.J. The Frequency of Peri-Implant Diseases: A Systematic Review and Meta-Analysis. *J. Periodontol.* **2013**, *84*, 1586–1598. [CrossRef]
10. Lee, C.-T.; Huang, Y.-W.; Zhu, L.; Weltman, R. Prevalences of peri-implantitis and peri-implant mucositis: Systematic review and meta-analysis. *J. Dent.* **2017**, *62*, 1–12. [CrossRef]
11. Belibasakis, G.N. Microbiological and immuno-pathological aspects of peri-implant diseases. *Arch. Oral Biol.* **2014**, *59*, 66–72. [CrossRef] [PubMed]
12. Lindhe, J.; Berglundh, T.; Ericsson, I.; Liljenberg, B.; Marinello, C. Experimental breakdown of peri-implant and periodontal tissues. A study in the beagle dog. *Clin. Oral Implant. Res.* **1992**, *3*, 9–16. [CrossRef] [PubMed]
13. Becker, S.T.; Beck-Broichsitter, B.E.; Graetz, C.; Dmd, C.E.D.; Wiltfang, J.; Häsler, R. Peri-Implantitis versus Periodontitis: Functional Differences Indicated by Transcriptome Profiling. *Clin. Implant Dent. Relat. Res.* **2014**, *16*, 401–411. [CrossRef] [PubMed]
14. Fransson, C.; Lekholm, U.; Jemt, T.; Berglundh, T. Prevalence of subjects with progressive bone loss at implants. *Clin. Oral Implant. Res.* **2005**, *16*, 440–446. [CrossRef]
15. Roos-Jansaker, A.-M.; Renvert, H.; Lindahl, C.; Renvert, S. Nine- to fourteen-year follow-up of implant treatment. Part III: Factors associated with peri-implant lesions. *J. Clin. Periodontol.* **2006**, *33*, 296–301. [CrossRef] [PubMed]
16. Tatakis, D.N. Interleukin-1 and bone metabolism: A review. *J. Periodontol* **1993**, *64*, 416–431.
17. Nicklin, M.; Weith, A.; Duff, G.W. A Physical Map of the Region Encompassing the Human Interleukin-1α, Interleukin-1β, and Interleukin-1 Receptor Antagonist Genes. *Genomics* **1994**, *19*, 382–384. [CrossRef] [PubMed]
18. Dinarello, C.A. Biologic basis for interleukin-1 in disease. *Blood* **1996**, *87*, 2095–2147. [CrossRef]
19. Liao, J.; Li, C.; Wang, Y.; Ten, M.; Sun, X.; Tian, A.; Zhang, Q.; Liang, X. Meta-analysis of the association between common interleukin-1 polymorphisms and dental implant failure. *Mol. Biol. Rep.* **2014**, *41*, 2789–2798. [CrossRef]
20. Dominici, R.; Cattaneo, M.; Malferrari, G.; Archi, D.; Mariani, C.; Grimaldi, L.; Biunno, I. Cloning and functional analysis of the allelic polymorphism in the transcription regulatory region of interleukin-1α. *Immunogenetics* **2002**, *54*, 82–86. [CrossRef]
21. Laine, M.L.; Leonhardt, A.; Roos-Jansaker, A.-M.; Pena, A.S.; Van Winkelhoff, A.J.; Winkel, E.G.; Renvert, S. IL-1RN gene polymorphism is associated with peri-implantitis. *Clin. Oral Implant. Res.* **2006**, *17*, 380–385. [CrossRef] [PubMed]
22. Hamdy, A.A.; Ebrahem, M.A. The effect of interleukin-1 allele 2 genotype (IL-1a(-889) and IL-1b(+3954)) on the individual's susceptibility to peri-implantitis: Case-control study. *J. Oral Implant.* **2011**, *37*, 325–334. [CrossRef] [PubMed]
23. Melo, R.F.; Lopes, B.M.V.; Shibli, J.A.; Junior, E.M.; Marcantonio, R.A.C.; Galli, G.M.T. Interleukin-1β and Interleukin-6 Expression and Gene Polymorphisms in Subjects with Peri-Implant Disease. *Clin. Implant Dent. Relat. Res.* **2012**, *14*, 905–914. [CrossRef] [PubMed]
24. He, K.; Jian, F.; He, T.; Tang, H.; Huang, B.; Wei, N. Analysis of the association of TNF-α, IL-1A, and IL-1B polymorphisms with peri-implantitis in a Chinese non-smoking population. *Clin. Oral Investig.* **2020**, *24*, 693–699. [CrossRef] [PubMed]
25. Lachmann, S.; Kimmerle-Müller, E.; Axmann, D.; Scheideler, L.; Weber, H.; Haas, R. Associations between peri-implant crevicular fluid volume, concentrations of crevicular inflammatory mediators, and composite IL-1A ?889 and IL-1B +3954 genotype: A cross-sectional study on implant recall patients with and without clinical signs of peri-implantitis. *Clin. Oral Implant. Res.* **2007**, *18*, 212–223. [CrossRef]
26. Saremi, L.; Shafizadeh, M.; Esmaeilzadeh, E.; Ghaffari, M.E.; Mahdavi, M.H.; Amid, R.; Kadkhodazadeh, M. Assessment of IL-10, IL-1ß and TNF-α gene polymorphisms in patients with peri-implantitis and healthy controls. *Mol. Biol. Rep.* **2021**, *48*, 2285–2290. [CrossRef]
27. Dereka, X.; Mardas, N.; Chin, S.; Petrie, A.; Donos, N. A systematic review on the association between genetic predisposition and dental implant biological complications. *Clin. Oral Implant. Res.* **2012**, *23*, 775–788. [CrossRef]
28. Mohammadi, H.; Roochi, M.M.; Sadeghi, M.; Garajei, A.; Heidar, H.; Meybodi, A.A.; Dallband, M.; Mostafavi, S.; Mostafavi, M.; Salehi, M.; et al. Association between *Interleukin-1* Polymorphisms and Susceptibility to Dental Peri-Implant Disease: A Meta-Analysis. *Pathogens* **2021**, *10*, 1600. [CrossRef]
29. Jin, Q.; Teng, F.; Cheng, Z. Association between common polymorphisms in IL-1 and TNFα and risk of peri-implant disease: A meta-analysis. *PLoS ONE* **2021**, *16*, e0258138. [CrossRef]
30. Lefebvre, C.; Glanville, J.; Briscoe, S.; Littlewood, A.; Marshall, C.; Metzendorf, M.-I.; Noel-Storr, A.; Rader, T.; Shokraneh, F.; Thomas, J.; et al. Chapter 4: Searching for and selecting studies. In *Cochrane Handbook for Systematic Reviews of Intervention*; Version 6.2.; Higgins, J.P.T., Thomas, J., Chandler, J., Cumpston, M., Li, T., Page, M.J., Welch, V.A., Eds.; Cochrane: London, UK, 2019. Available online: www.training.cochrane.org/handbook (accessed on 2 April 2022).
31. Moola, S.; Munn, Z.; Tufanaru, C.; Aromataris, E.; Sears, K.; Sfetcu, R.; Currie, M.; Qureshi, R.; Mattis, P.; Lisy, K.; et al. Chapter 7: Systematic reviews of etiology and risk. In *Joanna Briggs Institute Reviewer's Manual*; Aromataris, E., Munn, Z., Eds.; The Joanna Briggs Institute: Adelaide, SA, USA, 2017. Available online: https://reviewersmanual.joannabriggs.org/ (accessed on 2 April 2022).
32. Wallace, B.C.; Dahabreh, I.J.; Trikalinos, T.A.; Lau, J.; Trow, P.; Schmid, C.H. Closing the Gap between Methodologists and End-Users: R as a Computational Back-End. *J. Stat. Softw.* **2012**, *49*, 1–15. [CrossRef]

33. Schünemann, H.J.; Vist, G.E.; Higgins, J.P.T.; Santesso, N.; Deeks, J.J.; Glasziou, P.; Akl, E.A.; Guyatt, G.H. Chapter 15: Interpreting results and drawing conclusions. In *Cochrane Handbook for Systematic Reviews of Intervention*; Version 6.2.; Higgins, J.P.T., Thomas, J., Chandler, J., Cumpston, M., Li, T., Page, M.J., Welch, V.A., Eds.; Cochrane: London, UK, 2019. Available online: www.training.cochrane.org/handbook (accessed on 2 April 2022).
34. Garcia-Delaney, C.; Sanchez-Garces, M.; Figueiredo, R.; Sánchez-Torres, A.; Escoda, C.G. Clinical significance of interleukin-1 genotype in smoking patients as a predictor of peri-implantitis: A case-control study. *Med. Oral Patol. Oral Y Cir. Buccal* **2015**, *20*, e737–e743. [CrossRef] [PubMed]
35. Petkovic-Curcin, A.; Zeljic, K.; Cikota-Aleksic, B.; Dakovic, D.; Tatic, Z.; Magic, Z. Association of Cytokine Gene Polymorphism with Peri-implantitis Risk. *Int. J. Oral Maxillofac. Implant.* **2017**, *3*, e241–e248. [CrossRef] [PubMed]
36. Cafiero, C.; Spagnuolo, G.; Marenzi, G.; Martuscelli, R.; Colamaio, M.; Leuci, S. Predictive Periodontitis: The Most Promising Salivary Biomarkers for Early Diagnosis of Periodontitis. *J. Clin. Med.* **2021**, *10*, 1488. [CrossRef] [PubMed]
37. Huynh-Ba, G.; Lang, N.P.; Tonetti, M.S.; Zwahlen, M.; Salvi, G.E. Association of the compositeIL-1genotype with peri-implantitis: A systematic review. *Clin. Oral Implant. Res.* **2008**, *19*, 1154–1162. [CrossRef]
38. Feloutzis, A.; Lang, N.P.; Tonetti, M.S.; Bürgin, W.; Brägger, U.; Buser, D.; Duff, G.W.; Kornman, K.S. IL-1 gene polymorphism and smoking as risk factors for peri-implant bone loss in a well-maintained population. *Clin. Oral Implant. Res.* **2003**, *14*, 10–17. [CrossRef] [PubMed]
39. Gruica, B.; Wang, H.-Y.; Lang, N.P.; Buser, D. Impact of IL-1 genotype and smoking status on the prognosis of osseointegrated implants. *Clin. Oral Implant. Res.* **2004**, *15*, 393–400. [CrossRef] [PubMed]
40. Kornman, K.S.; Crane, A.; Wang, H.-Y.; Giovlne, F.S.; Newman, M.G.; Pirk, F.W.; Wilson, T.G.; Higginbottom, F.L.; Duff, G.W. The interleukin-1 genotype as a severity factor in adult periodontal disease. *J. Clin. Periodontol.* **1997**, *24*, 72–77. [CrossRef]
41. Armitage, G.C.; Wu, Y.; Wang, H.-Y.; Sorrell, J.; di Giovine, F.S.; Duff, G.W. Low Prevalence of a Periodontitis-Associated Interleukin-1 Composite Genotype in Individuals of Chinese Heritage. *J. Periodontol.* **2000**, *71*, 164–171. [CrossRef]
42. Andreiotelli, M.; Koutayas, S.O.; Madianos, P.N.; Strub, J.R. Relationship between interleukin-1 genotype and peri-implantitis: A literature review. *Quintessence Int.* **2008**, *39*, 289–298.

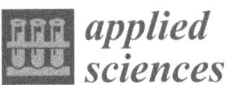

Article

Salivary Interleukin-6, Interleukin-1β, and C-Reactive Protein as a Diagnostic Tool for Plaque-Induced Gingivitis in Children

Ayshe Salim [1], Sirma Angelova [2], Bogdan Roussev [1], Todorka Sokrateva [1], Yoana Kiselova-Kaneva [1,*], Stefan Peev [3] and Diana Ivanova [1]

1. Department of Biochemistry, Molecular Medicine and Nutrigenomics, Faculty of Pharmacy, Medical University of Varna, 9000 Varna, Bulgaria
2. Department of Pediatric Dentistry, Faculty of Dental Medicine, Medical University of Varna, 9000 Varna, Bulgaria
3. Department of Periodontology and Dental Implantology, Faculty of Dental Medicine, Medical University of Varna, 9000 Varna, Bulgaria
* Correspondence: yoana.kiselova@mu-varna.bg

Abstract: Plaque-induced gingivitis (PIG) is one of the most widely distributed oral disorders in children. We aimed to identify the diagnostic value of interleukin-6 (IL-6), interleukin-1β (IL-1β), and c-reactive protein (CRP) in the unstimulated whole saliva of children with different degrees of PIG. The study included 45 healthy children (aged between 4–14 years). The participants were divided into four groups according to their Silness–Löe plaque index and Löe–Silness gingival index. ELISA methods for the quantification of salivary IL-6, IL-1β, and CRP were used. The highest levels of IL-6, IL-1β, and CRP were recorded in the group with severe gingivitis—14.96 pg/mL, 28.94 pg/mL, and 490.0 pg/mL, respectively—significantly exceeding those in the control group (9.506 pg/mL, 16.93 pg/mL and 254.4 pg/mL, respectively). Based on receiver operating characteristic (ROC) curve analysis, salivary IL-1β and CRP showed good diagnostic accuracy ($0.8 \leq AUC < 0.9$) and IL-6 showed fair diagnostic accuracy ($0.7 \leq AUC < 0.8$) with statistical significance to distinguish between children with a moderate degree of PIG and those with a severe degree of PIG. Sensitivity for IL-6, CRP, and IL-1β was 87.5% ($p < 0.05$), 87.5% ($p < 0.01$), and 75% ($p < 0.01$), respectively, and specificity was 63.16% ($p < 0.05$), 78.95% ($p < 0.01$), 83.33% ($p < 0.01$), respectively. Based on our results, we suggest salivary IL-1β and CRP as potential diagnostic tools that can be used to differentiate between moderate and severe PIG.

Keywords: plaque-induced gingivitis; salivary biomarkers; IL-6; IL-1β and CRP; children

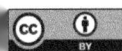

1. Introduction

Contemporary diagnostic methods increasingly rely on the potential of saliva as a promising diagnostic medium. The advantages of saliva sampling are the high abundance of different biomolecules and the non-invasive painless collection procedure. Saliva is rich in biomolecules of local and systemic origin which can serve as promising diagnostic markers, especially for oral-dental diseases [1–3]. Various studies report potential salivary markers for the diagnosis of several oral diseases—dental caries, diseases of the dental apparatus of an inflammatory and destructive nature, periodontitis, and gingivitis [4,5].

One of the most widely occurring oral disorders among children and adults is plaque-induced gingivitis (PIG) [6–11]. Frequent consumption of sugar-containing foods and beverages, especially among children, is associated with intensive plaque formation and accumulation. Another factor that increases plaque accumulation is poor oral hygiene. PIG is characterized by gingival inflammation provoked by plaque accumulation and the pathogenicity of microflora within the dental plaque. Hallmarks of gingival inflammation include increased vascular permeability and cell migration of mainly neutrophils, monocytes, and macrophages from the peripheral blood to gingival crevicular fluid. Gingival crevicular fluid is in constant and intensive interaction with saliva [12]. In parallel, adaptive immunity is mobilized through the activated influx of T and B into the inflammatory site. These cells trigger a specific inflammatory response with the local production of a significant amount of pro-inflammatory factors, namely interleukin 1β (IL-1β) and interleukin 6 (IL-6) [13,14]. The levels of these cytokines reflect the degree of gingival inflammation [15,16]. The C-reactive protein (CRP) is established as a reliable marker for the diagnosis of periodontal disorders [17]. To date, some of the most studied markers in saliva, with regard to gingivitis and periodontitis, are certain pro-inflammatory factors, due to their role in the pathogenic mechanisms of disease progression [18–20]. Kim et al. (2021) confirmed the prognostic value of salivary IL-1β for the diagnosis of periodontal disease and its use as a reliable salivary biomarker [20].

These findings reveal the potential use of IL-6, IL-1β, and CRP as local prognostic and diagnostic markers for gingival inflammation disorders in children, such as PIG. The application of these salivary biomarkers in children will be useful for disease monitoring and control, together with other parameters used in the clinical practice— Silness–Löe plaque index (PLI) and Löe–Silness gingival index (GI) [21]. Depending on the severity of gingival inflammation, PIG is characterized as mild, moderate, or severe [21]. The individual immune response and reactivity differ in each of the stages of this oral-dental disorder [21]. We hypothesized that the salivary levels of the examined pro-inflammatory factors IL-6, IL-1β, and CRP would correspond to the degree of clinical manifestation of PIG in children and that their diagnostic and prognostic significance would be high.

The identification and implementation of distinct inflammatory biomarkers such as IL-6, IL-1β, and CRP in saliva potentially provide novel prognostic, diagnostic, and preventive approaches for children suffering from, or at risk of developing, this periodontal disease. The use of saliva as a non-invasive diagnostic medium for the quantification of these inflammatory markers is important, especially for the youngest patients. The aim of our study was to assess the diagnostic and prognostic value of IL-6, IL-1β, and CRP levels in the unstimulated whole saliva of children with different degrees of PIG.

2. Materials and Methods

2.1. Study Design

This is a pilot prospective study. Declarations of informed consent were signed by the parents of the children or their legal guardians. The study was approved by the Ethics Committee of the Medical University of Varna (protocol No. 82/28.03.2019).

Participants in the study were recruited during their primary visit to the University Dental Medicine Center of the Medical University of Varna based on the inclusion and exclusion criteria.

Inclusion criteria:

1. Informed consent signed by the parent or guardian of each participant;
2. Age between 4–14 years;
3. No acute or chronic disease reported;
4. No medicine intake, including homeopathic remedies;
5. No known allergic reactions.

Exclusion criteria:

1. Children who are not collaborative during the examination and/or sample collection procedures;
2. Children with reported acute or chronic disease at the time of examination;
3. Children taking any treatment (anti-inflammatory, antibiotics, anti-allergy drugs, or homeopathic remedies);
4. Children with established allergic reactions;
5. Children displaying an open bite and mouth breathing;

This pilot prospective study included 45 children (26 girls and 19 boys) with no acute or chronic disease reported (aged between 4–14 years). For all participants, the clinical indices of PLI and GI were recorded and applied for the evaluation of the accumulation of dental plaque (Silness–Löe plaque index—PLI), assessment of gingival conditions, and registration of the qualitative changes in gingival tissues (Löe–Silness gingival index—GI).

The plaque index (PLI) is applied for the evaluation of dental plaque accumulation. This index is registered for Ramfjörd teeth 16, 22, 24, 36, 42 and 44. In children with primary and mixed dentition, in the case of missing representative teeth, the PLI is registered for mesially situated teeth. The recording of the PLI index is conducted by an atraumatic periodontal probe on the vestibular, oral, mesial, and distal surfaces along the site of contact with the marginal gingiva. The degree of dental plaque accumulation is recorded by the scores 0, 1, 2, and 3. The criteria are as follows: 0—no dental plaque on the examined tooth surface; 1—low levels of dental plaque on the peak of the probe; 2—moderate levels of dental plaque scratched by the probe; 3—a considerable, macroscopically visible accumulation of dental plaque on the tooth surface. The sum of all of the registered figures is divided by the total number of examined surfaces. The values of PLI in the interval from 0.1 to 1.1 indicate a condition that is "excellent with a tendency to have very good and good oral hygiene". PLI values between 1.2 and 2.0 indicate a condition that is "good, with a tendency to have satisfactory oral hygiene". PLI values from 2.1 to 3.0 are descriptive of a condition that is "satisfactory, with a tendency to have poor oral hygiene".

The GI is utilized to evaluate the severity of gingivitis. This index records the marginal and interproximal tissues separately on the bases of 0 to 3. The same Ramfjörd teeth applied for the assessment for PLI are applied for the recording of GI, with the following criteria: 0—normal gingiva; 1—mild-inflammation hyperemia and slight edema, without bleeding on probing; 2—moderate-inflammation hyperemia, edema, and provoked bleeding; 3—severe-inflammation hyperemia, considerable edema, and spontaneous bleeding. The assessment of bleeding was applied by atraumatic sampling along the site of the soft tissue of the gingival sulcus. To calculate the GI, the values of the four walls of the gingival tissues encircling the tooth were summed up and divided by four. The sum of these values was divided by the total number of examined sites. By the application of the GI, the diagnostic scores were determined as follows: GI = 0—normal gingiva; GI levels from 0.1 to 1.0—mild degree of gingivitis; GI values from 1.1 to 2.0—moderate degree of gingivitis; GI values from 2.1 to 3.0—severe degree of gingivitis [21].

The participants were divided into four groups according to their PLI and GI [21]: a control group without gingival inflammation (GI = 0; n = 6); a group with a mild degree of PIG ($0.1 < GI \leq 1$; n = 12); a group with a moderate degree of PIG ($1.1 \leq GI \leq 2$; n = 19); a group with a severe degree of PIG ($2.1 \leq GI \leq 3$; n = 8).

Clinical index determination and saliva sample collection were carried out on the day of dental examination and recruitment during the primary visit.

In summary, the study design is presented in Figure 1.

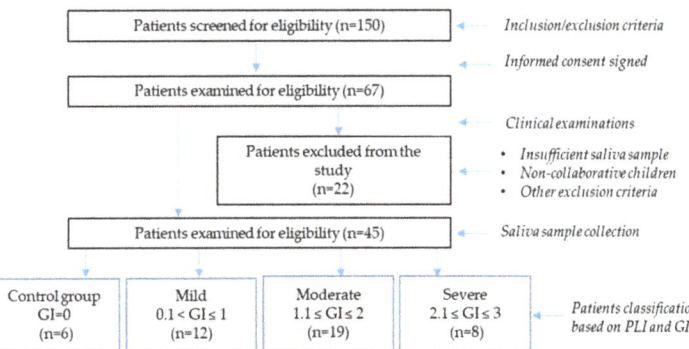

Figure 1. Study design.

2.2. Sample Size Calculation

The calculation of the sample size was carried out according to El-Patal et al. (2022) [22]. The calculated sample size was equal to 64 children with a power of 80% and $\alpha = 0.05$ using the SD (σ) with a margin of error of (E) = 0.8. In reality, the number of participants in our study was 44, because this is a pilot study and future investigations may proceed.

2.3. Salivary Sample Collection and Analysis

The collection of unstimulated whole saliva was conducted in sterile DNase- and RNase-free collection tubes, and the samples were frozen immediately on dry ice and stored at $-80\ °C$ until analysis. Saliva specimen collection was performed between 9.00 a.m. and 11.30 a.m. All the participants in the study were instructed to brush their teeth just before the sample collection. Enzyme-linked immunosorbent assays (ELISA) with monoclonal antibodies were used to determine the levels of IL-6, IL-1β, and CRP in saliva (Shanghai Sunred Biological Technology Co., Ltd., Shanghai, China). The respective absorptions were measured at 450 nm using a microtiter plate reader, Synergy 2, BioTek, Santa Clara, CA, USA.

2.4. Statistical Analysis

Statistical methods of descriptive statistics, an unpaired *t*-test, Spearman's correlation and receiver operating characteristic (ROC) analysis were applied. The significance level was established at $p < 0.05$. GraphPad prism version 5 (Boston, MA, USA) was used to perform the statistical analysis.

3. Results

3.1. Clinical Indicators for Plaque-Induced Gingivitis

All the examined clinical indicators were characterized by considerably higher values in the groups with gingivitis, compared to the control group ($p < 0.05$) (Table 1).

Table 1. Clinical indicators of PIG.

Clinical Indicators	Control Group n = 6	Mild-Degree n = 12	Moderate-Degree n = 18	Severe-Degree n = 8	*p* Value *t*-Test
PLI	0.74 ± 0.25	1.2 ± 0.12	1.64 ± 0.29	1.98 ± 0.21	$p < 0.05$
GI	0 ± 0	0.75 ± 0.24	1.38 ± 0.17	2.19 ± 0.09	$p < 0.05$

Data are expressed as mean ± SD; abbreviations: PLI (Silness–Löe plaque index), and GI (Löe–Silness gingival index); significance level established at $p < 0.05$.

The control group was represented by 4 girls and 2 boys. Two of the children had stable primary dentition. In four subjects, a state of mixed dentition was recorded. The mean age of the representatives in the group equaled 7 years and 5 months.

The group with a mild degree of gingivitis was represented by 5 girls and 7 boys. Two of the children had stable primary dentition. In ten subjects, a state of mixed dentition was recorded. The mean age of the representatives in the group equaled 7 years and 6 months.

The group with a moderate degree of gingivitis was represented by 11 girls and 8 boys. There were no children with stable primary dentition. In thirteen subjects, a state of mixed dentition was recorded. Five children had permanent dentition. The mean age of the representatives in the group equaled 7 years and 8 months.

The group with a severe degree of gingivitis was represented by 6 girls and 2 boys. There was one child with stable primary dentition. In seven subjects, a state of mixed dentition was recorded. The mean age of the representatives in the group equaled 8 years and 4 months.

3.2. Salivary Levels of IL-6, IL-1β, and CRP in Children with Different Degrees of Plaque-Induced Gingivitis

In the present study, we examined the concentrations of IL-6, IL-1β, and CRP in unstimulated whole saliva from children with different degrees of PIG. The mean levels of IL-6, IL-1β, and CRP were higher in children with gingivitis compared to those of children in the control group (ns). The highest mean concentrations of IL-6, IL-1β, and CRP were recorded in the group with a severe degree of PIG, which were 14.96 pg/mL, 28.94 pg/mL, and 490.0 pg/mL, respectively. These values are considerably higher compared to those in the control group (9.506 pg/mL; 16.93 pg/mL; 254.4 pg/mL) (ns) (Figure 2). The mean concentration of IL-6 was elevated 1.57-fold, that of IL-1β was elevated 1.71-fold, and that of CRP was elevated 1.93-fold among the children with a severe degree of PIG compared to the control group. A statistically significant difference was established only between the groups with a moderate and severe degree of gingivitis for all three investigated markers ($p < 0.05$) (Figure 2). We assume that the relatively small number of representatives did not allow the establishment of a statistical significance between the other groups. The levels of these pro-inflammatory biomarkers had the lowest mean values among the children with a moderate degree of gingivitis compared to those in the other groups and the controls (ns) (Figure 2). The statistically significant differences in the mean concentrations of IL-6 ($p = 0.0208$), IL-1β ($p = 0.009$), and CRP ($p = 0.0131$) between the moderate and severe degrees of PIG are presented in Figure 2.

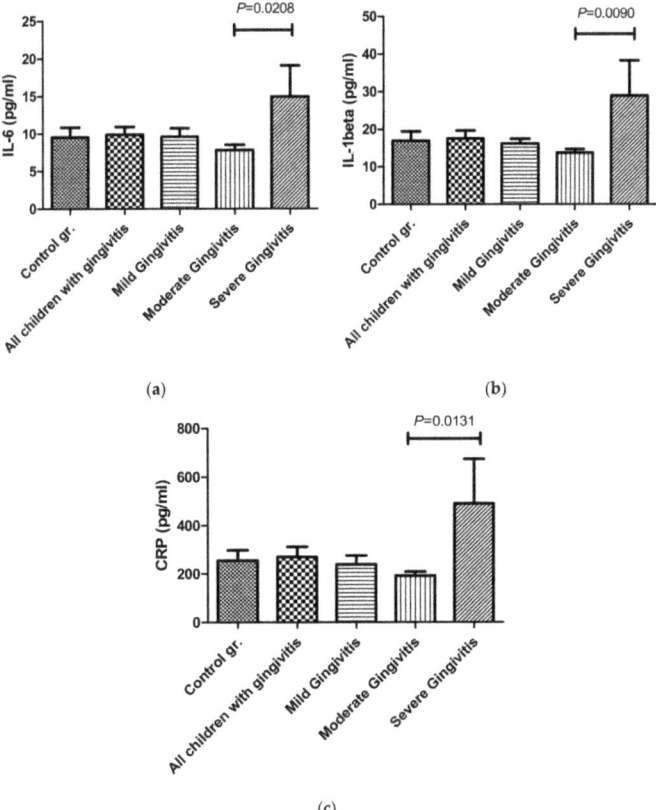

Figure 2. Mean concentrations of (**a**) IL-6, (**b**) IL-1β, and (**c**) CRP in the saliva of children with different degrees of PIG, the group with all of the children with plaque-induced gingivitis and healthy controls. Data expressed as mean ± SD. Significance level established at $p < 0.05$. Abbreviations: IL-6—interleukin-6, IL-1β—interleukin-1β, and CRP—C-reactive protein.

A positive significant correlation was observed between the investigated pro-inflammatory salivary biomarkers among all the participants with gingivitis. The Spearman's rank correlation coefficients between IL-6 and IL-1β equaled 0.7576 ($p < 0.0001$); those between IL-6 and CRP equaled 0.9272 ($p < 0.0001$); and those between IL-1β and CRP equaled 0.7546 ($p < 0.0001$) (Figure 3).

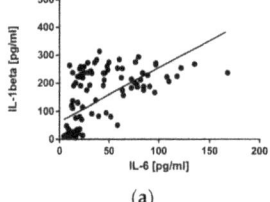
(a)

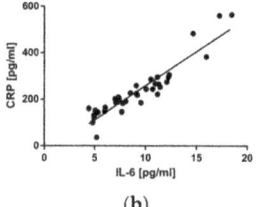
(b)

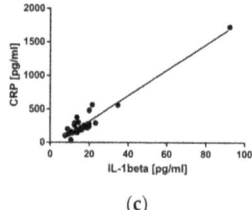
(c)

Figure 3. Spearman's correlations between (**a**) IL-6/IL-1β, (**b**) IL-6/CRP and (**c**) IL-1 β/CRP in the saliva of children with PIG. Abbreviations: IL-6—interleukin-6, IL-1β—interleukin-1β, and CRP—C-reactive protein.

3.3. Diagnostic Accuracy of Salivary IL-6, IL-1β, and CRP

Based on the ROC curve analysis, salivary IL-1β and CRP showed good diagnostic accuracy ($0.8 \leq AUC < 0.9$) and IL-6 showed fair diagnostic accuracy ($0.7 \leq AUC < 0.8$), as categorized by Nahm et al. (2022) [23]. Statistical significance was found to distinguish children with moderate PIG from children with a severe degree of PIG (Table 2, Figure 4). At the optimal cut-off values, based on the largest Youden's index, IL-6, IL-1β, and CRP demonstrated sensitivity values ranging from 75% to 87.5% and specificity values ranging from 63.16% to 83.33% (Table 3). Sensitivity for IL-6, CRP, and IL-1β was 87.5% ($p = 0.0384$), 87.5% ($p = 0.0093$), and 75% ($p = 0.0071$), respectively, and specificity was 63.16% ($p = 0.0384$), 78.95% ($p = 0.0093$), and 83.33% ($p = 0.0071$), respectively. IL-6 and CRP showed the highest sensitivity (87.5%) and IL-1β showed the highest specificity (83.33%), distinguishing between children with moderate PIG and children with a severe degree of PIG ($p < 0.05$) (Table 3).

Table 2. ROC logistic regression analysis of salivary IL-6, IL-1β, and CRP levels comparing the groups of children with different degrees of plaque-induced gingivitis.

	Mild–Moderate Degree of Gingivitis AUC (95% CI)	p-Value	Mild–Severe Degree of Gingivitis AUC (95% CI)	p-Value	Moderate–Severe Degree of Gingivitis AUC (95% CI)	p-Value
IL-6	0.6250	0.2478	0.6354	0.3159	0.7566	0.0384
IL-1β	0.6620	0.1385	0.6979	0.1427	0.8368	0.0071
CRP	0.6272	0.2396	0.6719	0.2031	0.8224	0.0093

The significance level was established at $p < 0.05$. Abbreviations: ROC—Receiver Operating Characteristic; AUC—Area Under the Curve; CI—Confidence Interval.

Table 3. ROC logistic regression analysis of salivary IL-6, IL-1β, and CRP as potential diagnostic biomarkers to differentiate children with a moderate degree of PIG from children with a severe degree of PIG.

	Cut-Off	AUC (95% CI)	Youden Index	Sensitivity%	Specificity%	p-Value
IL-6	8.385 pg/mL	0.7566	0.5066	87.50	63.16	0.0384
IL-1β	16.99 pg/mL	0.8368	0.5833	75.00	83.33	0.0071
CRP	223.8 pg/mL	0.8224	0.6645	87.50	78.95	0.0093

Significance level established at $p < 0.05$. Abbreviations: AUC—Area Under the Curve; CI—Confidence Interval.

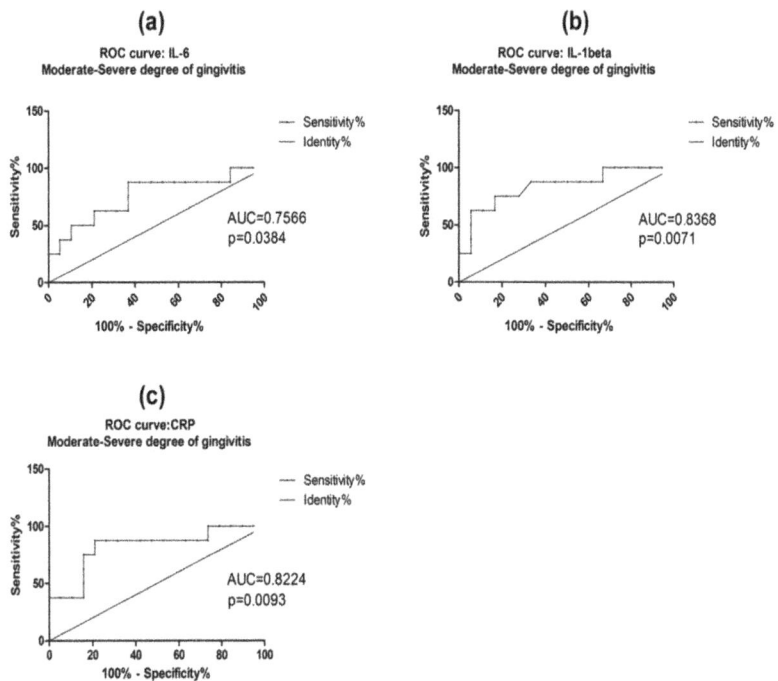

Figure 4. ROC curves of (**a**) IL-6, (**b**) IL-1β, and (**c**) CRP as potential diagnostic biomarkers for differentiating children with a moderate degree of PIG from children with a severe degree of PIG. Significance level established at $p < 0.05$. Abbreviations: ROC—receiver operating characteristic; AUC—area under the curve; IL-6—interleukin-6; IL-1β—interleukin-1β; CRP—C-reactive protein.

We estimated the fair diagnostic accuracy ($0.7 \leq AUC < 0.8$) of the investigated salivary pro-inflammatory biomarkers in distinguishing children without PIG from those with a severe degree of PIG (ns) (Table 4) [23]. IL-6 and CRP showed the highest sensitivity (87.5%) and IL-1β showed the highest specificity (83.33%), with $p = 0.1968$ (Table 5). Salivary IL-6, IL-1β, and CRP showed poor diagnostic capacity ($0.6 \leq AUC < 0.7$) to discriminate between children without PIG and those with a mild or moderate degree of PIG (ns) (Table 4) [23]. Our future research has to include a larger number of participants in all of the studied groups.

Table 4. ROC logistic regression analysis of salivary IL-6, IL-1β, and CRP levels comparing the control group with the groups with mild, moderate, and severe degrees of plaque-induced gingivitis.

	Control Group—Mild Degree of Gingivitis AUC (95% CI)	*p*-Value	Control Group—Moderate Degree of Gingivitis AUC (95% CI)	*p*-Value	Control Group—Severe Degree of Gingivitis AUC (95% CI)	*p*-Value
IL-6	0.5139	0.9254	0.6711	0.2148	0.7083	0.1968
IL-1β	0.5139	0.9254	0.6435	0.3015	0.7083	0.1968
CRP	0.5139	0.9254	0.6667	0.2267	0.7083	0.1968

Significance level established at $p < 0.05$. Abbreviations: ROC—receiver operating characteristic; AUC—area under the curve; CI—confidence interval; IL-6—interleukin-6; IL-1β—interleukin-1β; CRP—C-reactive protein.

Table 5. ROC logistic regression analysis of salivary IL-6, IL-1β, and CRP as potential diagnostic biomarkers for differentiating between children with a severe degree of PIG and those without plaque-induced gingival inflammation.

	Cut-Off	AUC (95% CI)	Youden Index	Sensitivity%	Specificity%	p-Value
IL-6	8.576 pg/mL	0.7083	0.5417	87.50	66.67	0.1968
IL-1β	16.62 pg/ml	0.7083	0.5833	75.00	83.33	0.1968
CRP	218.4 pg/ml	0.7083	0.5417	87.50	66.67	0.1968

Significance level established at $p < 0.05$. Abbreviations: ROC—receiver operating characteristic; AUC—area under the Curve; CI—confidence interval; IL-6—interleukin-6; IL-1β—interleukin-1β; CRP—C-reactive protein.

4. Discussion

Non-invasive and routine laboratory examination of potential salivary biomarkers such as IL-1β, IL-6, and CRP can be applied as a novel tool for the assessment of PIG severity in children, and could contribute towards practitioners' efforts in developing methods for the precise diagnosis, prognosis, treatment, and even prevention of PIG [1]. The precise diagnosis of the state of gingival inflammation in children is important for disease monitoring and control. In this study, we estimated that salivary IL-1β and CRP have good diagnostic accuracy and that IL-6 showed fair diagnostic accuracy in differentiating between children with moderate and children with a severe degree of PIG. These salivary markers may be implemented in the practice of precision dental medicine. The application of these markers in children with different degrees of PIG is important for the accurate diagnosis of the state of the disease, especially of a severe degree of PIG, and for adequate therapy and treatment to prevent the progression into periodontitis.

Etiologically, PIG is related to the accumulation of dental plaque, which has a tendency to increase the severity of pathological traits. The growth and maturation of dental plaque provoke inflammatory host tissue reactions. The conventional clinical parameters of the PLI and GI are applied for the evaluation of the degree of clinically manifested PIG [21]. The contemporary concept of personalized dental medicine is focused on the individual's specifics, including the progression of periodontal diseases. The sensitivity and severity of the host's immune response determine the course of inflammation on the systemic level and on the local level in the oral cavity.

The processes of the immune system that occur in response to the accumulation of bacterial biofilm are influenced by a great variety of pro- and anti-inflammatory cytokines and enzymes. Different studies have ascertained that immune cells in patients with diagnosed periodontal disorders release a greater amount of pro-inflammatory cytokines compared to cells in periodontally healthy individuals [21]. This corresponds to the higher salivary levels of the pro-inflammatory biomarkers of IL-6, IL-1β, and CRP among children suffering from PIG in comparison to controls, as established in our study. Other authors also report that the salivary concentration of IL-6 is increased among individuals with gingival inflammation [24,25].

We established a statistically significant difference in the mean levels of IL-6, IL-1β, and CRP between children with a moderate degree of PIG and those with a severe degree of PIG. The salivary levels of these pro-inflammatory biomarkers were significantly higher in the group with a severe degree of PIG compared to the group with a moderate degree of gingivitis. This is associated with the development of the inflammatory process that occurs in parallel to the progression of gingivitis. IL-1β and IL-6 are characterized as basic innate cytokines and serve as key inflammatory mediators under conditions of periodontal disorder [26,27]. IL-1β is secreted by monocytes, macrophages, and neutrophils. This pro-inflammatory cytokine is associated with the secretion of other mediators that provoke not only inflammatory alterations but also tissue damage [27,28]. Its function is related to the specifics of the clinical manifestation of PIG with the progression from moderate to severe degrees of PIG. The possible physiological feature connected to the decreased levels of IL-6, IL-1β, and CRP in the group with a moderate degree of PIG could be the shift in specific pathogenic microflora in the children with a severe degree of gingivitis, which would have led to an increase in the severity of the inflammatory response, increased gingival inflammation, and increased production of inflammatory mediators, such as IL-6 and IL-1β [21]. The qualitative and quantitative content of plaque is different as a result of plaque maturation [29,30]. The significant difference between moderate and severe PIG only seems reasonable because in patients with a low degree of PIG, host protective mechanisms (e.g., cell immunity) could still be not active enough. In patients with a moderate degree of PIG, the immunological mechanism differs from that of the severe form. The transition from a moderate to severe degree of gingivitis has been reported to be characterized by a shift from the innate immune response to the acquired immune response [31]. Macrophages, which predominate in the innate phase, have a reduced capacity for pro-inflammatory cytokine production compared to B-cells, which represent the acquired immune response [31].

We did not establish a statistical significance between IL-6, IL-1β, and CRP levels in the control group and the group with a mild degree of PIG because the PIG in the latter group was characterized as an initial phase of plaque-induced gingivitis. This initial phase of PIG is characterized by the formation of so-called initial lesions, where the appearance of gingival inflammation is low and characterized by hyperemia and slight edema, without bleeding upon probing [32]. The observed cytokine levels in the saliva in our study were also low, and not statistically different compared to those of the control group. The innate immune mechanisms are active during this stage and cytokine production is very low. The rate of collagen destruction also is low [32].

The moderate degree of gingivitis is characterized by hyperemia, edema, provoked bleeding, and the formation of early lesions. The inflammatory cells which are involved in this stage are lymphocytes and macrophages. The collagen degradation rate is higher than that in mild-degree PIG but lower than in severe-degree PIG [32]. The observed lowest levels of IL-6, IL-1β, and CRP in moderate-degree PIG could be due to the resolution of macrophages from M1 (classical) into M2 (alternative) phenotypes [33]. The M1 phenotype is the pro-inflammatory phenotype which is characterized by increased IL-6 production [34,35]. The M2 phenotype is involved in tissue repair and is characterized by decreased IL-6 production [36,37]. Probably, the anti-inflammatory M2 phenotype involved in active tissue repair is the distinctive immune response, a compensatory mechanism in moderate-degree PIG [36,37]. This explains the lowest cytokine levels that were found in moderate-degree PIG. Garaicoa-Pazmino et al. (2019) discuss in their study the transition of macrophages from M1 to M2 phenotypes in patients with gingivitis and periodontitis. Interestingly, they also did not find statistically significant differences between the M1 and M2 polarization of macrophages in healthy tissues and tissues with periodontitis [33]. The increased production of IL-6 and IL-1β demonstrated by the results of our study may have been related to the infiltration of T and B cells, which is typical for severe-degree PIG only. In severe gingivitis, the highest inflammatory response occurs through the increased local secretion of pro-inflammatory cytokines and other inflammatory molecules [32].

The established significant positive correlation between salivary levels of IL-6, IL-1β, and CRP among the participants with PIG is confirmed by several studies exploring the mechanism of interaction between these pro-inflammatory biomarkers. Bacterial lipopolysaccharide and IL-1β significantly increase IL-6 production in human gingival fibroblasts [27]. It was shown that the combined activity of IL-1β and IL-6 enhanced gingival inflammation and the risk of progression of periodontitis [27,38]. The established strong positive correlation between the pro-inflammatory cytokines IL-6 and IL-1β and the acute phase protein CRP described in our study has been widely explored and corroborated in the scientific literature [28,38]. Inflammatory stimuli such as IL-1β and IL-6 induce the synthesis of CRP from the liver. IL-6 and IL-1β act synergistically for the induction of CRP gene expression, as IL-1β alone has no effect [39]. These observations confirm the combined action of these molecules and their role in the development of inflammation [28,38,39].

The good diagnostic accuracy of these salivary biomarkers was confirmed by ROC curve analyses and the established AUC values in our study. IL-1β and CRP showed good diagnostic accuracy ($0.8 \leq$ AUC < 0.9) and IL-6 showed fair diagnostic accuracy ($0.7 \leq$ AUC < 0.8) with statistical significance in distinguishing between children with moderate PIG and children with a severe degree of PIG. the *t*-test analysis established a statistically significant difference between the levels of IL-1β, IL-6, and CRP in children with moderate and severe degrees of gingivitis. The trend of the considerable elevation of these inflammatory biomarkers parallel to the progression of PIG from a moderate to a severe degree could have been due to the action of the acquired immune system in the oral cavity. The rapid increase in the levels of these inflammatory parameters may be associated with the activation of enzymes involved in tissue destruction [40]. The results of our study are in line with the findings of other investigations in the field. The adoption of these inflammatory biomarkers in non-stimulated mixed saliva has the potential to serve as a prognostic tool for the progression of gingivitis from moderate to severe degrees before the clinical manifestation of the advanced inflammation of gingival tissues. Namely, the combined application of IL-6, IL-1β, and CRP, interpreted in the context of recording clinical indices and the evaluation of clinical findings and symptoms, can serve as prognostic and diagnostic indicators of the risk of PIG progression. This is key to the development of adequate, personalized prophylactic measures and the efficient control and minimization of the risk of the progression of PIG in later periods. The poor control and inefficient, sporadic treatment of PIG in children can be a predisposing factor for the initiation of periodontitis in adulthood. Many authors accentuate the late impact of gingivitis in children in terms of its effect on the gingival sulcus, which facilitates the establishment of the disease and the colonization of the site by periodontal pathogenic microflora [1]. On an epidemiological basis, strong evidence exists that shows the progression of gingivitis to periodontitis in adults [1]. In our study, we accentuated the relationship between clinical parameters for the wide-spread oral disorder of PIG and for inflammatory biomarkers in non-stimulated saliva. In light of the trending advancement of non-invasive and simple methods of assessing inflammation status, our results concerning the diagnostic potential of IL-6, IL-1β, and CRP as biomarkers for differentiating between moderate and severe degrees of clinical manifestation of PIG, can be useful for the development of gingivitis prevention strategies. Pediatric and dental practitioners should take into account the fact that the clinical manifestation of the severe forms of gingivitis in primary, mixed, and permanent dentition correlates with the degree of inflammatory cell infiltration into gingival tissues. It has been established that the chronic inflammation of periodontal tissues in childhood can provoke local tissue destruction, which could later develop into periodontitis [1]. Our findings are also relevant to the prophylaxis and limitations of favorable conditions that predispose gingivitis to periodontitis progression in later years. Non-invasive and routine laboratory biomarkers such as IL-1β and CRP with new applications in the diagnosis of the degree of PIG in children may add to the efforts of practitioners in the precise diagnosis, prognosis, treatment, and even prevention of the progression of PIG [1].

The main limitation of this study is the relatively small number of representatives in the examined groups, which will be taken into account in future work. Based on scientific sources, we do assume that under conditions in which there is a larger number of participants, we would obtain statistically significant results when comparing all the study groups, including the control.

This is a pilot study and future investigations may proceed. The search for non-invasive informative biomarkers is expected to provide fast and reliable diagnostics, especially in children. In this aspect, saliva appears to be a suitable matrix for further studies in dental medicine and oral biology.

5. Conclusions

Based on our results, we suggest salivary IL-1β and CRP as potential diagnostic tools to differentiate between moderate and severe degrees of plaque-induced gingivitis. Given the therapeutic approaches that differ depending on the severity of the disease, these markers could be implemented in personalized dental clinical practice.

Author Contributions: Conceptualization, S.A., Y.K.-K., D.I., S.P., A.S., B.R. and T.S.; methodology, B.R., A.S. and S.A.; validation, S.A., A.S. and B.R.; formal analysis, A.S., S.A., B.R. and T.S.; resources, S.A.; data curation, A.S., S.A. and B.R.; writing—original draft preparation, S.A., A.S., B.R. and T.S.; writing—review and editing, D.I., Y.K.-K. and S.P.; visualization, A.S., S.A., B.R. and T.S.; supervision, D.I., S.P. and Y.K.-K.; All authors have read and agreed to the published version of the manuscript.

Funding: This research was funded by Fund "Science" MU-Varna, Bulgaria, project number 18036, FN-12/11.02.2019.

Institutional Review Board Statement: The study was conducted in accordance with the Declaration of Helsinki, and approved by the Ethics Committee of Medical University Varna (protocol no. 82/28.03.2019).

Informed Consent Statement: Informed consent was given and a declaration of informed consent was signed by parents or legal guardians of children accompanying each child participating in the research.

Data Availability Statement: Not applicable.

Conflicts of Interest: The authors declare no conflict of interest.

References

1. Bimstein, E.; Huja, P.E.; Ebersole, J.L. The potential lifespan impact of gingivitis and periodontitis in children. *J. Clin. Pediatr. Dent.* **2013**, *38*, 95–99. [CrossRef] [PubMed]
2. Modéer, T.; Wondimu, B. Periodontal diseases in children and adolescents. *Rev. Dent. Clin. N. Am.* **2000**, *44*, 633–658. [CrossRef]
3. Murakami, S.; Mealey, B.L.; Mariotti, A.; Chapple, I.L.C. Dental plaque-induced gingival conditions. *J. Periodontol.* **2018**, *89*, 17–27. [CrossRef]
4. Ahmadi-Motamayel, F.; Goodarzi, M.T.; Mahdavinezhad, A.; Jamshidi, Z.; Darvishi, M. Salivary and serum antioxidant and oxidative stress markers in dental caries. *Caries Res.* **2018**, *52*, 565–569. [CrossRef]
5. Kaczor-Urbanowicz, K.E.; Trivedi, H.M.; Lima, P.O.; Camargo, P.M.; Giannobile, W.V.; Grogan, T.R.; Gleber-Netto, F.O.; Whiteman, Y.; Li, F.; Lee, H.J.; et al. Salivary exRNA biomarkers to detect gingivitis and monitor disease regression. *J. Clin. Periodontol.* **2018**, *45*, 806–817. [CrossRef]
6. Jenkins, W.M.; Papapanou, P.N. Epidemiology of periodontal disease in children and adolescents. *Periodontol. 2000* **2001**, *26*, 16–32. [CrossRef]
7. Singh, A.K. Prevalence of gingivitis and periodontitis among schools children in Lucknow region of Uttar Pradesh, India. *IOSR J. Dent. Med. Sci.* **2014**, *13*, 21–23. [CrossRef]
8. Bossnjak, A.; Curilovic, Z.; Vuccicevic-Boras, V.; Plancak, D.; Jorgic-Srdjak, K.; Relja, T.; Bozic, D.; Varnica, H. Prevalence of gingivitis in 6- to 11-year-old Croatian children. *Eur. J. Med. Res.* **2003**, *8*, 313–317.
9. Leous, P.; Palianskaya, L.; Leous, L. Oral hygiene and gingival inflammation in 6–8-year-olds from a junior school in Minsk who participated in a supervised oral hygiene programme. *Oral Health Dent. Manag.* **2009**, *7*, 27–30.
10. Burt, B. Research, Science and Therapy Committee of the American Academy of Periodontology. Position paper: Epidemiology of periodontal diseases. *J. Periodontol.* **2005**, *76*, 1406–1419. [CrossRef]
11. Dye, B.A. Global periodontal disease epidemiology. *Periodontol. 2000* **2012**, *58*, 10–25. [CrossRef] [PubMed]
12. Yaghobee, S.; Khorsand, A.; Rasouli Ghohroudi, A.A.; Sanjari, K.; Kadkhodazadeh, M. Assessment of interleukin-1beta and interleukin-6 in the crevicular fluid around healthy implants, implants with peri-implantitis, and healthy teeth: A cross-sectional study. *J. Korean Assoc. Oral Maxillofac. Surg.* **2014**, *40*, 220–224. [CrossRef] [PubMed]
13. Amar, S.; Oyaisu, K.; Li, L.; Van Dyke, T. Moesin: A potential LPS receptor on human monocytes. *J. Endotoxin. Res.* **2001**, *7*, 281–286. [CrossRef] [PubMed]
14. Isola, G.; Polizzi, A.; Santonocito, S.; Alibrandi, A.; Williams, R.C. Periodontitis activates the NLRP3 inflammasome in serum and saliva. *J. Periodontol.* **2022**, *93*, 135–145. [CrossRef] [PubMed]
15. Gorska, R.; Gregorek, H.; Kowalski, J.; Laskus-Perendyk, A.; Syczewska, M.; Madaliński, K. Relationship between clinical parameters and cytokine profiles in inflamed gingival tissue and serum samples from patients with chronic periodontitis. *J. Clin. Periodontol.* **2003**, *30*, 1046–1052. [CrossRef]
16. Aurer, A.; Jorgić-Srdjak, K.; Plancak, D.; Stavljenić-Rukavina, A.; Aurer-Kozelj, J. Proinflammatory factors in saliva as possible markers for periodontal disease. *Coll. Antropol.* **2005**, *29*, 435–439.
17. Shojaee, M.; Fereydooni Golpasha, M.; Maliji, G.; Bijani, A.; Aghajanpour Mir, S.M.; Mousavi Kani, S.N. C-reactive protein levels in patients with periodontal disease and normal subjects. *Int. J. Mol. Cell Med.* **2013**, *2*, 151–155.
18. Belstrøm, D.; Damgaard, C.; Könönen, E.; Gürsoy, M.; Holmstrup, P.; Gürsoy, U.K. Salivary cytokine levels in early gingival inflammation. *J. Oral Microbiol.* **2017**, *9*, 1364101. [CrossRef]
19. Boronat-Catalá, M.; Catalá-Pizarro, M.; Bagán Sebastián, J.V. Salivary and crevicular fluid interleukins in gingivitis. *J. Clin. Exp. Dent.* **2014**, *2*, e175–e179. [CrossRef]

20. Kim, J.Y.; Kim, K.R.; Kim, H.N. The potential impact of salivary IL-1 on the diagnosis of periodontal disease: A pilot study. *Healthcare* **2021**, *9*, 729. [CrossRef]
21. Rebelo, M.A.; Queiroz, A.C. Gingival Indices: State of Art. In *Gingival Diseases—Their Aetiology, Prevention and Treatment*; Panagakos, F., Davies, R., Eds.; IntechOpen: Rijeka, Croatia, 2011; pp. 41–54. [CrossRef]
22. El-Patal, M.A.; Khalil, M.A.; Shipl, W.; Barakat, I.; Youssef, E.M.I.; El Attar, S.; Fathi, A.; Abdallah, A.A. Detection of soluble urokinase type plasminogen activator receptors in children with gingivitis and normal subjects. *BMC Oral Health.* **2022**, *22*, 436. [CrossRef] [PubMed]
23. Nahm, F.S. Receiver operating characteristic curve: Overview and practical use for clinicians. *Korean J. Anesthesiol.* **2022**, *75*, 25–36. [CrossRef] [PubMed]
24. Taylor, J.J.; Preshaw, P.M.; Donaldson, P.T. Cytokine gene polymorphism and immunoregulation in periodontal disease. *Periodontol. 2000* **2004**, *35*, 158–182. [CrossRef] [PubMed]
25. Lee, A.; Ghaname, C.B.; Braun, T.M.; Sugai, J.V.; Teles, R.P.; Loesche, W.J.; Kornman, K.S.; Giannobile, W.V.; Kinney, J.S. Bacterial and salivary biomarkers predict the gingival inflammatory profile. *J. Periodontol.* **2012**, *83*, 79–89. [CrossRef]
26. Syndergaard, B.; Al-Sabbagh, M.; Kryscio, R.J.; Xi, J.; Ding, X.; Ebersole, J.L.; Miller, C.S. Salivary biomarkers associated with gingivitis and response to therapy. *J. Periodontol.* **2014**, *85*, e295–e303. [CrossRef]
27. Naruishi, K.; Nagata, T. Biological effects of interleukin-6 on Gingival Fibroblasts: Cytokine regulation in periodontitis. *J. Cell Physiol.* **2018**, *233*, 6393–6400. [CrossRef]
28. Volanakis, J.E. Human C-reactive protein: Expression, structure, and function. *Mol. Immunol.* **2001**, *38*, 189–197. [CrossRef]
29. Marsh, P.D.; Moter, A.; Devine, D.A. Dental plaque biofilms: Communities, conflict and control. *Periodontol. 2000* **2011**, *55*, 16–35. [CrossRef]
30. Marsh, P.D. Are dental diseases examples of ecological catastrophes? *Microbiology* **2003**, *149*, 279–294. [CrossRef]
31. Cekici, A.; Kantarci, A.; Hasturk, H.; Van Dyke, T.E. Inflammatory and immune pathways in the pathogenesis of periodontal disease. *Periodontol. 2000* **2014**, *64*, 57–80. [CrossRef]
32. Rathee, M.; Jain, P. *Gingivitis*; StatPearls Publishing: Treasure Island, FL, USA, 2022.
33. Garaicoa-Pazmino, C.; Fretwurst, T.; Squarize, C.H.; Berglundh, T.; Giannobile, W.V.; Larsson, L.; Castilho, R.M. Characterization of macrophage polarization in periodontal disease. *J. Clin. Periodontol.* **2019**, *46*, 830–839. [CrossRef] [PubMed]
34. Yu, T.; Zhao, L.; Huang, X.; Ma, C.; Wang, Y.; Zhang, J.; Xuan, D. Enhanced activity of the macrophage m1/m2 phenotypes and phenotypic switch to m1 in periodontal infection. *J. Periodontol.* **2016**, *87*, 1092–1102. [CrossRef] [PubMed]
35. Martinez, F.O.; Gordon, S. The M1 and M2 paradigm of macrophage activation: Time for reassessment. *F1000Prime Rep.* **2014**, *6*, 13. [CrossRef] [PubMed]
36. Das, A.; Sinha, M.; Datta, S.; Abas, M.; Chaffee, S.; Sen, C.K.; Roy, S. Monocyte and macrophage plasticity in tissue repair and regeneration. *Am. J. Pathol.* **2015**, *185*, 2596–2606. [CrossRef] [PubMed]
37. Garlet, G.P.; Giannobile, W.V. Macrophages: The bridge between inflammation resolution and tissue repair? *J. Dent. Res.* **2018**, *97*, 1079–1081. [CrossRef] [PubMed]
38. Young, D.P.; Kushner, I.; Samols, D. Binding of C/EBPbeta to the C-reactive protein (CRP) promoter in Hep3B cells is associated with transcription of CRP mRNA. *J. Immunol.* **2008**, *181*, 2420–2427. [CrossRef]
39. Kida, Y.; Kobayashi, M.; Suzuki, T.; Takeshita, A.; Okamatsu, Y.; Hanazawa, S.; Hasegawa, K. Interleukin-1 stimulates cytokines, prostaglandin E2 and matrix metalloproteinase-1 production via activation of MAPK/AP-1 and NF-kappaB in human gingival fibroblasts. *Cytokine* **2005**, *29*, 159–168. [CrossRef]
40. Sawada, S.; Chosa, N.; Ishisaki, A.; Naruishi, K. Enhancement of gingival inflammation induced by synergism of IL-1β and IL-6. *Biomed. Res.* **2013**, *34*, 31–40. [CrossRef]

Disclaimer/Publisher's Note: The statements, opinions and data contained in all publications are solely those of the individual author(s) and contributor(s) and not of MDPI and/or the editor(s). MDPI and/or the editor(s) disclaim responsibility for any injury to people or property resulting from any ideas, methods, instructions or products referred to in the content.

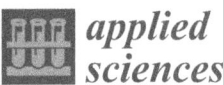

Article

Quantification of Salivary Nitric Oxide in Patients with Fixed Orthodontic Treatment

Ana-Madalina Raducanu [1], Sebastian Mihai [2], Ion Sandu [3,4,5,6,*], Andreea Anghel [7], Cristina Furnica [8,9,*], Raluca Ozana Chistol [8,10,*], Ciprian Adrian Dinu [11], Dana Tutunaru [11] and Kamel Earar [12]

1. MD Fixed Orthodontics SRL, 95 Ferdinand Blvd., 900709 Constanta, Romania
2. Faculty of Pharmacy, "Ovidius" University, 6 Capitan Aviator Al. Serbanescu St., 900470 Constanta, Romania
3. Academy of Romanian Scientists (AOSR), 54 Splaiul Independentei St., Sect. 5, 050094 Bucharest, Romania
4. Arheoinvest Platform, Alexandru Ioan Cuza University, 11 Carol I Blvd., 700506 Iasi, Romania
5. National Institute for Research and Development in Environmental Protection, 294 Splaiul Independentei Blvd., 6th District, 060031 Bucharest, Romania
6. Romanian Inventors Forum, 3 Sf. Petru Movila St., L11, III/3, 700089 Iasi, Romania
7. Faculty of Natural and Agricultural Sciences, "Ovidius" University, 24 Mamaia Blvd., 900527 Constanta, Romania
8. Faculty of Medicine, "Grigore T. Popa" University of Medicine and Pharmacy, 16 Universitatii St., 700115 Iasi, Romania
9. Institute of Forensic Medicine, 4 Buna Vestire St., 700455 Iasi, Romania
10. "Prof. Dr. George I.M. Georgescu" Cardiovascular Diseases Institute, 50 Carol I Blvd., 700503 Iasi, Romania
11. Department of Scientific Research, Dunarea de Jos University of Galati, 47 Domeneasca St., 800008 Galati, Romania
12. Department of Dental Medicine, Dunarea de Jos University of Galati, 47 Domeneasca St., 800008 Galati, Romania

* Correspondence: sandu_i03@yahoo.com (I.S.); cristina.furnica@umfiasi.ro (C.F.); raluca-ozana.chistol@umfiasi.ro (R.O.C.)

Abstract: Nitric oxide (NO) is considered a regulator of bone response to mechanical stress that mediates adaptive bone formation, the pathological effects of lipopolysaccharides (LPS), tumour necrosis factor (TNF), interleukin 1 (IL-1) and other cytokines; regulates leukocytes and epithelial cell adhesion; inhibits T cell proliferation; and enhances natural killer (NK) cell activity, as well as other immune-related processes. The aim of the current study was to test the potential use of salivary NO as a biomarker of bone response that is specific and sensitive to local changes, following the application of different types of dental appliances. Material and methods: Salivary NO was determined in 30 patients divided into three groups with 10 participants each: control (C), fixed metal braces group (M), and aligners group (A). Salivary NO was determined four times in each group (before the procedure, at 2 weeks, 30 days, and 60 days after the procedure) using ELISA and rapid semi-quantitative assay with Nitric Oxide Saliva Test Strips (Berkeley, CA, USA). The mean results were compared with the ANOVA test, and the Pearson correlation index was calculated. The results show a significant increase in salivary NO levels by both methods only in the metal braces group, which is suggestive of oxidative damage, increased invasiveness, and bone response to metal braces. In conclusion, our study showed that metal brackets lead to a significant temporary increase in oral oxidative stress as an adaptive reaction to the presence of foreign bodies in the oral cavity. The subsequent concentration decrease at 60 days suggests a normalization of the body's response to foreign bodies.

Keywords: nitric oxide; aligners; fixed apparatus; rapid strip testing; ELISA; dentistry; orthodontics

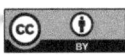

1. Introduction

Fixed orthodontic treatment is necessary in many types of dental anomalies. Positive aspects such as improved function, aesthetics, and self-esteem are also accompanied by side effects such as white spots, root resorption, pain (90% of cases), dental abrasions and microfractures, periodontal problems, and intra- and extra-oral lesions [1]. Lately, aligners have been developed as a less visible, less irritating, easier to clean and more comfortable treatment than conventional fixed therapy. The characteristics of the forces transmitted by the aligners depend largely on the properties of the materials used, their thickness and profile complexity, the degree of activation, and the use of accessory elements. Thermoplastic devices made of thicker materials produce a higher force, and thinner ones a lower force [2].

Nitric oxide (NO) is a pleiotropic biological mediator involved in intestinal motility, platelet aggregation and adhesion, bone tissue formation and destruction, apoptosis, neurotransmission, the regulation of vascular tone, and immunological functions [3,4]. It has a short in vivo half-life (a few seconds or less). Thus, levels of more stable metabolites such as nitrite (NO_2^-) and nitrate (NO_3^-) anions have been used for the indirect quantification of NO in biological fluids. Altered NO levels have been associated with septic status, sexual intercourse, infections, hypertension, exercise, type II diabetes mellitus, hypoxia, and cancer [4,5].

Since it is fat-soluble, NO is not stored but is synthesised de novo and diffuses freely across lipid membranes. NO has the potential to exert its effects on target cells through various mechanisms. For example, the NO-mediated activation of the enzyme guanylyl cyclase (GC) catalyses the formation of the secondary messenger $3',5'$-cyclic guanosine monophosphate (cGMP). cGMP is involved in several biological functions such as the regulation of smooth muscle contractility, cell survival, cell proliferation, axonal guidance, synapse plasticity, inflammation, and angiogenesis [5].

Nitric oxide is also considered a regulator of bone response to mechanical stress as it mediates adaptive bone formation (increased levels reduce osteoclastic activity and vice versa) and the pathological effects of lipopolysaccharides (LPS), tumour necrosis factor (TNF), interleukin 1 (IL-1) and other cytokines; regulates leukocytes and epithelial cell adhesion; inhibits T cell proliferation; and enhances natural killer (NK) cell activity, among other immune-related processes [6,7].

Given that any local oral change involves oxidative stress, we hypothesised that salivary nitric oxide may be a specific and sensitive marker for changes produced by orthodontic appliances.

Saliva is easy to collect and store and contains high quality DNA. However, research on its usage for diagnostic purposes is still in its early stages, and progress is limited by the lack of strict study protocols that allow a direct comparison of results from several independent laboratories [1].

The aim of the study is to quantify salivary NO levels by both rapid and specific methods and to demonstrate that it is a valid, specific, and sensitive biomarker for bone changes determined by the application of different types of braces. Moreover, the study aims to highlight the impact of fixed orthodontic equipment on the oxidative status of the oral cavity in comparison to thermoplastic aligners, as fixed bracers exert stronger forces and more friction on the oral soft tissue, which can cause inflammation, lesions, and a shift in the oxidative status of the oral cavity.

2. Material and Methods

2.1. Study Groups

We recruited 30 patients (Table 1) and divided them into 3 groups: control group (C), consisting of 6 women and 4 men (aged 18–30 years, mean 25.6 years); metal braces group (M), consisting of 5 women and 5 men (aged 16–30 years, mean 26.8 years); and the aligners group (A), with 8 women and 2 men (aged 18–30 years, mean 25.4 years).

Table 1. Inclusion and exclusion criteria.

Inclusion Criteria	Exclusion Criteria
• Age 16–30 years (radiologically confirmed growth peak—CS6 vertebral maturation stage). • Permanent teeth. • Candidate for orthodontic treatment; skeletal class I; no need for extractions, excessive extra expansion, or anchorage retaining appliances; and no history of trauma, bruxism, or parafunctions.	• Systemic diseases; • Large dental restorations, fixed or removable appliances; • Cleft lip or palate; • Anodontia; • Poor collaboration or oral hygiene; • Clinical or radiological periodontal damage; • Dental crowding over 6 mm; • Increased carious activity; • History of drug use; • Ongoing contraceptive medication; • Pregnancy; • Smoking; • Antibiotic treatment 6 months before harvesting; • Anti-inflammatory medication in the month before orthodontic treatment; • Active dental treatment at the beginning of application.

On the day of saliva sampling, the patients were asked not to brush their teeth with toothpaste (to avoid chemical interaction between saliva and toothpaste) and not to eat or drink water 30 min prior to sampling. All the patients were encouraged to maintain oral hygiene. After the fitting of dental braces, the patients were asked to use 500 mg of paracetamol in case of pain.

Written informed consent concerning saliva sampling and inclusion in the study was obtained in all cases. The study was approved by the Ovidius University Bioethics Committee in accordance with the principles of the Declaration of Helsinki (revised 2000, Edinburgh).

2.2. Application of Dental Braces

In the study, we used Micro Sprint metal braces produced by Forestadent Bernhard Förster GmbH (Pforzheim, Germany) and made of one-piece stainless steel. These braces are the smallest on the market and have a flat profile with no sharp edges to minimize the discomfort to the cheeks. All the springs initially used were 0.12 nickel-titanium (Ni-Ti), Alexander LTS shape produced by American Orthodontics (Murfreesboro, TN, USA). The composite (Enlight) and primer (Ortho Solo) were produced by Ormco (Orange, CA, USA). Briefly, the exposed dental crowns were dried, and a 37% phosphoric acid solution was applied for 30 s and then rinsed with distilled water. Brackets were applied according to the standard protocol.

In the case of aligners, prior impressions were made with Orthoprint alginate (Zhermack SpA, Rome, Italy). The material was prepared according to the manufacturer's instructions, placed in prefabricated spoons, and inserted into the oral cavity with gentle pressure from posterior to anterior so that the alginate could flow into depressions and record details as faithfully as possible. After removal and inspection, the impressions were washed with water, disinfected, and sent to the technical laboratory to manufacture the model [8]. The individualized aligners were produced by Scheu Dental GmbH (Am Burgberg, Germany) using polyethylene terephthalate glycol-copolyester, which meets the biocompatibility requirements for medical products.

2.3. Saliva Collection and Storage

Unstimulated saliva was collected in 4 time points: T0 before application; T1—at 2 weeks; T2—at 30 days; and T3—at 60 days after application. For saliva collection, patients rinsed the oral cavity with double distilled water; they were then asked to sit in a relaxed position with the head bent forward to promote fluid accumulation in the anterior part of the oral cavity. They were asked to swallow first, then for 5 min to spit into a tube-pan system without moving their tongue and cheeks. Each saliva sample was centrifuged immediately after collection at 14,000 rpm for 10 min, and the supernatant was transferred to sterile airtight tubes and stored without freeze–thaw cycles at $-20\,^\circ$C until analysis [9].

2.4. Detection and Quantification of Nitric Oxide by ELISA

The Total Nitric Oxide and Nitrate/Nitrite Parameter Assay Kit (R&D Systems Inc., Minneapolis, MN, USA) was used for an accurate quantitative determination of nitric oxide in the collected saliva. The determination of nitric oxide concentration is based on the enzymatic conversion of nitrate to nitrite by nitrate reductase, followed by the colorimetric detection of nitrite secondary to the Griess reaction. Treatment of the nitrate-containing saliva with the Griess reagent forms a pink-red azo dye through a two-step diazotization reaction—the acidic NO_2^- produced by a diazotizing agent reacts with sulfanilic acid to produce the diazonium ion, which reacts with N-(1-naphthyl)ethylenediamine in an azo coupling reaction to form the pink-red azo dye which absorbs light at 540–570 nm [8–10].

The kit requires two testing stages because NO- has a very short half-life (less than 0.1 s) and cannot be identified as such. The first step involves the quantification of endogenous nitrite. In the second step, nitrate is converted to nitrite using nitrate reductase, thus, quantifying total nitrite. The difference between total nitrite and endogenous nitrite matches the nitrate concentration representing the NO- level.

Prior to analysis, saliva was prepared according to the manufacturer's instructions, requiring double dilution with reagent diluent ($1\times$). All reagents were brought to room temperature prior to use. Double distilled water was used for the reconstruction and dilution of the reagents to avoid contamination with nitrates or nitrites. After completing all the steps according to the kit instructions, the samples were analysed by spectrophotometry (T Tecan Sunrise^{TM}, Männedorf, Switzerland) to quantify NO.

2.5. Determination of Total and Inducible Nitrite

All reagents and standards were prepared according to the procedures outlined above. A total of 50 µL of reaction diluent (1X) was placed in blank wells. A total of 50 µL of the test sample was added to the blank wells, over which 25 µL of NADH and 25 µL of nitrate reductase were added. The resulting solutions were mixed thoroughly, covered with adhesive tape, and incubated at 37 $^\circ$C for 30 min. After incubation, 50 µL of Griess Reagent I and 50 µL of Griess Reagent II were added to all wells, mixing by gently tapping the side of the plate. Afterwards, the plates were re-incubated for 10 min at room temperature. Finally, the absorbance of each well was read using a spectrophotometer equipped with a microplate reader (Tecan Sunrise^{TM}, Männedorf, Switzerland) at a wavelength of 540 nm.

2.6. Detection and Quantification of Nitric Oxide by Semi-Quantitative Method

A quick qualitative and semi-quantitative detection of salivary NO was performed with Nitric Oxide Saliva Test Strips (Berkeley, CA, USA) at similar time points for both the control and test groups: T0 before application; T1—at 2 weeks; T2—at 30 days; and T3—at 60 days. The strip was placed on the tongue for 10 s, folded and kept in contact for another 10 s. The result was compared with the colorimetric map available on the box for the semi-quantitative assessment (depleted, low, threshold, target, high). All the evaluations were carried out twice, with no differences between them.

2.7. Statistical Analysis

Microsoft Excel 360 software with Statistical Analysis Pack (Microsoft Corporation 2018) was used for the statistical evaluation. Endogenous nitrates were calculated by interpolation using the regression curve equation. The minimum accepted regression coefficient was 0.95 to ensure accurate mathematical interpolation. Total nitrates were calculated in a similar manner, and the concentration of inducible nitrates was computed as the difference between the total and endogenous nitrite concentration. Since the samples were diluted, the concentration was multiplied by the dilution factor.

The results were expressed as mean ± standard deviation. The mean values were compared using the ANOVA test. The Pearson correlation test was used to identify potential correlations between the analysed variables. A p-value < 0.05 was considered statistically significant.

3. Results

3.1. Quantification of Nitrite by ELISA

The mean molar concentrations of endogenous, total, and inducible nitrite quantified at the four time points through ELISA are detailed in Table 2.

Table 2. Mean endogenous, total, and inducible nitrite concentrations for the three study groups.

	T_0		T_1		T_2		T_3	
	μmol/L	SD	μmol/L	SD	μmol/L	SD	μmol/L	SD
			Endogenous nitrite					
Metal braces (M)	93.26	39.47	122.61	56.80	84.43	40.62	102.13	63.11
Aligners (A)	41.12	23.05	47.02	25.00	47.88	43.22	41.15	27.23
Control (C)	72.05	72.05	70.27	63.17	68.45	60.30	75.56	55.27
			Total nitrite					
Metal braces (M)	99.77	41.24	164.58	62.81	152.21	70.02	116.35	66.41
Aligners (A)	44.89	22.97	63.89	25.03	52.59	24.30	55.64	28.50
Control (C)	73.50	73.50	74.13	63.42	76.30	65.10	84.68	56.75
			Inducible nitrite					
Metal braces (M)	6.51	6.01	41.97	34.02	68.77	60.93	14.23	16.17
Aligners (A)	3.77	1.84	16.87	6.83	4.71	2.77	14.49	13.20
Control (C)	2.54	2.54	3.86	2.32	7.85	10.78	9.12	8.73

SD—standard deviation.

Total nitrite following the conversion of salivary nitrate registered significantly higher concentrations, especially at the T_1 and T_2 time points for patients with metal braces, compared to those with aligners and the control group ($p < 0.01$).

Inducible nitrite and the difference between total and endogenous nitrite registered an increase at T_1 and T_2 for groups A and M, with significantly higher values compared to the control group only for members of the M group ($p = 0.003$), while the A group displayed values close to the control group ($p = 0.45$).

3.2. Quantification of Nitrite by the Rapid Semi-Quantitative Method

Salivary nitrite concentrations determined using the rapid test are shown in Table 3.

Table 3. Salivary nitrite concentration by semi-quantitative method for the three study groups.

	T_0		T_1		T_2		T_3	
	μmol/L	SD	μmol/L	SD	μmol/L	SD	μmol/L	SD
Metallic braces (M)	92.00	37.95	146.00	85.40	143.00	53.14	103.00	55.59
Aligners (A)	38.00	37.95	47.00	43.47	38.00	37.95	38.00	37.95
Control (C)	91.51	91.51	83.37	43.37	68.48	68.48	47.43	47.43

SD—standard deviation.

Similar to the previous method, the patients with metal braces registered significantly higher values at T_1 and T_2 compared to those with aligners or in the control group ($p = 0.0021$). At T_3, nitrite concentrations approached the baseline ones for all patients.

The regression analysis proved a very good correlation between total nitrite concentration determined by the two methods at all time points (Figure 1).

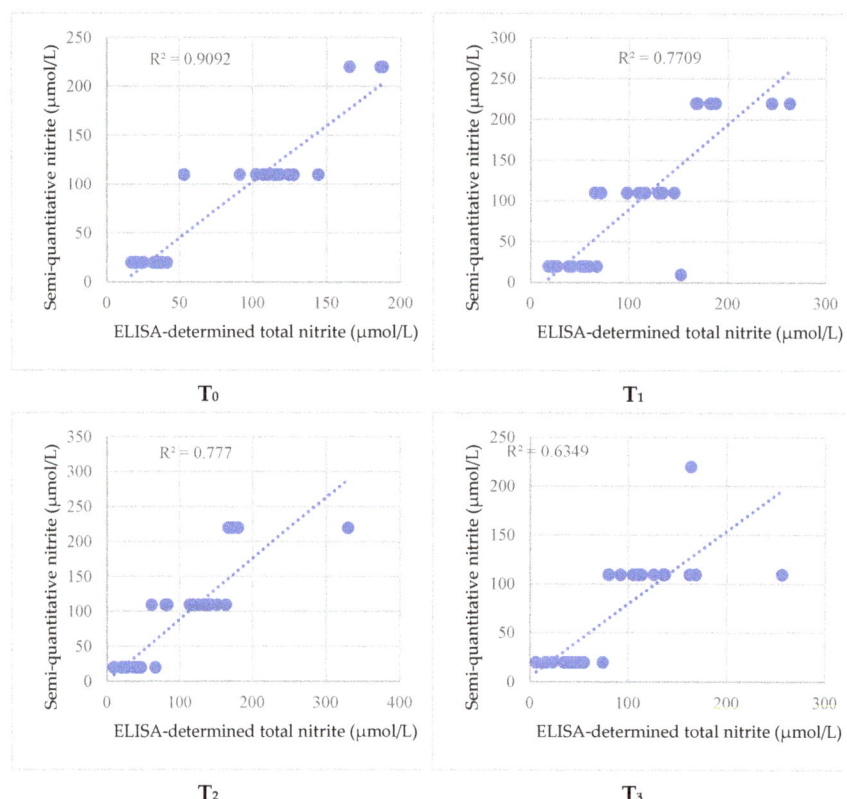

Figure 1. Correlations between total nitrite determined by ELISA and by the semi-quantitative method at T_0, T_1, T_2, T_3.

4. Discussions

In our study, the rapid test showed an increase in total nitrite in metal appliance wearers similar to ELISA for both T_1 and T_2 moments, as demonstrated by the statistical analysis. Moreover, the total nitrite concentration determined by the two methods (ELISA and Nitric Oxide Saliva Test Strips) displayed a strong correlation at all time points and for all three groups, suggesting that rapid testing could be used in daily practice as a substitute for a more expensive and laborious method with similar results.

Oxidative stress determined by free radicals mainly affects the cellular lipid component and is the subject of current research, although results are conflicting. This study also found a difference between the inducible nitrate levels in the metal bracers sub-group, compared to the sub-group treated with thermoplastic aligners, suggesting a higher impact of the metallic bracers on the oral cavity oxidative status. Nitric oxide is a free radical that plays an important role as a regulator of various physiological and pathological mechanisms in the body. In the oral cavity, it may act as a non-specific antimicrobial defence system by inhibiting bacterial growth or by enhancing macrophage-mediated cytotoxicity. There are two main transformation mechanisms: reduction in the enzyme reductase, released by certain bacteria, which converts nitrate (NO^{3-}) to nitrite (NO^{2-}); or by facilitated reduction by certain bacterial products resulting from the microflora of dental plaque, forming nitric oxide and nitric acid (which ionises to NO^{3-}). Enzymatically, it can also be produced from L-arginine by nitric oxide synthase (NOS), which has three isoforms: neuronal NOS (nNOS; Type I, NOS−1); inducible NOS (iNOS; Type II, NOS-2), which is present in various cells and tissues and is produced by immunocompetent cells—such as macrophages infected by the bacteria involved in regulating inflammatory reactions; and endothelial NOS (eNOS; Type III, NOS-3), which is found in vascular endothelial cells [11]. iNOS levels are significantly increased following tissue trauma (when cells are activated by external stimuli) and probably participates in the development of periodontal disease [11].

Regarding NO levels, Ka et al. showed similar mean values in patients with different oral cancers compared to orthodontic fixed appliances wearers [12]. Similarly, salivary NO levels in smokers are significantly higher than in non-smokers. In oral pathologies such as Behcet's disease and recurrent aphthous stomatitis, the elevated salivary values may guide the clinician as to the degree of severity and reflect serum values [11,13].

According to Shama et al., nitric oxide levels do not show considerable changes during one year of wearing orthodontic fixed appliances. Alarcon et al. demonstrated increases in NO levels from day 7 to day 30 since treatment initiation. In our study, total, endogenous, and inducible nitrite concentrations were determined in patients with fixed metal appliances and aligners and compared to a control group. The results revealed a statistically significant increase in total and inducible nitrite in the case of fixed metal appliances, compared to aligners and the control group. This elevation can be considered a physiological response to the presence of foreign bodies in the oral cavity [14,15]. A potential mechanism for the rise in inducible nitrates in the metal brackets sub-group is the interplay between the metal ions released by the device, and endogenous and bacterial metabolites that can lead to the formation of free radicals [16]. Furthermore, metal brackets have a more rigid and retentive surface that comes into intimate contact with oral soft tissues such as the cheeks, which can lead to the interaction of metal ions with surrounding cells, which, in turn, can lead to inflammation. Moreover, the normal movement of the oral cavity causes friction between the hard and irregular surface of the metal brackets, which can cause microlesions that can then cause an increase in oxidative stress and the production of free radicals [16]. Finally, during sleeping hours, both types of devices come into intimate contact with the oral mucosa, being pressed into it by the normal sleeping position. While the thermoplastic aligners have a smooth and regulated surface that is better tolerated by the oral mucosa, the metallic brackets can cause mechanical lesions to the mucosa that, ultimately, lead to inflammation. Aligner wearers registered similar values compared to the control group except for a non-significant increase in the inducible nitrite. Since inducible nitrite is a quantification of free radicals and, thus, a measure of oxidative stress [17], the results suggest the minimal invasiveness of aligner devices when compared to fixed metal devices. The level of oxidative stress expressed by the level of inducible nitrite returns to values close to baseline after a period of 60 days for both treatments.

Research investigating rapid nitrite quantification identified a positive correlation with salivary flow and caries incidence, especially in patients with high levels of daily stress [18,19].

A recent study assessed thermoplastic aligners that have self-ligating brackets with low friction and force exertion, regarding the oxidative stress of the oral cavity. The authors evaluated the patients at 30 and 90 days of treatment and highlighted an increase in oxidative stress in the first 30 days of treatment, followed by a return to base values after 90 days. The authors concluded that both methods impact salivary oxidative status similarly and note the importance of friction and other forces exerted on the saliva oxidative status [20].

Another recent study assessed the manifestation of oxidative stress in patients treated with fixed metallic appliances. The authors measured ROS in the patients' blood and the antioxidant defence (AD) and found that orthodontic treatments with fixed metal appliances can induce short-term systemic oxidative stress. This study highlights that fixed metallic appliances can cause microlesions that can lead to the formation of free radicals and shows that the shift of the oxidative status is traceable in other bodily fluids [21]. As microlesions form, there is a shift in the oxidative status of the oral cavity which favours the release of oxygen and nitrogen reactive species. As this phenomenon continues in time, it is possible that the oxidative status shift can be detected in other body fluids [21].

Additionally, metal brackets are also known to release nickel [22] and chromium [23]. This phenomenon further contributes to the shift of the oxidative status towards the formation of free radicals, further impacting all oxygen and nitrogen reactive species levels.

The alternatives to orthodontic treatment with vestibular appliances (those used in research) and aligners are the lingual technique and the self-ligation system. They also involve appliances with brackets bonded to the tooth using different mechanisms. We consider that aligners are the only real replacement of the classic system.

Limitations: A nitrate-rich diet together with the activity of commensal nitrate-reducing bacteria also increase salivary nitrate/nitrite levels by excretion or local production. The confounding effect of diet-derived nitrate could not be eliminated, as none of the patients followed a low-nitrate diet prior to saliva sampling. The small sample size was another limiting factor, as well as the overall lack of high-quality clinical trials working with saliva for the quantification of reactive oxygen and nitrogen species.

In our study, the rapid test showed an increase in total nitrite in metal appliances wearers similar to ELISA for both the T_1 and T_2 moments, as demonstrated by the statistical analysis. Moreover, total nitrite concentration determined by the two methods (ELISA and Nitric Oxide Saliva Test Strips) displayed a strong correlation at all time points and for all three groups, suggesting that rapid testing could be used in daily practice as a substitute to a more expensive and laborious method with similar results.

5. Conclusions

Metal brackets lead to a significant temporary increase in oral oxidative stress (total and inducible nitrites) as an adaptive reaction to the presence of foreign bodies in the oral cavity. The subsequent concentration decrease at 60 days indicates a normalization of the body's response to foreign bodies. Nevertheless, the tolerability and non-invasiveness of aligners are superior to metal brackets, as suggested by the lack of a significant increase in oxidative stress. Rapid tests could be used as a substitute to ELISA for nitrite quantification in daily practice.

Author Contributions: Conceptualization, A.-M.R., C.A.D. and R.O.C.; methodology, A.-M.R. and I.S.; software, S.M.; validation, A.-M.R., C.F. and R.O.C.; formal analysis, S.M., C.A.D. and I.S.; investigation, A.-M.R., D.T. and K.E.; resources, A.-M.R., D.T. and A.A.; data curation, A.A. and S.M.; writing—original draft preparation, A.-M.R. and K.E.; writing—review and editing, R.O.C. and C.F.; visualization, K.E., R.O.C. and C.F.; supervision, I.S. All authors have read and agreed to the published version of the manuscript.

Funding: This research received no external funding.

Institutional Review Board Statement: The study was conducted in accordance with the Declaration of Helsinki and approved by the the Ovidius University Bioethics Committee (17712/15.11.2018).

Informed Consent Statement: Informed consent was obtained from all subjects involved in the study.

Data Availability Statement: Data available on request due to restrictions e.g., privacy or ethical.

Conflicts of Interest: The authors declare no conflict of interest.

References

1. Mainali, A. Occurrence of Oral Ulcerations in Patients undergoing Orthodontic Treatment: A Comparative study. *Orthod. J. Nepal* **2013**, *3*, 32–35. [CrossRef]
2. Moshiri, M.; Eckhart, J.E.; McShane, P.; German, D.S. Consequences of poor oral hygiene during aligner therapy. *J. Clin. Orthod.* **2013**, *47*, 494–498. [PubMed]
3. Greabu, M.; Battino, M.; Mohora, M.; Totan, A.; Spinu, T.; Totan, C.; Didilescu, A.; Duţa, C. Could constitute saliva the first line of defence against oxidative stress? *Rom. J. Intern. Med.* **2007**, *45*, 209–213. [PubMed]
4. Tsikas, D. Methods of quantitative analysis of the nitric oxide metabolites nitrite and nitrate in human biological fluids. *Free Radic. Res.* **2005**, *39*, 797–815. [CrossRef] [PubMed]
5. Yugar-Toledo, J.C.; Tanus-Santos, J.E.; Sabha, M.; Sousa, M.G.; Cittadino, M.; Tácito, L.H.; Moreno, H., Jr. Uncontrolled hypertension, uncompensated type II diabetes, and smoking have different patterns of vascular dysfunction. *Chest* **2004**, *125*, 823–830. [CrossRef] [PubMed]

6. Tan, S.D.; Xie, R.; Klein-Nulend, J.; van Rheden, R.E.; Bronckers, A.L.; Kuijpers-Jagtman, A.M.; Von den Hoff, J.W.; Maltha, J.C. Orthodontic force stimulates eNOS and iNOS in rat osteocytes. *J. Dent. Res.* **2009**, *88*, 255–260. [CrossRef]
7. Wang, Y.; Liu, X.-F.; Cornish, K.G.; Zucker, I.H.; Patel, K.P. Effects of nNOS antisense in the paraventricular nucleus on blood pressure and heart rate in rats with heart failure. *Am. J. Physiol. Circ. Physiol.* **2005**, *288*, H205–H213. [CrossRef]
8. Miles, A.M.; Wink, D.A.; Cook, J.C.; Grisham, M.B. Determination of nitric oxide using fluorescence spectroscopy. *Methods Enzymol.* **1996**, *268*, 105–120. [CrossRef]
9. Malamud, D. Saliva as a Diagnostic Fluid. *Dent. Clin. N. Am.* **2011**, *55*, 159–178. [CrossRef]
10. R&D Systems Kit, E. Total Nitric Oxide and Nitrate/Nitrite Parameter Assay Kit [Internet]. Available online: https://www.rndsystems.com/products/total-nitric-oxide-and-nitrate-nitrite-parameter-assay-kit_kge001#product-citations (accessed on 14 December 2021).
11. Wang, Y.; Huang, X.; He, F. Mechanism and role of nitric oxide signaling in periodontitis. *Exp. Ther. Med.* **2019**, *18*, 3929–3935. [CrossRef]
12. Ka, F.; Castelino, R.L.; Babu, S.G.; Madi, M.; Shetty, S.R.; Balan, P.; Bhat, S. Status of Salivary Nitric Oxide Levels and Buccal Epithelial Cell DNA Damage in Potentially Malignant Disorders—A Biochemical Study. *J. Dent. Indones.* **2017**, *24*, 34–37. [CrossRef]
13. Menziletoglu, D.; Kucukkolbasi, H.; Dursun, R.; Kulaksizoglu, S.; Yilmaz, S. Evaluation of Serum and Salıva Nıtrıc Oxıde Levels ın Recurrent Aphthous Stomatıtıs and Behcet's Dısease. *SN Compr. Clin. Med.* **2019**, *1*, 334–338. [CrossRef]
14. Subramaniam, P.; Sharma, A.; Moiden, S. Analysis of salivary IgA, amylase, lactoferrin, and lysozyme before and after comprehensive dental treatment in children: A prospective study. *Contemp. Clin. Dent.* **2017**, *8*, 526–530. [CrossRef]
15. Yan, T.; Xie, Y.; He, H.; Fan, W.; Huang, F. Role of nitric oxide in orthodontic tooth movement (Review). *Int. J. Mol. Med.* **2021**, *48*, 168. [CrossRef] [PubMed]
16. Paithankar, J.G.; Saini, S.; Dwivedi, S.; Sharma, A.; Chowdhuri, D.K. Heavy metal associated health hazards: An interplay of oxidative stress and signal transduction. *Chemosphere* **2021**, *262*, 128350. [CrossRef]
17. Alves, R.C.C.; Ferreira, R.O.; Frazão, D.R.; Né, Y.G.d.S.; Mendes, P.F.S.; Marañón-Vásquez, G.; Royes, L.F.F.; Fagundes, N.C.F.; Maia, L.C.; Lima, R.R. The Relationship between Exercise and Salivary Oxidative Stress: A Systematic Review. *Antioxidants* **2022**, *11*, 1489. [CrossRef]
18. Al-Moosawi, R.I.K.; Qasim, A.A. The impact of dental environment stress on dentition status, salivary nitric oxide and flow rate. *J. Int. Soc. Prev. Community Dent.* **2020**, *10*, 163–170. [CrossRef]
19. Aksit-Bicak, D.; Emekli-Alturfan, E.; Ustundag, U.V.; Akyuz, S. Assessment of dental caries and salivary nitric oxide levels in children with dyspepsia. *BMC Oral Health* **2019**, *19*, 11. [CrossRef]
20. López-Mateos, C.M.; López-Mateos, M.L.M.; Aguilar-Salvatierra, A.; Gómez-Moreno, G.; Carreño, J.C.; Khaldy, H.; Menéndez-Núñez, M. Salivary Markers of Oxidative Stress in Patients Undergoing Orthodontic Treatment with Clear Aligners versus Self-Ligating Brackets: A Non-Randomized Clinical Trial. *J. Clin. Med.* **2022**, *11*, 3531. [CrossRef]
21. Kovac, V.; Poljsak, B.; Perinetti, G.; Primozic, J. Systemic Level of Oxidative Stress during Orthodontic Treatment with Fixed Appliances. *BioMed Res. Int.* **2019**, *2019*, 5063565. [CrossRef]
22. Sfondrini, M.F.; Cacciafesta, V.; Maffia, E.; Scribante, A.; Alberti, G.; Biesuz, R.; Klersy, C. Nickel release from new conventional stainless steel, recycled, and nickel-free orthodontic brackets: An in vitro study. *Am. J. Orthod. Dentofac. Orthop.* **2010**, *137*, 809–815. [CrossRef] [PubMed]
23. Sfondrini, M.F.; Cacciafesta, V.; Maffia, E.; Massironi, S.; Scribante, A.; Alberti, G.; Biesuz, R.; Klersy, C. Chromium Release from New Stainless Steel, Recycled and Nickel-free Orthodontic Brackets. *Angle Orthod.* **2009**, *79*, 361–367. [CrossRef] [PubMed]

 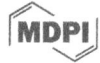

Review
Probiotics in Oral Health and Disease: A Systematic Review

Perrine Saïz, Nuno Taveira * and Ricardo Alves

Centro de Investigação Interdisciplinar Egas Moniz (CiiEM), Instituto Universitário Egas Moniz, 2829-511 Monte de Caparica, Portugal; perrinesaiz.psz@gmail.com (P.S.); ralves@egasmoniz.edu.pt (R.A.)
* Correspondence: ntaveira@ff.ulisboa.pt; Tel.: +351-966147563

Abstract: Purpose: Probiotics may exclude or antagonize oral pathogens and be useful to prevent oral dysbiosis and treat oral diseases. The objective of this review was to assess the benefits of probiotics in oral health and disease, and in dental practice; Methods: Primary articles published between January 2012 and 30 December 2020 with full text available were searched in PubMed, ClinicalTrials.gov, ScienceDirect, Google Scholar, B-on, and SciELO; Results: The electronic search identified 361 references of which 91 (25.2%) met all the inclusion criteria. In total, data from 5374 participants with gingivitis, periodontitis, peri-implantitis, caries, orthodontic conditions, halitosis, or oral conditions associated with chemo-radiotherapy were included. Despite major inconsistencies between clinical trials, probiotics have been found to contribute to reduce *S. mutans* counts (*L. paracasei* SD1), reduce probing depth in chronic periodontitis (*B. animalis* subsp. *lactis* DN-173010 with *L. reuteri*), reduce levels of volatile sulfur compounds and halitosis (*L. salivarius* WB21), treat oral mucositis and improve the quality of life of patients undergoing cancer chemo-radiotherapy (*L. brevis* CD2). Combinations of probiotic bacteria tend to lead to higher clinical efficacy than any individual probiotic agent; Conclusion: Oral probiotics influence favorably the oral microbiota and provide benefits to the oral ecosystem in periodontal diseases, cariology, halitosis, orthodontics and management of oral mucositis resulting from cancer treatment. However, the use of probiotics in dental practice or in self-management preventive strategies requires additional well controlled clinical trials to determine the most effective probiotic combinations, the most appropriate probiotic vehicle, and the frequency of administration.

Keywords: probiotics; oral microbiota; oral health; oral diseases; dental practice

Citation: Saïz, P.; Taveira, N.; Alves, R. Probiotics in Oral Health and Disease: A Systematic Review. *Appl. Sci.* **2021**, *11*, 8070. https://doi.org/10.3390/app11178070

Academic Editor: Bruno Chrcanovic

Received: 15 July 2021
Accepted: 26 August 2021
Published: 31 August 2021

Publisher's Note: MDPI stays neutral with regard to jurisdictional claims in published maps and institutional affiliations.

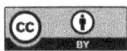

Copyright: © 2021 by the authors. Licensee MDPI, Basel, Switzerland. This article is an open access article distributed under the terms and conditions of the Creative Commons Attribution (CC BY) license (https://creativecommons.org/licenses/by/4.0/).

1. Introduction

The oral cavity is a dynamic ecosystem, with environmental changes and permanent interactions in which commensal bacteria limit the colonization of pathogenic microorganisms. The oral microbiota is heterogeneous and diverse, and its imbalance leads to the onset of major oral diseases such as periodontitis and dental caries [1]. Conventional treatment of these diseases involves removal of the bacterial plaque by mechanical means and antimicrobial drug therapy which may have limited efficacy due to drug resistance [2]. It is necessary to look for alternatives and adjuvants to conventional therapeutic and prevention approaches and probiotics may play an important role in this context.

According to the World Health Organization (WHO) and the Food and Agriculture Organization of the United Nations (FAO), probiotics are "living microorganisms that, when administered in adequate amounts, confer benefits to host health" [3]. Probiotic-based intervention strategies are widely used for intestinal diseases but not yet for oral diseases due to the limited scientific evidence of usefulness. Probiotics can outcompete pathogenic bacteria and increase the proportion of beneficial bacteria in the mouth thereby contributing for the prevention and therapy of oral diseases [4–6]. In order to be effective in the oral cavity, probiotics must support oral environmental conditions, adhere to and colonize oral surfaces, inhibit oral pathogens [7,8], and/or delay colonization by pathogenic strains [5]. Furthermore, they must not ferment the sugars in order to avoid the pH decrease and demineralization of the enamel, they should hamper the organization of the extracellular matrix responsible for biofilm formation, limit the production of cytotoxic products by pathogenic bacteria, and beneficially alter the biochemical parameters that influence the dental plaque (e.g., salivary components, buffer capacity) (Figure 1) [9]. In addition, oral probiotics must be safe for the host [10,11].

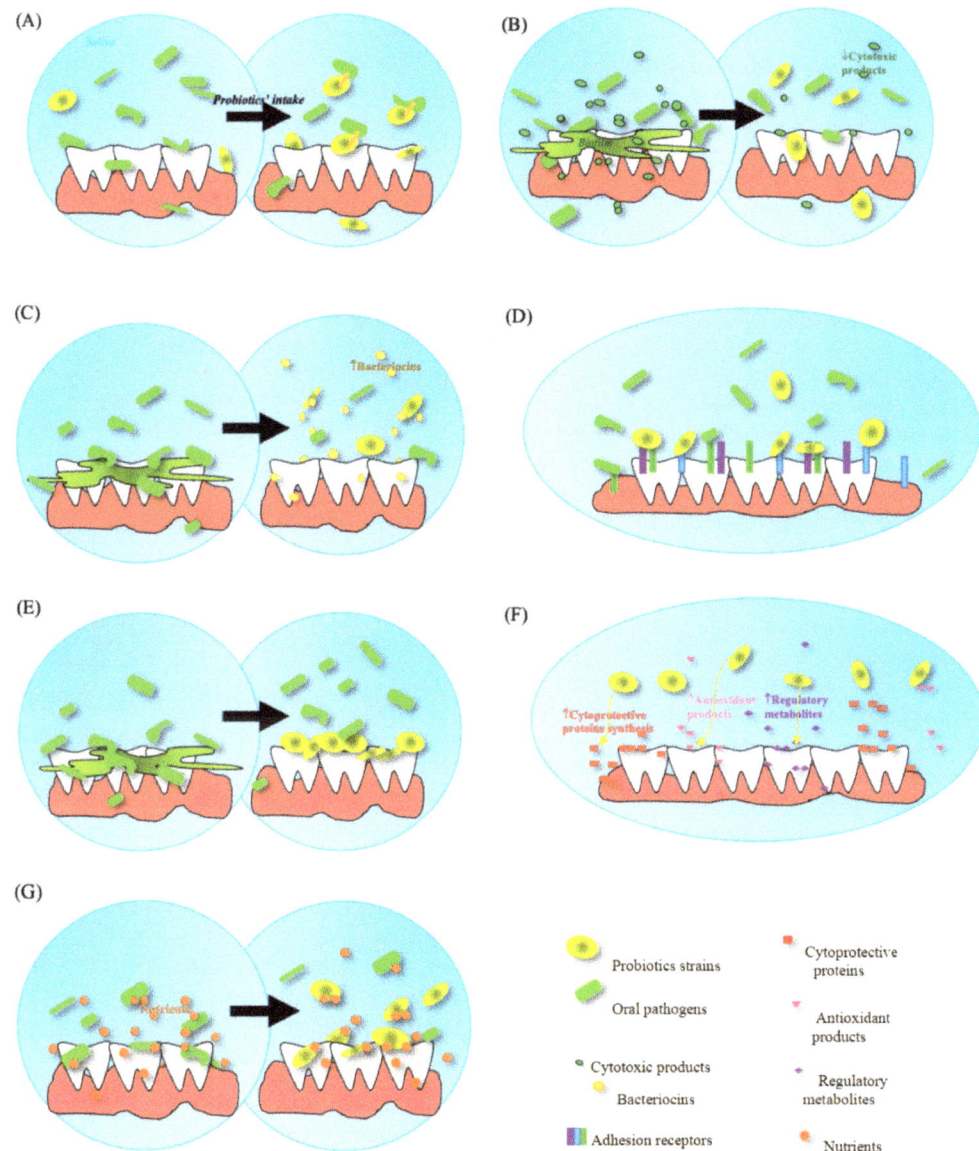

Figure 1. Potential mechanisms of action of probiotics in oral health and disease: (**A**) direct interaction with pathogens to prevent pathogen colonization; (**B**) antagonistic activity on pathogens cytotoxic metabolites, oral biofilm, and extracellular matrix; (**C**) synthesis of antibacterial agents (e.g., bacteriocins) against oral pathogens; (**D**) alter adhesion, aggregation, colonization, and proliferation of pathogens in oral tissues due to mechanisms of exclusion and competition; (**E**) coating oral tissues to protect oral surfaces from pathogens action; (**F**) maintain oral ecosystem balance by synthetizing cytoprotective proteins, antioxidant products, and regulatory metabolites on surface of oral cells; (**G**) competition for nutrients.

The therapeutic and prophylactic potential of probiotics has been explored with promising results in major oral diseases like periodontitis and dental caries [12–15]. However, questions remain regarding the best probiotic species or strains for each oral disease or condition and for each population or individual [16], and regarding the most appropriate probiotic vehicles, dose, and frequency of administration. To determine the usefulness of probiotics in current dental practice we make a critical review of clinical studies assessing the potential benefits of probiotics in oral health and disease.

2. Material and Methods

2.1. Protocol

This systematic review used the Preferred Reporting Items for Systematic reviews and Meta-analysis (PRISMA) guidelines [17]. The PRISMA checklist is available as a Supplementary file (Table S1).

2.2. Focused Question and Eligibility Criteria

The following question was set: "Is there scientific evidence that the use of probiotics confers benefits to human oral health?" The PICOS criteria that allowed the elaboration of the research question are presented in Table S2.

The eligibility criteria of the studies to be included in the review were:

1. Types of study: randomized clinical trials, without any information of blinding, blind (single, double, or triple), placebo controlled, or non-placebo controlled (compared to another intervention), including cross-over studies.
2. Type of participants: of any age (adults, children, the elderly), without gender restriction, healthy or not.
3. Type of intervention: use of any probiotic (alone or in combination).
4. Considering any dosage regimen, vehicle of delivery or frequency of intervention. Comparators may consist of placebo or other active intervention without probiotics (with or without prebiotic/synbiotic vs. placebo/other intervention). Prebiotics are a group of nutrients that are degraded by gut microbiota. Synbiotic is a mixture of pre- and probiotics. Studies including an auxiliary to the active treatment were analyzed.
5. Primary outcomes: clinical, microbiological, immunological, and biochemical parameters.
6. Secondary outcomes: any adverse effects, rate of adherence, quality of life.

2.3. Search Strategy and Study Selection

The bibliographic search was carried out in the following electronic databases PubMed, ClinicalTrials.gov, ScienceDirect, Google Scholar, B-on, SciELO using the keywords "probiotics", "dental practice", "oral health", "oral diseases" and "oral microbiota" and the conjugation of these keywords. Articles published between January 2012 and 30 December 2020 with full text available were selected. Duplicate references, articles available in 2011 published in 2012, theses, reviews, and articles related to oral probiotics intake with only systemic repercussion were excluded. Further research was done after reading the references of all relevant articles. The full texts of all articles corresponding to the inclusion criteria were obtained and examined for final inclusion. The selection process was included in a PRISMA flow diagram (Figure S1).

3. Results

The electronic search identified 361 references. After removing the duplicates, 308 references were selected for eligibility based on the titles and abstracts, excluding in vitro studies, animal studies, and ongoing and unpublished clinical trials. After searching in the references, 28 additional articles were identified. For the full text review, 129 articles were selected. Of these, 38 clinical trials were excluded because oral health was not the focus of the study, because the study design was unclear, there was no information about allocation, the intake of probiotics was evaluated in animals, and studies were performed in vitro. The 91 randomized controlled trials (RTCs) included in the review involve data from

5374 participants with gingivitis ($n = 14$), periodontitis ($n = 21$), peri-implantitis ($n = 8$), carie ($n = 23$), orthodontic conditions ($n = 6$), halitosis ($n = 4$), oral conditions associated with chemo-radiotherapy ($n = 6$) and changes in the oral ecosystem ($n = 9$). Sample sizes range from 10 and 321 participants. The duration of interventions varied between 7 days and up to 2 years. There were 59 studies performed in adults, 24 in children, and 8 in more than one age group. Regarding the probiotic/s administered, 53 studies have implemented a combination of probiotics and 37 have administered a single probiotic. Two studies used symbiotic/prebiotic (1 with a single probiotic and 1 with a combination). The concentrations of the probiotics were not reported in 29 studies and one study did not specify the probiotic that was used. In two studies the duration of administration of probiotic(s) was not given. Adverse effects were reported in 13 trials.

Regarding the study design, there are 11 cross-over trials, 80 placebo-controlled trials and 11 trials compared with another intervention. Regarding the blinding, there are 18 studies without indication of blinding, five single blinding, 61 double-blind, six triple-blind and one with no blinding. The primary results of the studies are mainly focused on clinical, microbiological, and immunological parameters. No data were analyzed regarding financing, for-profit bias, and location of studies.

4. Discussion

4.1. Impact of Probiotics in the Oral Microbiota

The community of microorganisms that colonizes the mouth and forms the dental plaque mainly plays a protective role against pathogens. Dental plaque consists of bacterial cells (mainly streptococci and lactobacilli), bacterial metabolites/products/toxins, salivary polymers/proteins, and food debris [1]. Probiotic lactobacilli may inhibit the adhesion of pathogenic bacteria to the oral tissues, reducing the amount of biofilm formed (Figure 1). On the other hand, lactobacilli probiotics may potentiate dental plaque acidogenicity and increase the load of acid tolerant bacteria such as *S. mutans* and viridans streptococci, making the dental biofilm more pathogenic [18]. The following 9 trials studied the impact of probiotics in the oral ecosystem (Table S3). In Thakkar et al. [19], dental plaque accumulation in children was significantly reduced after 14 days of tablet consumption containing *L. acidophilus, L. rhamnosus, Bifidobacterium longum* and *S. boulardii*, and after three weeks of intervention. In a study by Burton et al. [20], administration of *Streptococcus salivarius* M18 to children for 3 months caused a significant decrease in dental plaque scores. Non-target microorganisms, *S. salivarius, Lactobacillus* spp., hemolytic streptococci and *Candida* spp. levels were not changed during the study. Despite a high adhesion rate (>80%), only 22% of the children were colonized by *S. salivarius* M18 and this lasted until 4 months after discontinuation. *S. mutans* counts were reduced, especially in colonized children, suggesting that *S. salivarius* M18 may have anti-carie activity and that colonization helps the probiotic effect.

A significant reduction of salivary *Aggregatibacter actynomycetancomitans, P. gingivalis* and *Streptococcus mutans* counts, and total number of microorganisms was achieved in children after 2-weeks ingestion of Petit-Suisse (cream cheese) with *L. casei* [21]. However, the reduction of total number of microorganisms and *Streptococcus mutans* was attributed to Petit-Suisse alone as it occurred in both the probiotic and control groups.

A significant decrease in *S. mutans* counts and in the total number of microorganisms occurred after once daily consumption of fermented milk containing *L. rhamnosus* SD11 in adults during 4-weeks and after 4-weeks discontinuation [22]. In contrast, *Lactobacillus* spp. counts increased significantly at week 4 in all patients, and the probiotic was detected up to 8 weeks in 80% of the individuals. In a study by Toiviainen et al. [23], a combination of *L. rhamnosus* GG and *B. lactis* BB-12 administered over 4 weeks to adults caused no change in the salivary *S. mutans* or *Lactobacillus* spp. counts. Similarly, *L. reuteri* DSM 17938 and ATCC PTA 5289 administered during 2–12 weeks to adults had no impact on salivary *S. mutans* count and microbial profile and diversity [24–26]. Administration of *L. rhamnosus* GG or *L. reuteri* D2112 and PTA 5289, also did not impact salivary *S. mutans* count [18].

However, there was a significant increase in lactobacilli in volunteers taking *L. reuteri* but not *L. rhamnosus*.

In summary, most probiotic strains analyzed in these trials are safe, as they do not significantly and definitively affect the commensal oral microbiota, and some can transiently colonize the dental surfaces and have the potential to prevent dental caries.

4.2. Probiotics in Periodontology

Periodontitis is caused by periodontopathogenic bacteria (*Porphyromonas gingivalis, Treponema denticola, Tannerella forsythia* and *Aggregatibacter actinomycetancomitans*) that are organized in biofilms at the supragingival and subgingival levels in susceptible hosts [1,27]. Treatment consists of the mechanical removal of pathogenic biofilm and the use of antiseptics or antibiotics [28]. The main objective of the treatments is to avoid recolonization by pathogenic bacteria. Probiotics as adjuvants to mechanical treatment could modify and occupy the subgingival niche susceptible to recolonization by pathogenic bacteria and allow a new equilibrium with the oral environment (Figure 1) [7]. Probiotics could also alter the bacterial profile of the biofilm adjacent to implants [29]. In addition, they could act as immunomodulators in the oral cavity by decreasing pro-inflammatory cytokines IL-1β, TNF-α and matrix metalloproteinases (MMP) levels, and increasing IL-10, TGF-β1 and tissue inhibitor of metalloproteinases (TIMP) levels [30–32].

4.2.1. Probiotics in Gingival Health and Gingivitis

Fourteen randomized clinical trials related to the use of probiotics in gingivitis and gingival health were analyzed (Table S4). In a study by Kuru et al. [33], 4-week use of yogurt supplemented with *Bifidobacterium animalis subsp. lactis* DN-173010 had a positive effect on gingival inflammatory parameters after a 5-day non-brushing period. In a study by Yousuf et al. [9], plaque index (PI) and gingival index (GI) scores were reduced in adolescents after two weeks administration of a probiotic combination containing *Bifidobacterium longum, Lactobacillus acidophilus, Bifidobacterium bifidum, Bifidobacterium lactis* and acid lactic *bacillus*. Dhawan and Dhawan [11] showed a significant reduction of PI up to 4 weeks with the probiotic combination *Lactobacillus sporogenes, Streptococcus faecalis* PC, *Clostridium butyrium* TO-A, and *Bacillus mesentericus* TO-A in patients with gingivitis. In studies by Desmukh et al. [34] and Nadkerny et al. [7], individuals with gingival health and gingivitis were administered with a probiotic combination for two weeks. Control group used chlorhexidine. The probiotic combination reduced gingival inflammation and plaque accumulation in the same way as chlorhexidine in both studies suggesting it could serve as an adjuvant in plaque control. Alkaya et al. [35] tested three modes of application of *Bacillus subtilis, Bacillus megaterium,* and *Bacillus pumulus* in patients with gingivitis after mechanical therapy and no significant difference was observed between the probiotic and placebo groups.

Similar negative results were obtained by Keller et al. [36] when using *Lactobacillus rhamnosus* and *Lactobacillus curvatus* tablets in patients with gingivitis.

Contrasting results were obtained when using *Lactobacillus reuteri* (DSM17938 and ATCC PTA 5289) probiotic for gingivitis. In a study by Hallstrom et al. [30], there were no clinical, microbiological, and immunological benefits in women with experimental gingivitis. In a study by Iniesta et al. [37], there was a significant reduction in salivary counts of total anaerobes after 4 weeks of intervention, and *Prevotella intermedia* counts after 4 and 8 weeks in patients with gingivitis relative to the placebo group. *Porphyromonas gingivalis* counts also decreased significantly in a subgingival sample up to 4 weeks. However, there was no difference between PI and GI scores in the test and placebo groups. In contrast, Sabatini et al. [4] showed a significant reduction in PI and GI scores in patients with controlled diabetes type II after 30 days on probiotic. Likewise, Schagenhauf et al. [38] showed a significant reduction of clinical parameters and a complete resolution of sites with mild inflammation in pregnant women. The results suggest that *L. reuteri*-based probiotics may help to manage gingivitis in individuals more susceptible to oral infections.

Lee et al. [39] evaluated the effects of *Lactobacillus brevis* CD2 in experimental gingivitis. Significant differences at the bleeding on probing (BOP) level were found on day 10 in favor of the probiotic group but no longer on day 14 suggesting that this strain can delay the onset of gingivitis over a short period of time. Consistent with this, there was a progressive increase in nitric oxide (NO), an inflammatory mediator, in the gingival crevicular fluid (GCF) of the placebo group unlike the probiotic group in which there was no change.

Alanzi et al. [40] evaluated the 4-weeks administration of probiotic tablets containing *Lactobacillus rhamnosus*, *Bifidobacterium lactis* on adolescents with gingival health. There was a significant reduction in *Aggregatibacter actynomycetancomitans* and *F. nucleatum* counts in saliva and plaque, and *P. gingivalis* count in plaque in the probiotic group. GI scores also improved in the probiotic group. In Montero et al. [41] administration of tablets containing *Lactobacillus plantarum, Lactobacillus brevis*, and *Peiococcus acidilactici* for 6-weeks to patients with gingivitis led to a significant reduction of severe gingival inflammation scores when compared to placebo. In addition, the average number of sites per patient with moderate inflammation was reduced from 56 to 4 after the probiotic intervention period. There was a decrease in *T. forsythia* counts which the authors correlated with the decrease of severe inflammation scores.

Overall, these studies suggest that long term use of some probiotics may aid in oral hygiene, promote gingival health, and help to treat gingivitis. This effect is more significant when there is no mechanical removal of the plaque [4,7,9,11,38,40] than when the plaque is removed [35]. Additional long-term studies are needed in larger population across all age ranges and ethnic groups to obtain more consistent clinical results, and to determine if probiotics need to colonize the oral cavity to cause a beneficial effect.

4.2.2. Probiotics in Periodontitis

The uncontrolled expansion of periodontopathogenic bacteria (*Porphyromonas gingivalis, Treponema denticola, Tannerella forsythia, Filifactor alocis, Parvimonas micra, Aggregatibacter actinomycetemcomitans* and species of *Fusobacterium and Prevotella*) along with dysregulation of the immune barriers and tissue damage leads to periodontitis [1]. Remodeling of the periodontal extracellular matrix depends on the balance between proteolytic enzymes responsible for the degradation and remodeling of extracellular matrix proteins (MMPs), present in saliva, dental plaque and GCF and tissue inhibitors of MMPs, TIMP-1 and TIMP-2 [42,43]. In case of periodontal diseases, an imbalance in the ratio of MMPs/TIMPs (e.g., TIMP-1 reduction and MMP 8–9 increase) leads to periodontal destruction.

The conventional treatment of periodontitis involves the mechanical removal of the subgingival plaque. Scaling and root planing (SRP) is the standard control method and can be complemented by the addition of antibiotics which can lead to development of resistance, modifications of the commensal flora and risk of dysbiosis [28]. On the other hand, bacterial plaque is difficult to remove in low access sites, and remaining bacteria can cause periodontitis relapse and can invade adjacent tissues (i.e., mucosa, tongue, tonsils) and cause new infections [1].

Probiotics were proposed as adjuncts to the mechanical therapy of periodontitis aiming at restoring the commensal microbiota and reduce inflammation and tissue damage [44,45]. For this review, 21 randomized clinical trials related to the implementation of probiotics in periodontal conditions were selected (Table S5). Most trials have used species of *Lactobacillus* because it is a commensal bacterium that antagonizes *P. gingivalis* [10,46].

In Vicario et al. [10], tablets containing *L. reuteri* ATCC 55,730 and *L. reuteri* ATCCPTA 5289 were administered to patients with chronic periodontitis for 30 days. All clinical parameters improved significantly in the test group, suggesting a possible synergy between the strains used. In a study by Imran et al. [47], ingestion of milk with *Lactobacillus casei* for one month provided no clinical benefit to patients with chronic periodontitis in spite of a significant decrease in *P. gingivalis* counts in the first months after the intervention. *Aggregatibacter actynomycetancomitans* and *P. intermedia* counts showed no significant reduction.

Iwasaki et al. [48] evaluated the use for 12 weeks of heat-killed *Lactobacillus plantarum* in patients undergoing supportive periodontal therapy. Mechanical control of plaque was performed and improved clinical parameters in both the test and placebo groups. A significant decrease in favor of the probiotic group was observed at 12 weeks in bleeding on probing (BOP), number of teeth with periodontal pocket depth (PD) >4 mm and number of sites with PD >4 mm, suggesting that this probiotic can prevent a possible recurrence and/or disease progression.

Grusovin et al. [8] evaluated for 12 months the effects of a *Lactibacillus reuteri* DSM 17938 and PTA 5389 probiotic combination in patients treated for a stage III-IV periodontitis, grade C. In the probiotic group, there was a higher reduction of mean PD throughout the study, higher clinical attachment level (CAL) gain at 6 months, and higher reduction of BOP at 6 and 9 months.

In a study by Penala et al. [46], probiotics *L. salivarius* and *L. reuteri* were evaluated as an adjunct to SRP in the treatment of patients with chronic periodontitis. The test group received subgingival delivery of probiotics and probiotic mouthwash for 14 days. A significant difference in favor of the test group was observed after 3 months in the number of moderate periodontal pockets. Moreover, there was a significant reduction in the benzoyl-DL arginine-naphthylamide (BANA) test for detecting digesting peptidase in the test group after 1 month, compared to the placebo group, but the difference was no longer observed at 3 months.

Chandra et al. [49] tested a subgingival combination of probiotics *Saccharomyces boulardii* with a prebiotic (fructo-oligosaccharide) in patients with chronic periodontitis as adjuvant to SRP. Despite a short-term colonization by *Saccharomyces boulardii* (until day 7), there was significant clinical improvement (as measured by the reduction of PI, GI, CAL, and PD) in the test group at 3 and 6 months after the mechanical treatment. The results suggest that *S. boulardii* may be a good auxiliary agent in the treatment of chronic periodontitis.

In a study by Boyeena et al. [50], the effects of a probiotic combination were compared to the application of tetracycline fibers directly in the periodontal pocket after mechanical removal of the plaque. Use of probiotics caused a significant reduction of BOP and PD when compared to the tetracycline fibers. The combination of both approaches showed a significant improvement of BOP and PD when compared to tetracycline fibers alone illustrating the benefits of using tetracycline fibers and probiotics to treat periodontitis.

Shah et al. [51] tested *L. brevis*, with or without doxycycline, for the treatment of patients with aggressive periodontitis after mechanical plaque removal. After 2 weeks, there was a significantly higher reduction of PD in patients on *L. brevis* and doxycycline relative to the other patients. At 2 months *Lactobacillus* spp. count (CFU/mL) increased significantly in patients on *L. brevis* and all patients had significantly improved clinical parameters when compared to baseline.

In a study by Morales et al. [52], the effects of daily administration of *Lactobacillus rhamnosus* SP1 or azithromycin tablets for 3 months were studied as an adjunct to SRP in patients with chronic periodontitis. Clinical and microbiological outcomes (as determined by the presence and levels of *Tannerella forsythia*, *Porphyromonas gingivalis* and *Aggregatibacter actinomycetemcomitans*) improved over the study period but there were no significant differences between groups.

Yuki et al. [53] compared the effects of consumption for 90 days of yogurt containing *L. rhamnosus* L820 with placebo yogurt in individuals with mental deficiency and periodontal disease. The PMA (papillary-marginal-attached) score was significantly reduced in the probiotic group at 90 days suggesting that *L. rhamnosus* L820 may have a beneficial effect on periodontal disease as an adjunct to mechanical oral hygiene.

Ikram et al. [44] compared *L. reuteri* with metronidazole as adjuvant to SRP in patients with chronic periodontitis. There was a significant improvement in the clinical parameters at all evaluation periods with no difference between groups, indicating that the efficacy of probiotic and antibiotic was similar.

In a study by Laleman et al. [54], the use of *Streptococcus oralis* KJ3, *Streptococcus uberis* KJ2, and *Streptococcus rattus* JH14 was not effective as adjunctive treatment of periodontitis despite lower PI at the end of the monitoring period (24 weeks) and the decrease of salivary *P. intermedia* at 12 weeks.

Murugesan et al. [55] evaluated the efficacy of co-administration of doxycycline and synbiotic tablet (consisting of prebiotic *Streptococcus faecalis* T-110 JPC and probiotics *Clostridium butyricum* TO-A, *Bacillus mesentericus* TO-A and *L. sporogenes*) as adjuvant to SRP in patients with periodontitis. Four weeks after the end of the intervention, a significant reduction of PD, CAL and BOP was observed in the test group indicating that this prebiotic-probiotic mixture can be a complement to the mechanical removal and doxycycline to improve clinical parameters, reduce bacterial load and repopulate the treated niche.

Three different trials studied the impact of *L. reuteri* in patients with chronic periodontitis using comparable study design (administration for 3 weeks of probiotic tablets containing *L. reuteri* compared to placebo) and obtained similar results [5,31,56]. Most clinical and microbiological parameters (as evidenced by a delay of recolonization up to 6 months) were significantly improved during the study period and the probiotic groups had fewer patients at high risk of disease progression and more patients at low risk. In one study the probiotic was found until day 90 in 11 patients and was no longer found on day 180, indicating temporary colonization [31].

Residual periodontal pockets are associated with an increased risk of periodontal disease progression and therefore require additional treatment. The effect of probiotic combination *L. reuteri* ATCC PTA 5289 and DSM 17938 as an adjunct to the SRP treatment of residual pockets was evaluated in patients with chronic periodontitis previously treated [57]. The use of *L. reuteri* after re-instrumentation did not affect colonization by periodontopathogens. While no significant clinical improvement was observed after 12-week consumption of probiotics and after 12 weeks of discontinuation, at 24 weeks after discontinuation PD was significantly reduced in moderate and deep pockets, and more pockets were sealed in the probiotic group. Taken together, these studies suggest that probiotic *L. reuteri* may serve as an effective complement to mechanical therapy in the treatment of chronic and relapsing periodontitis.

In a study by Sajedinejad et al. [45], use of *L. salivarius* NK02 in mouthwash for 28 days significantly improved clinical parameter (reduced PD, GI, and BOP) in patients with chronic periodontitis. In addition, *Aggregatibacter actynomycetancomitans* counts in saliva and gingival crevicular fluid were significantly reduced in the test group which also presented more commensal bacteria than the placebo group.

Bifidobacterium animalis subsp. lactis HN019 was evaluated for 30 days in patients with chronic periodontitis [58]. The probiotic colonized the subgingival flora for 60 days. There was a significant reduction of IL-1β at the end of 30–90 days, and IL-8 at the end of 30 days as compared to the control group. Likewise, there was a higher reduction of periodontopathogens (*P. gingivalis*, *T. denticola*, *F. nucleatum sub* spp. *vincentii*) in the test group up to 90 days. Clinical parameters improved significantly in the test group as determined by CAL and PD (in moderate and deep pockets at 90 days), and the risk of disease progression was also lower in the test group relative to the control group.

In a study by Butera et al. [59], the use of probiotics combinations for 6 months as an adjunct to SRP in patients with periodontitis improved clinical parameters in both probiotics groups (group 2: toothpaste with *Bifidobacterium* and *Lactobacillus* and group 3: toothpaste + chewing-gum with *L. reuteri*, *L. salivarius*, and *L. plantarum*), except for adherent gingiva and RG. Hence, BOP, PI, number of bleeding sites, pathological site, and sulcus bleeding index improved significantly at month 3 in both groups (also at month 6 in group 3). PD and CAL also improved significantly at month 3 in both groups. There was a significant reduction of orange complex pathogens *P. intermedia* and *F. nucleatum* between 3 and 6 months in both probiotics groups. Overall, group 3 presented better and more durable effects than group 2 suggesting a synergistic effect between the probiotic strains present in toothpaste and chewing-gum.

4.2.3. Probiotics in Peri-Implant Diseases

Peri-implant mucositis is a reversible soft tissue inflammation around the implants with no bone loss, caused by bacteria biofilm [60]. Its evolution leads to peri-implantitis, characterized by bone resorption and potential implant loss, increased levels of IL-6, IL-1β, and IL-8 and increased GCF volume [61]. The mechanical control of the biofilm and the use of antiseptics and antibiotics may be insufficient for the complete cure. Probiotics may aid in the formation of a new protective biofilm compatible with peri-implant health.

Eight randomized clinical trials investigating the effects of different species of *Lactobacillus* in peri-implant inflammation in otherwise healthy adults were analyzed (Table S6). Laleman et al. [62], studied the use of *L. reuteri* ATCC PTA 5289 and DSM 17938 in initial peri-implantitis. After SRP, probiotics were administered in drops directly to the site of peri-implantitis and afterwards in lozenges consumed for 12 weeks twice a day. There were no clinical and microbiological benefits from the administration of the probiotics. Similar negative results were obtained by Lauritano et al. [63], who evaluated the daily consumption of *L. reuteri* tablets for 28 days in patients with peri-implant mucositis, by Peña et al. [64] who studied the addition for 1 month of *L. reuteri* DSM 17938 and ATCC PTA in patients with peri-implant mucositis who received mechanical therapy and 0.12% chlorhexidine 15 days before the start of probiotic intervention, by Galofré et al. [65] who also evaluated the effects of administration of *L. reuteri* DSM 17938 and ATCC PTA 5289 in patients with peri-implant mucositis and peri-implantitis for 30 days, and by Hallström et al. [29] who administered *L. reuteri* DSM 17938 and ATCC PTA 5289 in patients with peri-implant mucositis for 3 months. Mongardini et al. [66] also found no clinical benefits after 14-days administration of *L. plantarum* and *L. brevis* on patients with experimental peri-implant mucositis.

In contrast, Flichy-Fernández et al. [67] found that administration of *L. reuteri* DSM 17938 and ATCC PTA 5289 for 30 days was useful to treat and prevent peri-implant mucositis. At the end of the study, a single patient developed mucositis and most (17 of 23) of the patients with mucositis were cured. Accordingly, PI, GI, PD and GCF volume were significantly reduced in the probiotic group when compared with placebo. IL-6 and IL-8 levels were also significantly reduced in the mucositis group taking the probiotics. The severity of peri-implant mucositis was also reduced significantly in a more recent trial using a probiotic combination (*L. reuteri* DSM 26866, *L. rhamnosus* DSM 21690, *L. bulgaricus* DSM21690, and *Bifidobacterium animalis* ssp. *lactis* DSM 17741) [68]. Clinical parameters (as determined by PI, GI, BOP, and PD) improved significantly in the test group relative to the control group after 1 month of consumption of probiotics. Salivary flow increased after 1 month in test group, with a significant difference between groups. Immunological parameters (salivary cytokines Il-1β, Il-4, TNF-α) decreased significantly at 1 and 6 months after the start of the intervention. Finally, the pathogenic species *Prevotella intermedia*, *Treponema denticola*, *Aggregatibacter actinomycetemcomitans*, *Porphyromonas gingivalis*, and *Fusobacterium nucleatum*, decreased after 1 month of probiotic consumption. The positive results obtained in these two trials may be related with a better removal of the subgingival plaque prior to the application of probiotics. On the other hand, the lack of results in the remaining trials may be related with small sample sizes and short administration times [69]. Clearly, further standardized clinical trials are indispensable to determine the usefulness of probiotics in prevention, management, and treatment of gingival, periodontal and peri-implant conditions, and to develop practical recommendations and adequate clinical protocols.

4.3. Probiotics in Cariology

Dental caries is a multifactorial disease, related to acidogenic and acid tolerant bacteria such as *S. mutans* and *Lactobacillus* spp. [70]. These bacteria produce acids from fermentation of carbohydrates that demineralize dental tissues. The prevention of dental caries involves the administration of fluoride, the use of sealants and modification of dietary habits (lower consumption of sucrose) [71]. The treatment and control of dental caries requires mechanical removal of the carious lesions which should be combined with an antimicrobial in the case of high-risk children. Probiotics have been proposed as an adjunct method to dental caries management strategies as they adhere to oral tissues, prevent adhesion/colonization/proliferation of caries pathogens and formation of pathogenic biofilm, produce inhibitors of cell adhesion and antibacterial agents, and consume nutrients before caries pathogens can use them (Figure 1) [33,72–75].

Seventeen clinical trials evaluated the effect of different probiotics on cariology in children and infants (Table S7). Overall, it was easier to modify the immature dental biofilm of children through colonization with probiotics than the established biofilm of adults. Six trials in adults assessed whether permanent integration of probiotics into the mature biofilm can be achieved in a cariogenic environment.

In a study by Rodriguez et al. [76], administration of *L. rhamnosus* SP1 strain in milk to children for 10 months led to a lower prevalence of dental caries relative to the placebo group (54.5% vs. 65.8%), lower incidence of cavitated lesions (9.7% vs. 24.3%), and lower incidence of new lesions. Administration of tablets containing *Streptococcus uberis* KJ2TM, *Streptococcus oralis* KJ3TM and *Streptococcus rattus* JH145TM to children for 3 months, caused a significant reduction in dental caries at the end of one year with prevention of enamel demineralization [77]. In a study by Di Pierro et al. [78], *Streptococcus salivarius* M18 probiotic in tablets was evaluated for 90 days in children with high risk of caries. There was a significant reduction in the overall cariogram result. In the probiotic group, PI and *S. mutans* counts were significantly reduced indicating that the consumption of this probiotic may help to prevent the development of new caries in high-risk children.

The daily and triweekly consumption of probiotic milk containing *L. paracasei* SD1 on *Streptococcus mutans* and lactobacilli counts in saliva and plaque samples was evaluated in preschool children for 6 months [79]. Probiotic administration reduced *S. mutans* counts and increased total lactobacilli counts in the saliva and plaque samples that persisted at least 6 months after discontinuation. Similar results were obtained by Pahumunto et al. [72] after 3-months consumption of milk containing *L. paracasei* SD1, and by Teanpaisan et al. [75] after 6-months consumption. In the latter study, there was colonization by the probiotic strain already at month 3 which decreased progressively with time to undetectable levels at month 12. Overall, the results suggest that in children with high risk of caries, daily consumption of probiotic *L. paracasei* SD1 may be recommended to control the amount of *S. mutans* responsible for the initial process of tooth decay.

Stensson et al. [80] administered *L. reuteri* as drops to pregnant women (from the 9th month of pregnancy) and their infants (up to 1 year old). At 9 years of age, the infants in the test group showed significant improvements in GI and dental caries prevalence relative to placebo (82% children free of carious lesions vs. 58%). *L. reuteri* was detected in only two children from each group. Diet, oral hygiene, fluoride supplementation and socioeconomic factors were similar in both groups at baseline but were not documented at the end of the study preventing the identification of potential contributors for the benefit of probiotics in dental caries development in early age.

In a study by Campus et al. [81], administration of *L. brevis* CD2 lozenges for 6 weeks in children led to significant reduction in salivary *S. mutans* mean counts ($\log_{10}$ CFU/mL), a significant reduction in the dental plaque pH, and a significant reduction in gingival bleeding at week 6. The benefits were also significant 2 weeks after probiotic discontinuation.

Bhalla et al. [82] evaluated *Bifidobacterium animalis subsp. lactis* BB-12 administered in curds to children. A significant reduction in the *S. mutans* count in saliva occurred after 1 h of ingestion and after 7 days of intervention. In a study by Sudhir et al. [83], *L. acidophilus* administered in curds to children for 30 days led to a significant reduction in the *S. mutans* count in saliva in the test group. A probiotic combination of *L. acidophilus* LA5 and *B. lactis* BB12 also caused a significant reduction of salivary *S. mutans* counts in children at days 7 and 30 after ingestion [73]. However, after 6 months of discontinuation, *S. mutans* values returned to the initial values indicating that the colonization was temporary. Tablet consumption of *L. reuteri* DSM 17938 and ATCC PTA 5289 for 28 days also caused a significant reduction in salivary *S. mutans* and *Lactobacillus* spp. counts in children [84]. In contrast, *L. paracasei* F19 given as a dietary supplement for 9 months had no significant effect at the microbiological and clinical levels at 3, 6 and 9 years of age [74]. Consistent with this, the probiotic did not colonize the oral flora. Likewise, in Taipale et al. [85], *Bifidobacterium animalis subsp. lactis* BB-12, administered by slow release or tablet from the age of 1–2 months to 2 years, had no significant effect in the occurrence of dental caries in children with low caries risk up to 4 years old when compared to xylitol and sorbitol. Administration in children of *L. rhamnosus* and *Bifidobacterium longum* in milk for 9 months [86] or *Bifidobacterium lactis* in yogurt for two weeks [87] also caused no significant impact on *S. mutans* counts, dental caries prevalence, or pH and plaque accumulation. Finally, in Cildir et al. [88], *L. reuteri* administration in drops for 25 days in children with cleft palate (population with higher food retention, and higher levels of dental caries and cariogenic bacteria than healthy children) caused no significant reduction in salivary *S. mutans* and *Lactobacillus* spp. levels.

In adults, consumption of yogurt with *L. acidophilus* LA5 and/or *Bifidobacterium lactis* BB12 for 2 weeks caused a significant temporary reduction of *S. mutans* count in saliva after 2 weeks [89,90]. This effect was lost 2 weeks after discontinuation. Similar results were obtained in adults who consumed white cheese with *L. casei* LAFTI L26 for 2 weeks [91]. Administration for 4 weeks of *L. paracasei* SD1 in milk allowed a significant reduction of *S. mutans* quantities at all monitoring times [92]. *Lactobacillus* spp. count increased significantly in most (75%) of the patients up to week 4 suggestive of probiotic colonization. Ingestion of ice cream containing *B. infantis* for 28 days, caused a significant reduction in *S. mutans* counts when compared to baseline and to the control group [93]. There was no effect in *Lactobacillus* spp. levels.

The topical application of *Streptococcus dentisani* in an adhesive gel on dental surfaces in single and multiple doses was evaluated in healthy adults [94]. There was a significant increase of the number of *S. dentisani* in dental plaque at day 14 after the first application which was no longer observed on day 28. In dental plaque samples, *S. mutans* count decreased significantly in the single dose group on day 28.

In summary, *L. acidophilus*, *L. reuteri*, *S. dentisani*, *S. salivarius*, *B. lactis* and *L. paracasei* may be effective as an adjunct method to restorative treatment in children at any risk of caries especially when used in conjunction with changes in dietary habits. Dairy products (yogurt, milk) appear to be the favorite vehicles for oral probiotics in children. Besides being easy to ingest, they contain essential nutrients: calcium, phosphorus, vitamin, protein, casein phosphopeptides that promote enamel remineralization, neutralize acids, participate in buffering, and interfere with the acidity of the probiotics *Lactobacillus* spp. or *Bifidobacterium* spp. The mixture of probiotic(s) with dairy products induces a synergistic effect. The heterogeneity of the trials (variability in study design, range of administration, strains used, dosage, vehicle) likely explains variations in results and prevents significant comparisons. Overall, however, these studies suggest that short term consumption of probiotics may reduce cariogenic bacteria counts, prevent dental plaque formation, and thus control the progression of dental caries. These effects seem to require the temporary colonization of the oral ecosystem which may lead to the exclusion of bacterial pathogens (Figure 1). However, probiotics are unable to definitively eliminate pathogenic bacteria and a reduction in salivary counts does not imply a reduction of bacterial plaque virulence [24]. Future trials should not only evaluate the cariogenic bacteria counts but also the dental caries progression/incidence because, as already mentioned, virulence and counting are not synonymous [72,75,81].

4.4. Probiotics in Orthodontics

The orthodontic treatment causes dysbiosis of the oral microbiome due to difficulty in hygienizing the orthodontic appliance [95]. Probiotics may be useful as supplements to hinder bacterial colonization and render the dental biofilm less virulent in patients with fixed or removable orthodontic appliances. Six studies related to the effect of probiotics on orthodontics were analyzed (Table S8).

Jose et al. [96] found a significant reduction of *S. mutans* levels in dental plaque around the bracket evaluated after probiotic (undisclosed composition) administration with curd or toothpaste. In a study by Ritthagol et al. [97], four weeks ingestion of milk containing *L. paracasei* SD1 in adolescents with non-syndromic lip-palatine cleft led to a significant increase of salivary *Lactobacillus* spp. count and decrease of *S. mutans* count at all times of evaluation when compared with baseline data. *L. paracasei* SD1 temporarily colonized the oral microbiota, being detected in saliva up to 4 weeks after cessation. The results suggest that this probiotic may help to prevent caries after orthodontic treatment in this population.

The effectiveness of 14-days milk consumption of *L. casei* or *L. reuteri* lozenges was investigated in young adults undergoing orthodontic treatment [98]. Periodontal condition was improved in both probiotic groups, better results being observed in the *L. reuteri* group. Alp and Baka [99] assessed the effect of a systemic probiotic (*Lactococcus lactis* subsp, *Leuconostoc* spp., *Lactobacillus* spp. and *S. thermophilus* and yeasts isolated from cereal grains) or local intervention (bacteriocin extracted from lactic acid bacteria), for 6 weeks on salivary microbial colonization in orthodontic patients. There was a significant reduction in *S. mutans* count at weeks 3 and 6 in both intervention groups. *Lactobacillus* spp. counts decreased significantly at week 3 in the probiotic group and at week 6 in the local intervention group. In contrast, in a study by Pinto et al. [100] there were no oral benefits after two-weeks consumption of yogurt containing *B. animalis subsp. lactis* DN-173010, and in Gizani et al. [101] there were no clinical and microbiological advantages to the use of *L. reuteri* lozenges in patients with maxillary orthodontic appliance. In summary, daily consumption of some but not all probiotics may help to prevent caries and improve periodontal condition in patients on orthodontic treatment.

4.5. Probiotics in Halitosis

Halitosis has multiple etiologies, and may be caused by ingestion of certain foods, poor oral hygiene, periodontitis, respiratory infections, tobacco consumption, genetic predisposition, dry mouth and oral microbiome dysbiosis [102]. Volatile sulfur compounds (VCS) responsible for halitosis include hydrogen sulfide, methyl mercaptan and dimethyl sulfide. In the oral cavity, these substances essentially result from the metabolic activity of oral microorganisms [102]. Several factors contribute to the production of these compounds, such as higher prevalence of gram-negative anaerobic bacteria, alkaline salivary pH, low redox potential, and the presence of sulfuric substrates (cysteine and methionine) [103,104]. Four studies have looked at the impact of probiotics in reducing halitosis by decreasing the density of the bacteria responsible by VCS production (Table S9).

Lee et al. [105] assessed the effect of consumption of *Weissella cibaria* tablets for 8 weeks on halitosis in healthy adults. *W. cibaria* counts were higher in the probiotic group at 4 and 8 weeks, and there was a significant reduction in VCS levels at week 4, and a significant reduction in bad breath improvement (BBI) score at week 8. The results suggest that *W. cibaria* tablets can be a useful oral hygiene product to control bad breath.

Streptococcus salivarius M18 has also been shown to reduce halitosis in patients with orthodontic treatment [106]. This required a month of consumption of two probiotic lozenges per day. Only *Rothia* spp. levels were significantly reduced in the probiotic group. The VCS score decreased significantly throughout the study in the probiotic group and placebo groups after 1 month but, after 3 months of follow-up, the VCS levels returned to the baseline value in the placebo group whereas in the probiotic group the VCS levels decreased significantly. A reduction in halitosis levels was also observed 1 and 3 months after ingestion of *L. salivarius* and *L. reuteri* for 14 days in patients with chronic periodontitis and halitosis [46]. In a similar study performed with *L. salivarius* WB21 only, VCS levels were significantly reduced and there was a significant reduction of PD [107]. Also, bacteria known to produce malodourous compounds like *F. nucleatum* were reduced in the probiotic group. Finally, in Keller et al. [108] *L. reuteri* reduced the organoleptic scores in patients who had a subjective feeling of bad breath.

In summary, regular consumption of probiotics *L. salivarius*, *S. salivarius*, *W. cibaria* or *L. reuteri* may complement mechanical oral care in controlling halitosis.

4.6. Probiotics in Oral Wound Healing and Oral Mucositis Related with Cancer Therapy

Wound healing in the oral mucosa involves several inflammatory mediators/molecules and is impacted by several factors such as age, dietary habits, and the oral microbiome [109,110]. Cancer therapy affects salivary quality and reduce salivary glycoproteins that cover and protect oral mucosa against microorganism's adherence and irritation. In addition, it induces oral mucositis that may favor the emergence of opportunistic infections, fever, anorexia, hemorrhage, severe pain, dysphagia and dysgeusia [111]. Oral glutamine has been recommended to mitigate radiotherapy-induced oral mucositis in head and neck cancer patients but other effective interventions are needed [112]. As mentioned previously, probiotics may participate indirectly in re-epithelization and tissue regeneration due to their potential to: (1) influence immune-regulating factors (e.g., kB nuclear factor, toll-like receptors in dendritic cells), (2) modulate inflammatory mediator levels (e.g., cytokines such as IL-1β, TNF-α, IL-6 and IL-15 and chemokines such as IL-8); and (3) induce the production of proteolytic enzymes involved in tissue remodeling (MMPs).

A few clinical trials have investigated the role of topical administration of probiotics in oral wound healing and in the treatment of oral mucositis in patients undergoing chemo-radiotherapy (Table S10). In a study by Twetman et al. [113], the application of *L. reuteri* in adults with healthy mucosa one week before standardized biopsy of the oral mucosa and one week later showed no improvement in healing. However, patients in the probiotic group had lower pain, less erythema/edema and the fibrin more rapidly covered the wound. There was no change in the levels of MMP1-3 and IFN-α2, IFN-β and IFN-γ in the wound exudate during the first healing week [114].

Walivaara et al. [115] evaluated the effects of *L. reuteri* supplements administered 3 times a day for 2 weeks on the healing of wounds after surgical extraction of lower third molars. Probiotic had no effect on the healing process as determined by extra-oral swelling, level of salivary oxytocin, and presence of bacteria. However, in patients on probiotic the subjective perception of pain, discomfort and swelling was significantly reduced and leading to improved quality of life during the healing process.

Limaye et al. [116] assessed the safety and tolerability of a 1, 3 or 6 mouthwash/day containing *Lactococcus lactis* (AG013, a strain that produces human trefoil factor 1) in patients newly diagnosed with advanced squamous cell head and neck cancer who were to start chemotherapy. The mean number of days with oral mucositis was reduced by 35% in the probiotic group, and there were fewer emergency visits (36% vs. 60%). The placebo patients had at least 2 days with oral mucositis while 29% of those taking AG013 had oral mucositis for 0 or 1 day. *Lactococcus lactis* AG013 was detected in mucosa and saliva shortly after the mouthwash, and up to 14 days after the mouthwash in equivalent number in the test groups. The probiotic was safe as there was no infection in neutropenic patients.

In a study by Jiang et al. [117], a significant improvement in oral mucositis was observed in patients with nasopharyngeal carcinoma undergoing chemoradiotherapy taking a probiotic combination of *Bifidobacterium longum*, *Lactobacillus lactis*, and *Enterococcus faecium*. Finally, Sharma et al. [118] evaluated the effect of *L. brevis* CD2 taken in lozenges in patients with squamous cell carcinoma of head and neck submitted to chemo-radiotherapy. The incidence and severity of oral mucositis was reduced in the probiotic group. In the probiotic group, more patients completed the cancer treatment, and fewer patients needed adjuvant medications to control the pain associated with mucositis. In summary, while probiotics seem to have no direct effect on oral wound healing, they can contribute to attenuate oral mucositis and improve quality of life in patients undergoing cancer therapy.

5. Conclusions

The use of probiotic bacteria is an expanding area of research in dentistry. Oral probiotics are safe, influence favorably the oral microbiota and provide benefits to the oral ecosystem in periodontal diseases, cariology, halitosis, orthodontics and management of oral mucositis resulting from cancer treatment. The areas in which probiotics should be further developed are endodontics, dental traumatology, and healing of chronic oral wounds.

Probiotics likely act without colonization or by transient colonization of the oral cavity, so a daily intake is advised. In addition, synergistic combinations of probiotic bacteria should lead to higher clinical efficacy than any individual probiotic agent.

Before recommending probiotic use in daily dental practice and considering probiotics as a self-management preventive strategy or adjuvant/alternative therapy, additional large-scale, long-term, randomized, placebo-controlled clinical trials studies are needed to determine the most effective probiotic strain combinations, the most suitable probiotic vehicles, and the most appropriate dosage and frequency of administration. Further research is also needed on product compliance and acceptance by different age groups. Finally, a better understanding of the mechanisms of action of probiotics and of the host response to probiotics is needed. Algorithms matching person-specific data and known factors interfering with probiotic efficacy will allow the identification of the optimal probiotic modality for stratified populations or individuals [16].

Supplementary Materials: The following are available online at https://www.mdpi.com/article/10.3390/app11178070/s1, Figure S1: Preferred Reporting Items for Systematic Reviews and Meta-Analysis (PRISMA) flow diagram, Table S1: PRISMA checklist, Table S2: PICOS criteria, Table S3: Characteristics of clinical trials of probiotics in the oral ecosystem, Table S4: Characteristics of clinical trials of probiotics in gingivitis and gingival health, Table S5: Characteristics of clinical trials of probiotics in periodontal diseases, Table S6: Characteristics of clinical trials of probiotics in peri-implantitis, Table S7: Characteristics of clinical trials of probiotics in cariology, Table S8: Characteristics of clinical trials of probiotics in orthodontics, Table S9: Characteristics of clinical trials of probiotics in halitosis, Table S10: Characteristics of clinical trials of probiotics in oral wound healing and treatment of oral mucositis related to cancer treatment.

Author Contributions: Conceptualization, P.S., N.T. and R.A.; formal analysis, P.S., N.T. and R.A.; investigation, P.S., N.T. and R.A.; data curation, P.S., N.T. and R.A.; writing—original draft preparation, P.S., N.T. and R.A.; writing—review and editing, P.S., N.T. and R.A.; supervision, N.T.; project administration, N.T.; funding acquisition, N.T. All authors have read and agreed to the published version of the manuscript.

Funding: This work was funded by national funds through the FCT-Foundation for Science and Technology, I.P., under the project UIDB/04585/2020.

Conflicts of Interest: The authors declare no conflict of interest. The funders had no role in the design of the study; in the collection, analyses, or interpretation of data; in the writing of the manuscript, or in the decision to publish the results.

References

1. Willis, J.R.; Gabaldon, T. The Human Oral Microbiome in Health and Disease: From Sequences to Ecosystems. *Microorganisms* **2020**, *8*, 308. [CrossRef] [PubMed]
2. Haque, M.; Sartelli, M.; Haque, S.Z. Dental Infection and Resistance-Global Health Consequences. *Dent. J.* **2019**, *7*, 22. [CrossRef] [PubMed]
3. FAO/OMS. Food Safety and Quality: Probiotics 2006. Available online: http://www.fao.org/food/food-safety-quality/a-z-index/probiotics/en/ (accessed on 1 July 2021).
4. Sabatini, S.; Lauritano, D.; Candotto, V.; Silvestre, F.J.; Nardi, G.M. Oral probiotics in the management of gingivitis in diabetic patients: A double blinded randomized controlled study. *J. Biol. Regul. Homeost. Agents* **2017**, *31*, 197–202.
5. Tekce, M.; Ince, G.; Gursoy, H.; Dirikan Ipci, S.; Cakar, G.; Kadir, T.; Yilmaz, S. Clinical and microbiological effects of probiotic lozenges in the treatment of chronic periodontitis: A 1-year follow-up study. *J. Clin. Periodontol.* **2015**, *42*, 363–372. [CrossRef] [PubMed]

6. Keller, M.K.; Brandsborg, E.; Holmstrom, K.; Twetman, S. Effect of tablets containing probiotic candidate strains on gingival inflammation and composition of the salivary microbiome: A randomised controlled trial. *Benef. Microbes.* **2018**, *9*, 487–494. [CrossRef]
7. Nadkerny, P.V.; Ravishankar, P.L.; Pramod, V.; Agarwal, L.A.; Bhandari, S. A comparative evaluation of the efficacy of probiotic and chlorhexidine mouthrinses on clinical inflammatory parameters of gingivitis: A randomized controlled clinical study. *J. Indian Soc. Periodontol.* **2015**, *19*, 633–639. [CrossRef]
8. Grusovin, M.G.; Bossini, S.; Calza, S.; Cappa, V.; Garzetti, G.; Scotti, E.; Gherlone, E.F.; Mensi, M. Clinical efficacy of Lactobacillus reuteri-containing lozenges in the supportive therapy of generalized periodontitis stage III and IV, grade C: 1-year results of a double-blind randomized placebo-controlled pilot study. *Clin. Oral. Investig.* **2020**, *24*, 2015–2024. [CrossRef] [PubMed]
9. Yousuf, A.; Sidiq, M.; Ganta, S.; Nagaraj, A.; Vishnani, P.; Jan, I. Effect of Freeze Dried Powdered Probiotics on Gingival Status and Plaque Inhibition: A Randomized, Double-blind, Parallel Study. *Contemp. Clin. Dent.* **2017**, *8*, 116–121. [CrossRef]
10. Vicario, M.; Santos, A.; Violant, D.; Nart, J.; Giner, L. Clinical changes in periodontal subjects with the probiotic Lactobacillus reuteri Prodentis: A preliminary randomized clinical trial. *Acta Odontol. Scand.* **2013**, *71*, 813–819. [CrossRef]
11. Dhawan, R.; Dhawan, S. Role of probiotics on oral health: A randomized, double-blind, placebo-controlled study. *J. Interdiscip. Dent.* **2013**, *3*, 71. [CrossRef]
12. Seminario-Amez, M.; Lopez-Lopez, J.; Estrugo-Devesa, A.; Ayuso-Montero, R.; Jane-Salas, E. Probiotics and oral health: A systematic review. *Med. Oral. Patol. Oral. Cir. Bucal.* **2017**, *22*, e282–e288. [CrossRef] [PubMed]
13. Laleman, I.; Teughels, W. Probiotics in the dental practice: A review. *Quintessence Int.* **2015**, *46*, 255–264. [CrossRef]
14. Pujia, A.M.; Costacurta, M.; Fortunato, L.; Merra, G.; Cascapera, S.; Calvani, M.; Gratteri, S. The probiotics in dentistry: A narrative review. *Eur. Rev. Med. Pharmacol. Sci.* **2017**, *21*, 1405–1412. [CrossRef]
15. Sivamaruthi, B.S.; Kesika, P.; Chaiyasut, C. A Review of the Role of Probiotic Supplementation in Dental Caries. *Probiotics Antimicrob Proteins* **2020**, *12*, 1300–1309. [CrossRef]
16. Veiga, P.; Suez, J.; Derrien, M.; Elinav, E. Moving from probiotics to precision probiotics. *Nat. Microbiol.* **2020**, *5*, 878–880. [CrossRef]
17. Moher, D.; Liberati, A.; Tetzlaff, J.; Altman, D.G.; Group, P. Preferred reporting items for systematic reviews and meta-analyses: The PRISMA statement. *PLoS Med.* **2009**, *6*, e1000097. [CrossRef] [PubMed]
18. Marttinen, A.; Haukioja, A.; Karjalainen, S.; Nylund, L.; Satokari, R.; Ohman, C.; Holgerson, P.; Twetman, S.; Soderling, E. Short-term consumption of probiotic lactobacilli has no effect on acid production of supragingival plaque. *Clin. Oral. Investig.* **2012**, *16*, 797–803. [CrossRef] [PubMed]
19. Thakkar, P.K.; Imranulla, M.; Naveen Kumar, P.G.; Prashant, G.M.; Sakeenabi, B.; Sushanth, V.H. Effect of probiotic mouthrinse on dental plaque accumulation: A randomized controlled trial. *Dent. Med Res.* **2013**, *1*, 6.
20. Burton, J.P.; Drummond, B.K.; Chilcott, C.N.; Tagg, J.R.; Thomson, W.M.; Hale, J.D.F.; Wescombe, P.A. Influence of the probiotic Streptococcus salivarius strain M18 on indices of dental health in children: A randomized double-blind, placebo-controlled trial. *J. Med. Microbiol.* **2013**, *62*, 875–884. [CrossRef]
21. Sarmento, E.G.; Cesar, D.E.; Martins, M.L.; de Oliveira Gois, E.G.; Furtado Martins, E.M.; da Rocha Campos, A.N.; Del'Duca, A.; de Oliveira Martins, A.D. Effect of probiotic bacteria in composition of children's saliva. *Food Res. Int.* **2019**, *116*, 1282–1288. [CrossRef]
22. Rungsri, P.; Akkarachaneeyakorn, N.; Wongsuwanlert, M.; Piwat, S.; Nantarakchaikul, P.; Teanpaisan, R. Effect of fermented milk containing Lactobacillus rhamnosus SD11 on oral microbiota of healthy volunteers: A randomized clinical trial. *J. Dairy Sci.* **2017**, *100*, 7780–7787. [CrossRef]
23. Toiviainen, A.; Jalasvuori, H.; Lahti, E.; Gursoy, U.; Salminen, S.; Fontana, M.; Flannagan, S.; Eckert, G.; Kokaras, A.; Paster, B.; et al. Impact of orally administered lozenges with Lactobacillus rhamnosus GG and Bifidobacterium animalis subsp. lactis BB-12 on the number of salivary mutans streptococci, amount of plaque, gingival inflammation and the oral microbiome in healthy adults. *Clin. Oral. Investig.* **2015**, *19*, 77–83. [CrossRef] [PubMed]
24. Keller, M.K.; Hasslof, P.; Dahlen, G.; Stecksen-Blicks, C.; Twetman, S. Probiotic supplements (Lactobacillus reuteri DSM 17938 and ATCC PTA 5289) do not affect regrowth of mutans streptococci after full-mouth disinfection with chlorhexidine: A randomized controlled multicenter trial. *Caries Res.* **2012**, *46*, 140–146. [CrossRef] [PubMed]
25. Romani Vestman, N.; Chen, T.; Lif Holgerson, P.; Ohman, C.; Johansson, I. Oral Microbiota Shift after 12-Week Supplementation with Lactobacillus reuteri DSM 17938 and PTA 5289; A Randomized Control Trial. *PLoS ONE* **2015**, *10*, e0125812. [CrossRef] [PubMed]
26. Keller, M.K.; Twetman, S. Acid production in dental plaque after exposure to probiotic bacteria. *BMC Oral. Health* **2012**, *12*, 44. [CrossRef]
27. Hajishengallis, G. Periodontitis: From microbial immune subversion to systemic inflammation. *Nat. Rev. Immunol.* **2015**, *15*, 30–44. [CrossRef]
28. Socransky, S.S.; Haffajee, A.D.; Teles, R.; Wennstrom, J.L.; Lindhe, J.; Bogren, A.; Hasturk, H.; van Dyke, T.; Wang, X.; Goodson, J.M. Effect of periodontal therapy on the subgingival microbiota over a 2-year monitoring period. I. Overall effect and kinetics of change. *J. Clin. Periodontol.* **2013**, *40*, 771–780. [CrossRef]
29. Hallstrom, H.; Lindgren, S.; Widen, C.; Renvert, S.; Twetman, S. Probiotic supplements and debridement of peri-implant mucositis: A randomized controlled trial. *Acta Odontol. Scand.* **2016**, *74*, 60–66. [CrossRef] [PubMed]

30. Hallstrom, H.; Lindgren, S.; Yucel-Lindberg, T.; Dahlen, G.; Renvert, S.; Twetman, S. Effect of probiotic lozenges on inflammatory reactions and oral biofilm during experimental gingivitis. *Acta Odontol. Scand.* **2013**, *71*, 828–833. [CrossRef]
31. Ince, G.; Gursoy, H.; Ipci, S.D.; Cakar, G.; Emekli-Alturfan, E.; Yilmaz, S. Clinical and Biochemical Evaluation of Lozenges Containing Lactobacillus reuteri as an Adjunct to Non-Surgical Periodontal Therapy in Chronic Periodontitis. *J. Periodontol.* **2015**, *86*, 746–754. [CrossRef]
32. Jasberg, H.; Tervahartiala, T.; Sorsa, T.; Soderling, E.; Haukioja, A. Probiotic intervention influences the salivary levels of Matrix Metalloproteinase (MMP)-9 and Tissue Inhibitor of metalloproteinases (TIMP)-1 in healthy adults. *Arch. Oral. Biol.* **2018**, *85*, 58–63. [CrossRef] [PubMed]
33. Kuru, B.E.; Laleman, I.; Yalnizoglu, T.; Kuru, L.; Teughels, W. The Influence of a Bifidobacterium animalis Probiotic on Gingival Health: A Randomized Controlled Clinical Trial. *J. Periodontol.* **2017**, *88*, 1115–1123. [CrossRef] [PubMed]
34. Deshmukh, M.A.; Dodamani, A.S.; Karibasappa, G.; Khairnar, M.R.; Naik, R.G.; Jadhav, H.C. Comparative Evaluation of the Efficacy of Probiotic, Herbal and Chlorhexidine Mouthwash on Gingival Health: A Randomized Clinical Trial. *J. Clin. Diagn. Res.* **2017**, *11*, ZC13–ZC16. [CrossRef]
35. Alkaya, B.; Laleman, I.; Keceli, S.; Ozcelik, O.; Cenk Haytac, M.; Teughels, W. Clinical effects of probiotics containing Bacillus species on gingivitis: A pilot randomized controlled trial. *J. Periodontal. Res.* **2017**, *52*, 497–504. [CrossRef]
36. Keller, M.K.; Kragelund, C. Randomized pilot study on probiotic effects on recurrent candidiasis in oral lichen planus patients. *Oral. Dis.* **2018**, *24*, 1107–1114. [CrossRef] [PubMed]
37. Iniesta, M.; Herrera, D.; Montero, E.; Zurbriggen, M.; Matos, A.R.; Marin, M.J.; Sanchez-Beltran, M.C.; Llama-Palacio, A.; Sanz, M. Probiotic effects of orally administered Lactobacillus reuteri-containing tablets on the subgingival and salivary microbiota in patients with gingivitis. A randomized clinical trial. *J. Clin. Periodontol.* **2012**, *39*, 736–744. [CrossRef]
38. Schlagenhauf, U.; Jakob, L.; Eigenthaler, M.; Segerer, S.; Jockel-Schneider, Y.; Rehn, M. Regular consumption of Lactobacillus reuteri-containing lozenges reduces pregnancy gingivitis: An RCT. *J. Clin. Periodontol.* **2016**, *43*, 948–954. [CrossRef]
39. Lee, J.K.; Kim, S.J.; Ko, S.H.; Ouwehand, A.C.; Ma, D.S. Modulation of the host response by probiotic Lactobacillus brevis CD2 in experimental gingivitis. *Oral. Dis.* **2015**, *21*, 705–712. [CrossRef]
40. Alanzi, A.; Honkala, S.; Honkala, E.; Varghese, A.; Tolvanen, M.; Soderling, E. Effect of Lactobacillus rhamnosus and Bifidobacterium lactis on gingival health, dental plaque, and periodontopathogens in adolescents: A randomised placebo-controlled clinical trial. *Benef. Microbes.* **2018**, *9*, 593–602. [CrossRef]
41. Montero, E.; Iniesta, M.; Rodrigo, M.; Marin, M.J.; Figuero, E.; Herrera, D.; Sanz, M. Clinical and microbiological effects of the adjunctive use of probiotics in the treatment of gingivitis: A randomized controlled clinical trial. *J. Clin. Periodontol.* **2017**, *44*, 708–716. [CrossRef]
42. Checchi, V.; Maravic, T.; Bellini, P.; Generali, L.; Consolo, U.; Breschi, L.; Mazzoni, A. The Role of Matrix Metalloproteinases in Periodontal Disease. *Int. J. Environ. Res. Public Health* **2020**, *17*, 4923. [CrossRef]
43. Kim, J.Y.; Kim, H.N. Changes in Inflammatory Cytokines in Saliva after Non-Surgical Periodontal Therapy: A Systematic Review and Meta-Analysis. *Int. J. Environ. Res. Public Health* **2020**, *18*, 194. [CrossRef] [PubMed]
44. Ikram, S.; Hassan, N.; Baig, S.; Borges, K.J.J.; Raffat, M.A.; Akram, Z. Effect of local probiotic (Lactobacillus reuteri) vs systemic antibiotic therapy as an adjunct to non-surgical periodontal treatment in chronic periodontitis. *J. Investig. Clin. Dent.* **2019**, *10*, e12393. [CrossRef]
45. Sajedinejad, N.; Paknejad, M.; Houshmand, B.; Sharafi, H.; Jelodar, R.; Shahbani Zahiri, H.; Noghabi, K.A. Lactobacillus salivarius NK02: A Potent Probiotic for Clinical Application in Mouthwash. *Probiotics Antimicrob Proteins* **2018**, *10*, 485–495. [CrossRef] [PubMed]
46. Penala, S.; Kalakonda, B.; Pathakota, K.R.; Jayakumar, A.; Koppolu, P.; Lakshmi, B.V.; Pandey, R.; Mishra, A. Efficacy of local use of probiotics as an adjunct to scaling and root planing in chronic periodontitis and halitosis: A randomized controlled trial. *J. Res. Pharm Pract* **2016**, *5*, 86–93. [CrossRef]
47. Imran, F.; Das, S.; Padmanabhan, S.; Rao, R.; Suresh, A.; Bharath, D. Evaluation of the efficacy of a probiotic drink containing Lactobacillus casei on the levels of periodontopathic bacteria in periodontitis: A clinico-microbiologic study. *Indian J. Dent. Res.* **2015**, *26*, 462–468. [CrossRef]
48. Iwasaki, K.; Maeda, K.; Hidaka, K.; Nemoto, K.; Hirose, Y.; Deguchi, S. Daily Intake of Heat-killed Lactobacillus plantarum L-137 Decreases the Probing Depth in Patients Undergoing Supportive Periodontal Therapy. *Oral. Health Prev. Dent.* **2016**, *14*, 207–214. [CrossRef]
49. Chandra, R.V.; Swathi, T.; Reddy, A.A.; Chakravarthy, Y.; Nagarajan, S.; Naveen, A. Effect of a Locally Delivered Probiotic-Prebiotic Mixture as an Adjunct to Scaling and Root Planing in the Management of Chronic Periodontitis. *J. Int. Acad. Periodontol.* **2016**, *18*, 67–75. [PubMed]
50. Boyeena, L.; Koduganti, R.R.; Panthula, V.R.; Jammula, S.P. Comparison of efficacy of probiotics versus tetracycline fibers as adjuvants to scaling and root planing. *J. Indian Soc. Periodontol.* **2019**, *23*, 539–544. [CrossRef]
51. Shah, M.P.; Gujjari, S.K.; Chandrasekhar, V.S. Evaluation of the effect of probiotic (inersan(R)) alone, combination of probiotic with doxycycline and doxycycline alone on aggressive periodontitis—A clinical and microbiological study. *J. Clin. Diagn. Res.* **2013**, *7*, 595–600. [CrossRef]

52. Morales, A.; Gandolfo, A.; Bravo, J.; Carvajal, P.; Silva, N.; Godoy, C.; Garcia-Sesnich, J.; Hoare, A.; Diaz, P.; Gamonal, J. Microbiological and clinical effects of probiotics and antibiotics on nonsurgical treatment of chronic periodontitis: A randomized placebo- controlled trial with 9-month follow-up. *J. Appl. Oral. Sci.* **2018**, *26*, e20170075. [CrossRef]
53. Yuki, O.; Furutani, C.; Mizota, Y.; Wakita, A.; Mimura, S.; Kihara, T.; Ohara, M.; Okada, Y.; Okada, M.; Nikawa, H. Effect of bovine milk fermented with Lactobacillus rhamnosus L8020 on periodontal disease in individuals with intellectual disability: A randomized clinical trial. *J. Appl. Oral. Sci.* **2019**, *27*, e20180564. [CrossRef] [PubMed]
54. Laleman, I.; Yilmaz, E.; Ozcelik, O.; Haytac, C.; Pauwels, M.; Herrero, E.R.; Slomka, V.; Quirynen, M.; Alkaya, B.; Teughels, W. The effect of a streptococci containing probiotic in periodontal therapy: A randomized controlled trial. *J. Clin. Periodontol.* **2015**, *42*, 1032–1041. [CrossRef] [PubMed]
55. Murugesan, G.; Sudha, K.M.; Subaramoniam, M.K.; Dutta, T.; Dhanasekar, K.R. A comparative study of synbiotic as an add-on therapy to standard treatment in patients with aggressive periodontitis. *J. Indian Soc. Periodontol.* **2018**, *22*, 438–441. [CrossRef] [PubMed]
56. Szkaradkiewicz, A.K.; Stopa, J.; Karpinski, T.M. Effect of oral administration involving a probiotic strain of Lactobacillus reuteri on pro-inflammatory cytokine response in patients with chronic periodontitis. *Arch. Immunol. Ther. Exp.* **2014**, *62*, 495–500. [CrossRef] [PubMed]
57. Teughels, W.; Durukan, A.; Ozcelik, O.; Pauwels, M.; Quirynen, M.; Haytac, M.C. Clinical and microbiological effects of Lactobacillus reuteri probiotics in the treatment of chronic periodontitis: A randomized placebo-controlled study. *J. Clin. Periodontol.* **2013**, *40*, 1025–1035. [CrossRef] [PubMed]
58. Invernici, M.M.; Salvador, S.L.; Silva, P.H.F.; Soares, M.S.M.; Casarin, R.; Palioto, D.B.; Souza, S.L.S.; Taba, M., Jr.; Novaes, A.B., Jr.; Furlaneto, F.A.C.; et al. Effects of Bifidobacterium probiotic on the treatment of chronic periodontitis: A randomized clinical trial. *J. Clin. Periodontol.* **2018**, *45*, 1198–1210. [CrossRef] [PubMed]
59. Butera, A.; Gallo, S.; Maiorani, C.; Molino, D.; Chiesa, A.; Preda, C.; Esposito, F.; Scribante, A. Probiotic Alternative to Chlorhexidine in Periodontal Therapy: Evaluation of Clinical and Microbiological Parameters. *Microorganisms* **2020**, *9*, 69. [CrossRef]
60. Heitz-Mayfield, L.J.A.; Salvi, G.E. Peri-implant mucositis. *J. Clin. Periodontol* **2018**, *45* Suppl. 20, S237–S245. [CrossRef]
61. Ting, M.; Craig, J.; Balkin, B.E.; Suzuki, J.B. Peri-implantitis: A Comprehensive Overview of Systematic Reviews. *J. Oral. Implantol.* **2018**, *44*, 225–247. [CrossRef]
62. Laleman, I.; Pauwels, M.; Quirynen, M.; Teughels, W. The usage of a lactobacilli probiotic in the non-surgical therapy of peri-implantitis: A randomized pilot study. *Clin. Oral. Implants. Res.* **2020**, *31*, 84–92. [CrossRef] [PubMed]
63. Lauritano, D.; Carinci, F.; Palmieri, A.; Cura, F.; Caruso, S.; Candotto, V. Reuterinos((R)) as adjuvant for peri-implant treatment: A pilot study. *Int. J. Immunopathol. Pharmacol.* **2019**, *33*, 2058738419827745. [CrossRef] [PubMed]
64. Pena, M.; Barallat, L.; Vilarrasa, J.; Vicario, M.; Violant, D.; Nart, J. Evaluation of the effect of probiotics in the treatment of peri-implant mucositis: A triple-blind randomized clinical trial. *Clin. Oral. Investig.* **2019**, *23*, 1673–1683. [CrossRef]
65. Galofre, M.; Palao, D.; Vicario, M.; Nart, J.; Violant, D. Clinical and microbiological evaluation of the effect of Lactobacillus reuteri in the treatment of mucositis and peri-implantitis: A triple-blind randomized clinical trial. *J. Periodontal. Res.* **2018**, *53*, 378–390. [CrossRef] [PubMed]
66. Mongardini, C.; Pilloni, A.; Farina, R.; Di Tanna, G.; Zeza, B. Adjunctive efficacy of probiotics in the treatment of experimental peri-implant mucositis with mechanical and photodynamic therapy: A randomized, cross-over clinical trial. *J. Clin. Periodontol.* **2017**, *44*, 410–417. [CrossRef]
67. Flichy-Fernandez, A.J.; Ata-Ali, J.; Alegre-Domingo, T.; Candel-Marti, E.; Ata-Ali, F.; Palacio, J.R.; Penarrocha-Diago, M. The effect of orally administered probiotic Lactobacillus reuteri-containing tablets in peri-implant mucositis: A double-blind randomized controlled trial. *J. Periodontal. Res.* **2015**, *50*, 775–785. [CrossRef]
68. Ahmedbyli, D.R.; Seyidbekov, O.S.; Dirikan, I.S.; Mamedov, F.Y.; Ahmedbeyli, R.M. Efficacy of probiotic application in the treatment and prevention of peri-implant mucositis. *Stomatologiia* **2019**, *98*, 20–24. [CrossRef]
69. Zhao, R.; Hu, H.; Wang, Y.; Lai, W.; Jian, F. Efficacy of Probiotics as Adjunctive Therapy to Nonsurgical Treatment of Peri-Implant Mucositis: A Systematic Review and Meta-Analysis. *Front. Pharmacol.* **2020**, *11*, 541752. [CrossRef] [PubMed]
70. Baker, J.L.; Morton, J.T.; Dinis, M.; Alvarez, R.; Tran, N.C.; Knight, R.; Edlund, A. Deep metagenomics examines the oral microbiome during dental caries, revealing novel taxa and co-occurrences with host molecules. *Genome Res.* **2021**, *31*, 64–74. [CrossRef]
71. Pitts, N.B.; Zero, D.T.; Marsh, P.D.; Ekstrand, K.; Weintraub, J.A.; Ramos-Gomez, F.; Tagami, J.; Twetman, S.; Tsakos, G.; Ismail, A. Dental caries. *Nat. Rev. Dis. Primers* **2017**, *3*, 17030. [CrossRef]
72. Pahumunto, N.; Piwat, S.; Chankanka, O.; Akkarachaneeyakorn, N.; Rangsitsathian, K.; Teanpaisan, R. Reducing mutans streptococci and caries development by Lactobacillus paracasei SD1 in preschool children: A randomized placebo-controlled trial. *Acta Odontol. Scand.* **2018**, *76*, 331–337. [CrossRef] [PubMed]
73. Ashwin, D.; Ke, V.; Taranath, M.; Ramagoni, N.K.; Nara, A.; Sarpangala, M. Effect of Probiotic Containing Ice-cream on Salivary Mutans Streptococci (SMS) Levels in Children of 6–12 Years of Age: A Randomized Controlled Double Blind Study with Six-months Follow Up. *J. Clin. Diagn. Res.* **2015**, *9*, ZC06-09. [CrossRef]
74. Hasslof, P.; West, C.E.; Videhult, F.K.; Brandelius, C.; Stecksen-Blicks, C. Early intervention with probiotic Lactobacillus paracasei F19 has no long-term effect on caries experience. *Caries Res.* **2013**, *47*, 559–565. [CrossRef] [PubMed]

75. Teanpaisan, R.; Piwat, S.; Tianviwat, S.; Sophatha, B.; Kampoo, T. Effect of Long-Term Consumption of Lactobacillus paracasei SD1 on Reducing Mutans streptococci and Caries Risk: A Randomized Placebo-Controlled Trial. *Dent. J.* **2015**, *3*, 43–54. [CrossRef]
76. Rodriguez, G.; Ruiz, B.; Faleiros, S.; Vistoso, A.; Marro, M.L.; Sanchez, J.; Urzua, I.; Cabello, R. Probiotic Compared with Standard Milk for High-caries Children: A Cluster Randomized Trial. *J. Dent. Res.* **2016**, *95*, 402–407. [CrossRef]
77. Hedayati-Hajikand, T.; Lundberg, U.; Eldh, C.; Twetman, S. Effect of probiotic chewing tablets on early childhood caries–a randomized controlled trial. *BMC Oral. Health* **2015**, *15*, 112. [CrossRef] [PubMed]
78. Di Pierro, F.; Zanvit, A.; Nobili, P.; Risso, P.; Fornaini, C. Cariogram outcome after 90 days of oral treatment with Streptococcus salivarius M18 in children at high risk for dental caries: Results of a randomized, controlled study. *Clin. Cosmet. Investig. Dent.* **2015**, *7*, 107–113. [CrossRef] [PubMed]
79. Manmontri, C.; Nirunsittirat, A.; Piwat, S.; Wattanarat, O.; Pahumunto, N.; Makeudom, A.; Sastraruji, T.; Krisanaprakornkit, S.; Teanpaisan, R. Reduction of Streptococcus mutans by probiotic milk: A multicenter randomized controlled trial. *Clin. Oral. Investig.* **2020**, *24*, 2363–2374. [CrossRef]
80. Stensson, M.; Koch, G.; Coric, S.; Abrahamsson, T.R.; Jenmalm, M.C.; Birkhed, D.; Wendt, L.K. Oral administration of Lactobacillus reuteri during the first year of life reduces caries prevalence in the primary dentition at 9 years of age. *Caries Res.* **2014**, *48*, 111–117. [CrossRef]
81. Campus, G.; Cocco, F.; Carta, G.; Cagetti, M.G.; Simark-Mattson, C.; Strohmenger, L.; Lingstrom, P. Effect of a daily dose of Lactobacillus brevis CD2 lozenges in high caries risk schoolchildren. *Clin. Oral. Investig.* **2014**, *18*, 555–561. [CrossRef]
82. Bhalla, M.; Ingle, N.A.; Kaur, N.; Yadav, P. Mutans streptococci estimation in saliva before and after consumption of probiotic curd among school children. *J. Int. Soc. Prev. Community Dent.* **2015**, *5*, 31–34. [CrossRef] [PubMed]
83. Sudhir, R.; Praveen, P.; Anantharaj, A.; Venkataraghavan, K. Assessment of the effect of probiotic curd consumption on salivary pH and streptococcus mutans counts. *Niger. Med. J.* **2012**, *53*, 135–139. [CrossRef] [PubMed]
84. Alamoudi, N.M.; Almabadi, E.S.; El Ashiry, E.A.; El Derwi, D.A. Effect of Probiotic Lactobacillus reuteri on Salivary Cariogenic Bacterial Counts among Groups of Preschool Children in Jeddah, Saudi Arabia: A Randomized Clinical Trial. *J. Clin. Pediatr. Dent.* **2018**, *42*, 331–338. [CrossRef]
85. Taipale, T.; Pienihakkinen, K.; Alanen, P.; Jokela, J.; Soderling, E. Administration of Bifidobacterium animalis subsp. lactis BB-12 in early childhood: A post-trial effect on caries occurrence at four years of age. *Caries Res.* **2013**, *47*, 364–372. [CrossRef]
86. Villavicencio, J.; Villegas, L.M.; Arango, M.C.; Arias, S.; Triana, F. Effects of a food enriched with probiotics on Streptococcus mutans and Lactobacillus spp. salivary counts in preschool children: A cluster randomized trial. *J. Appl. Oral. Sci.* **2018**, *26*, e20170318. [CrossRef] [PubMed]
87. Nozari, A.; Motamedifar, M.; Seifi, N.; Hatamizargaran, Z.; Ranjbar, M.A. The Effect of Iranian Customary Used Probiotic Yogurt on the Children's Salivary Cariogenic Microflora. *J. Dent.* **2015**, *16*, 81–86.
88. Cildir, S.K.; Sandalli, N.; Nazli, S.; Alp, F.; Caglar, E. A novel delivery system of probiotic drop and its effect on dental caries risk factors in cleft lip/palate children. *Cleft Palate-Craniofac. J.* **2012**, *49*, 369–372. [CrossRef]
89. Bafna, H.P.; Ajithkrishnan, C.G.; Kalantharakath, T.; Singh, R.P.; Kalyan, P.; Vathar, J.B.; Patel, H.R. Effect of Short-term Consumption of Amul Probiotic Yogurt Containing Lactobacillus acidophilus La5 and Bifidobacterium Lactis Bb12 on Salivary Streptococcus mutans Count in High Caries Risk Individuals. *Int. J. Appl. Basic Med. Res.* **2018**, *8*, 111–115. [CrossRef]
90. Javid, A.Z.; Amerian, E.; Basir, L.; Ekrami, A.; Haghighi-zadeh, M.H. Effects of Short-term Consumption of Probiotic Yogurt on Streptococcus Mutans and lactobacilli Levels in 18-30 Years Old Students with Initial Stages of Dental Caries in Ahvaz City. *Nutr. Food Sci. Res.* **2015**, *2*, 6.
91. Mortazavi, S.; Akhlaghi, N. Salivary Streptococcus mutans and Lactobacilli levels following probiotic cheese consumption in adults: A double blind randomized clinical trial(*). *J. Res. Med. Sci.* **2012**, *17*, 57–66.
92. Teanpaisan, R.; Piwat, S. Lactobacillus paracasei SD1, a novel probiotic, reduces mutans streptococci in human volunteers: A randomized placebo-controlled trial. *Clin. Oral. Investig.* **2014**, *18*, 857–862. [CrossRef] [PubMed]
93. Nagarajappa, R.; Daryani, H.; Sharda, A.J.; Asawa, K.; Batra, M.; Sanadhya, S.; Ramesh, G. Effect of Chocobar Ice Cream Containing Bifidobacterium on Salivary Streptococcus mutans and Lactobacilli: A Randomised Controlled Trial. *Oral. Health Prev. Dent.* **2015**, *13*, 213–218. [CrossRef]
94. Ferrer, M.D.; Lopez-Lopez, A.; Nicolescu, T.; Salavert, A.; Mendez, I.; Cune, J.; Llena, C.; Mira, A. A pilot study to assess oral colonization and pH buffering by the probiotic Streptococcus dentisani under different dosing regimes. *Odontology* **2020**, *108*, 180–187. [CrossRef]
95. Wang, Q.; Ma, J.B.; Wang, B.; Zhang, X.; Yin, Y.L.; Bai, H. Alterations of the oral microbiome in patients treated with the Invisalign system or with fixed appliances. *Am. J. Orthod. Dentofacial Orthop.* **2019**, *156*, 633–640. [CrossRef] [PubMed]
96. Jose, J.E.; Padmanabhan, S.; Chitharanjan, A.B. Systemic consumption of probiotic curd and use of probiotic toothpaste to reduce Streptococcus mutans in plaque around orthodontic brackets. *Am. J. Orthod. Dentofacial Orthop.* **2013**, *144*, 67–72. [CrossRef]
97. Ritthagol, W.; Saetang, C.; Teanpaisan, R. Effect of Probiotics Containing Lactobacillus paracasei SD1 on Salivary Mutans Streptococci and Lactobacilli in Orthodontic Cleft Patients: A Double-Blinded, Randomized, Placebo-Controlled Study. *Cleft Palate-Craniofac. J.* **2014**, *51*, 257–263. [CrossRef] [PubMed]
98. Kohar, N.M.; Emmanuel, V.; Astuti, L. Comparison between probiotic lozenges and drinks towards periodontal status improvement of orthodontic patients. *Dent. J.* **2015**, *48*, 126–129. [CrossRef]

99. Alp, S.; Baka, Z.M. Effects of probiotics on salivary Streptecoccus mutans and Lactobacillus levels in orthodontic patients. *Am. J. Orthod. Dentofacial Orthop.* **2018**, *154*, 517–523. [CrossRef]
100. Pinto, G.S.; Cenci, M.S.; Azevedo, M.S.; Epifanio, M.; Jones, M.H. Effect of yogurt containing Bifidobacterium animalis subsp. lactis DN-173010 probiotic on dental plaque and saliva in orthodontic patients. *Caries Res.* **2014**, *48*, 63–68. [CrossRef]
101. Gizani, S.; Petsi, G.; Twetman, S.; Caroni, C.; Makou, M.; Papagianoulis, L. Effect of the probiotic bacterium Lactobacillus reuteri on white spot lesion development in orthodontic patients. *Eur. J. Orthod.* **2016**, *38*, 85–89. [CrossRef] [PubMed]
102. Hampelska, K.; Jaworska, M.M.; Babalska, Z.L.; Karpinski, T.M. The Role of Oral Microbiota in Intra-Oral Halitosis. *J. Clin. Med.* **2020**, *9*, 2484. [CrossRef]
103. Ye, W.; Zhang, Y.; He, M.; Zhu, C.; Feng, X.P. Relationship of tongue coating microbiome on volatile sulfur compounds in healthy and halitosis adults. *J. Breath Res.* **2019**, *14*, 016005. [CrossRef]
104. Monedeiro, F.; Milanowski, M.; Ratiu, I.A.; Zmyslowski, H.; Ligor, T.; Buszewski, B. VOC Profiles of Saliva in Assessment of Halitosis and Submandibular Abscesses Using HS-SPME-GC/MS Technique. *Molecules* **2019**, *24*, 2977. [CrossRef]
105. Lee, D.S.; Lee, S.A.; Kim, M.; Nam, S.H.; Kang, M.S. Reduction of Halitosis by a Tablet Containing Weissella cibaria CMU: A Randomized, Double-Blind, Placebo-Controlled Study. *J. Med. Food* **2020**, *23*, 649–657. [CrossRef]
106. Benic, G.Z.; Farella, M.; Morgan, X.C.; Viswam, J.; Heng, N.C.; Cannon, R.D.; Mei, L. Oral probiotics reduce halitosis in patients wearing orthodontic braces: A randomized, triple-blind, placebo-controlled trial. *J. Breath Res.* **2019**, *13*, 036010. [CrossRef]
107. Suzuki, N.; Yoneda, M.; Tanabe, K.; Fujimoto, A.; Iha, K.; Seno, K.; Yamada, K.; Iwamoto, T.; Masuo, Y.; Hirofuji, T. Lactobacillus salivarius WB21–containing tablets for the treatment of oral malodor: A double-blind, randomized, placebo-controlled crossover trial. *Oral. Surg. Oral. Med. Oral. Pathol. Oral. Radiol.* **2014**, *117*, 462–470. [CrossRef]
108. Keller, M.K.; Bardow, A.; Jensdottir, T.; Lykkeaa, J.; Twetman, S. Effect of chewing gums containing the probiotic bacterium Lactobacillus reuteri on oral malodour. *Acta Odontol. Scand.* **2012**, *70*, 246–250. [CrossRef] [PubMed]
109. Smith, P.C.; Martínez, C. Wound healing in the oral mucosa. In *Oral Mucosa in Health and Disease*; Bergmeier, L., Ed.; Springer: Cham, Switzerland, 2018.
110. Vanlancker, E.; Vanhoecke, B.; Sieprath, T.; Bourgeois, J.; Beterams, A.; De Moerloose, B.; De Vos, W.H.; Van de Wiele, T. Oral microbiota reduce wound healing capacity of epithelial monolayers, irrespective of the presence of 5-fluorouracil. *Exp. Biol. Med.* **2018**, *243*, 350–360. [CrossRef]
111. Lalla, R.V.; Brennan, M.T.; Gordon, S.M.; Sonis, S.T.; Rosenthal, D.I.; Keefe, D.M. Oral Mucositis Due to High-Dose Chemotherapy and/or Head and Neck Radiation Therapy. *J. Natl. Cancer Inst. Monogr.* **2019**, *2019*, lgz011. [CrossRef] [PubMed]
112. Davy, C.; Heathcote, S. A systematic review of interventions to mitigate radiotherapy-induced oral mucositis in head and neck cancer patients. *Support. Care Cancer* **2021**, *29*, 2187–2202. [CrossRef] [PubMed]
113. Twetman, S.; Keller, M.K.; Lee, L.; Yucel-Lindberg, T.; Pedersen, A.M.L. Effect of probiotic lozenges containing Lactobacillus reuteri on oral wound healing: A pilot study. *Benef. Microbes.* **2018**, *9*, 691–696. [CrossRef]
114. Twetman, S.; Pedersen, A.M.L.; Yucel-Lindberg, T. Probiotic supplements containing Lactobacillus reuteri does not affect the levels of matrix metalloproteinases and interferons in oral wound healing. *BMC Res. Notes* **2018**, *11*, 759. [CrossRef]
115. Walivaara, D.A.; Sjogren, I.; Gerasimcik, N.; Yucel-Lindberg, T.; Twetman, S.; Abrahamsson, P. Effects of Lactobacillus reuteri-containing lozenges on healing after surgical removal of mandibular third molars: A randomised controlled trial. *Benef. Microbes.* **2019**, *10*, 653–659. [CrossRef] [PubMed]
116. Limaye, S.A.; Haddad, R.I.; Cilli, F.; Sonis, S.T.; Colevas, A.D.; Brennan, M.T.; Hu, K.S.; Murphy, B.A. Phase 1b, multicenter, single blinded, placebo-controlled, sequential dose escalation study to assess the safety and tolerability of topically applied AG013 in subjects with locally advanced head and neck cancer receiving induction chemotherapy. *Cancer* **2013**, *119*, 4268–4276. [CrossRef] [PubMed]
117. Jiang, C.; Wang, H.; Xia, C.; Dong, Q.; Chen, E.; Qiu, Y.; Su, Y.; Xie, H.; Zeng, L.; Kuang, J.; et al. A randomized, double-blind, placebo-controlled trial of probiotics to reduce the severity of oral mucositis induced by chemoradiotherapy for patients with nasopharyngeal carcinoma. *Cancer* **2019**, *125*, 1081–1090. [CrossRef] [PubMed]
118. Sharma, A.; Rath, G.K.; Chaudhary, S.P.; Thakar, A.; Mohanti, B.K.; Bahadur, S. Lactobacillus brevis CD2 lozenges reduce radiation- and chemotherapy-induced mucositis in patients with head and neck cancer: A randomized double-blind placebo-controlled study. *Eur. J. Cancer* **2012**, *48*, 875–881. [CrossRef] [PubMed]

Article

Effect of the Passive Ultrasonic Irrigation and the Apical Diameter Size on the Debridement Efficacy of Infected Root Canals: A Multivariate Statistical Assessment of Histological Data

Marcela Alcota [1], Jimena Osorio [1], Claudia Díaz [1], Ana Ortega-Pinto [2], Cristián Peñafiel [2], Juan C. Rivera [3], Daniela Salazar [1], Germán Manríquez [4,5,6,*] and Fermín E. González [1,7,8,*]

[1] Department of Conservative Dentistry, Faculty of Dentistry, University of Chile, Santiago 8380492, Chile; malcota@u.uchile.cl (M.A.); jimeosoriom@gmail.com (J.O.); cdiaz@odontologia.uchile.cl (C.D.); dsalazar@odontologia.uchile.cl (D.S.)
[2] Department of Pathology and Oral Medicine, Faculty of Dentistry, University of Chile, Santiago 8380492, Chile; aortega@odontologia.uchile.cl (A.O.-P.); cpenafiel@odontologia.uchile.cl (C.P.)
[3] Private Practice, Cali 760042, Colombia; juancamiloriverac@hotmail.com
[4] Centre for Quantitative Analysis in Dental Anthropology (CA2), Faculty of Dentistry, University of Chile, Santiago 8380492, Chile
[5] Dental Sciences Research Institute, Faculty of Dentistry, University of Chile, Santiago 8380492, Chile
[6] Department of Anthropology, Faculty of Social Sciences, University of Chile, Santiago 8380492, Chile
[7] Laboratory of Experimental Immunology & Cancer, Faculty of Dentistry, University of Chile, Santiago 8380492, Chile
[8] Millennium Institute on Immunology and Immunotherapy, Faculty of Medicine, University of Chile, Santiago 8380453, Chile
* Correspondence: gmanriquezs@odontologia.uchile.cl (G.M.); fgonzalez@uchile.cl (F.E.G.)

Abstract: The removal of necrotic and vital pulp substrates and microorganisms and their toxins from the root canal system (RCS) has been found to be the basis for a successful endodontic treatment. In this study, our aim was to evaluate the effect of passive ultrasonic irrigation (PUI) on the elimination of the organic remnant tissue from infected, narrow and curved mandibular root canals during their instrumentation. For this purpose, mesiobuccal canals from mandibular first molars were instrumented with the RaCe rotary system, using PUI activation or conventional irrigation (CI) and two apical diameters (#25 and #35). The root canal cleanness of the samples was evaluated by microscopy and using a modified Langeland's ordinal scale. Parametric and non-parametric statistical analyses and principal coordinates analysis (PCoA) of the samples were performed. When PUI was used, there was a significant reduction of the organic remnant in the apical enlargement of 25 at 2 mm from the apex ($p < 0.001$). After pooling the groups, regardless of the depth of the observation (2 and 4 mm from the apex), the pair #35 + PUI vs. #25 + CI showed statistically significant differences ($p < 0.001$). The effect of PUI explained 65% of the overall variance when compared with the CI samples. The use of PUI reduced the organic material of narrow infected and curved root canals with an apical enlargement of #25 and #35. When PUI is not used, a biomechanical instrumentation up to a diameter $\geq$#35 is recommended.

Keywords: passive ultrasonic irrigation; apical enlargement; organic remnant

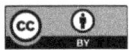

1. Introduction

Conventionally, the cleaning of the root canal system (RCS) is done with a chemical-mechanical preparation using endodontic instruments and irrigating the area profusely with disinfecting chemical solutions [1]. The basis for a successful endodontic treatment is the complete removal from the RCS [2] of both necrotic and vital pulp substrates, together with microorganisms and their toxins. In this context, the complexity of the morphology of the RCS makes their complete mechanical debridement a major challenge for clinicians. It has been shown that over 35% of the RCS surface remains untouched by endodontic instruments after instrumentation [3,4], highlighting the importance of efficient instrumentation and irrigation to ensure the proper chemical debridement and disinfection of the RCS.

One of the most important factors for the clinical success of an endodontic treatment is the proper preparation of the apical third of the root canal. Inappropriate preparation and disinfection of this portion can lead to the persistence of organic remnants (i.e., microorganisms and necrotic tissue). These, in turn, may cause periapical inflammation, disfavouring tissue repair and resulting in the consequent failure of the treatment, especially in non-vital and infected teeth [5,6].

When analysing the amount of enlargement needed in the preparation of the apical portion of infected root canals, several aspects must be considered, such as the action of the irrigant solutions [5,7], the bacterial penetration into dentinal tubules [5,8,9], and the irregular and complex morphology of the RCS [5,7,10,11].

It has been demonstrated that the higher the apical diameter the better disinfection of root canals, mainly because of the mechanical elimination of contaminated dentin and the penetration of the irrigant solution in the apical region [5,12]. Despite great advances in mechanised instrumentation systems and their alloys, in complex anatomies it is difficult to reach high apical diameters during instrumentation. Although these last-generation instruments may allow for higher diameter coverage, they may also lead to the risk of procedural mistakes, such as transportations and foramen deformation, among others. In these situations, the effect of the irrigant solution becomes fundamental in order to remove debris, dissolve remnant tissue and act as a lubricant [4,10,11].

On the other hand, as far as the irrigation of the root canal is concerned, it has been shown that PUI is more effective than CI for removing organic tissue, because of its ability to disintegrate more bacteria and dentin debris [13–17]. Recently, Lee et al. (2019) have demonstrated that a higher amount of organic remnant is eliminated using PUI during the ex vivo preparation of vital root canals when using instruments with low apical diameters [18]. However, they state that their conclusions are not completely applicable to infected root canals. Thus, our hypothesis states that PUI enhances the removal of dentin debris and organic remnant during the preparation of infected root canals, especially when instruments with low apical diameters are used.

The objective of this study was to evaluate the effect of PUI on the removal of the organic remnant tissue from narrow, infected and curved root canals during their instrumentation with apical enlargements of #25 and #35.

2. Materials and Methods

2.1. Sample Collection

Fifty-three mandibular molars were selected according to the following selection criteria:

Inclusion criteria: (i) recently extracted non-vital and infected mandibular molars; (ii) non-endodontically treated teeth; (iii) diagnosis of symptomatic apical periodontitis and chronic or acute apical abscesses; (iv) root canals with moderate curvature (between 10° and 25°) according to Schneider's criteria [19]; and (v) narrow and permeable mesiobuccal root canals of mandibular molars.

In order to measure the curvature by Schneider's criteria, X-rays of the roots were taken in the same direction of the curve [19]. For this purpose, the extracted teeth were positioned on a N°2 X-ray intraoral film with the crown-apical axis of the mesiobuccal root parallel to the film with the central ray tangent to the curve of the root. To determine the permeability of the root canals, we used canals where a #10 K-file was the highest instrument which reached patency.

Exclusion criteria: teeth with previous history of endodontic access or treatment; and fused, incompletely developed and straight or fractured roots.

2.2. Study Groups

The selected root canals with moderate curvatures were randomly divided into two groups: Group 1 consisting of 24 root canals instrumented by using RaCe rotary files (FKG Dentaire SA, La Chaux-de-Fonds, Switzerland) and using PUI; and group 2 consisting of 24 root canals instrumented with RaCe rotary files and using CI with syringes as control. Five non-instrumented root canals were used for assessing histological intraobserver error calibration. Groups 1 and 2 were further divided in two subgroups: 1A, in which an instrument with an apical diameter of #25 (n = 10) was used; 1B, in which an instrument with an apical diameter of #35 (n = 10) was used; 2A, in which an instrument with an apical diameter of #25 (n = 12) was used; and 2B, in which an instrument with an apical diameter of #35 (n = 12) was used.

2.3. Instrumentation Procedures

Immediately after extraction, the teeth were kept in a 10% formalin buffer solution for a week. The teeth were allocated into different groups by a randomised and alternate assignment following the sequence 1A, 1B, 2A, and 2B. Instrumentation procedures were performed by two experimented and calibrated operators (J.O. and C.D.). Teeth were endodontically accessed and patency achieved with a size 10 K-file (Dentsply Maillefer, Ballaigues, Switzerland). Coronal pre-flaring was accomplished with a size 20 K-file (Dentsply Maillefer) and PreRaCe file #30/0.06 taper to obtain straight line access to the canal and eliminate coronal curvature. A size 10 K-file (Dentsply Maillefer, Ballaigues, Switzerland) was passively introduced into each canal until its tip was visible at the apical foramen. The working length (WL) was established by subtracting 1 mm from the previous distance. The root canal preparation was performed using RaCe file #15/0.04 taper and RaCe file #25/0.04 taper for subgroups 1A y 2A, and an additional RaCe file #35/0.04 taper for subgroups 1B y 2B. During the instrumentation procedure, the root canals were irrigated before and after each instrument with 0.5 mL of NaOCl 5.25%, using a 27 G needle (Monoject) and positive pressure irrigation at WL -2 mm, followed by a final wash with 0.5 mL of EDTA for 2 min and 1 mL NaOCl 5.25%.

For group 1, the root canal preparation was finished using the same final protocol irrigation together with PUI. The file was passively inserted at WL -2 mm and activated for 30 s with a Varios 560 multifunctional ultrasonic scaler (NSK, Kanuma, Japan) with 2.5 power and ultrasonic tips with a diameter of #20. Attempts were made to maintain the file centred in the canal during activation. Each file was used and discarded after five samples. For group 2, the root canal preparation was finished using the same final protocol irrigation using CI with syringes. The RaCe rotary files were operated in a continuous rotation motion at 350 rpm and a torque of 2 Ncm by an electric motor model Endo-Mate TC (NSK, Kanuma, Japan).

2.4. Histological Procedures and Organic Remnant Analysis

After instrumentation, the teeth were fixed in 10% formalin, demineralised in a 5% Nitric Acid solution for 48 hrs and then moved to an Ana Morse solution for two weeks. Decalcified roots were included in paraffin and then perpendicular crosscut slices (5-micrometers thickness) were obtained. Four slides with 2–4 cuts each were prepared at 2 and 4 mm from the apex, stained with haematoxylin and eosin (H&E) and stored for further analysis. Therefore, at least eight cuts were made at both depths in each sample and the most representative section was chosen for further histological analysis.

During histological procedures, two teeth were lost in groups 1A and 1B, so the final sample size for these groups was ten teeth each. The root transversal samples were analysed with a light microscope Leica DM5000 (Leica Microsystems, Wetzlar, Germany) at different magnifications. Images were captured using LAS EZ 3.2.0. photo capture software. The root canal cleanness was evaluated by a single blinded and calibrated observer (A.O.) with a 0 to 3 score scale, similar to that used by Langeland et al. [20,21] in which we eliminated score 4 (i.e., the count of inflammatory cells in samples from animal models, which is not the case in this study). The score used was: 0 to refer to a root canal with organic remnant, predentin or debris in all the lumen of the histological sample; 1 to refer to a root canal with organic remnant in most parts of the lumen; 2 to refer to a relatively wide root canal with organic remnant in the margins; and 3 to refer to an absolutely clean root canal (Figure 1).

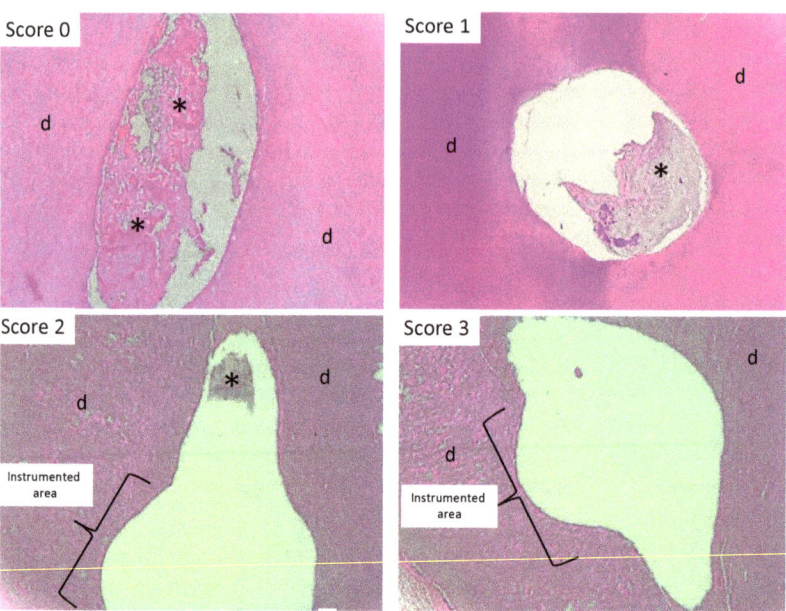

Figure 1. Representative images of the score scale used for the evaluation of root canal cleanness (based on Langeland et al.). Score 0: Root canal with organic remnant, predentin or debris in every histological sample. Score 1: Root canal with organic remnant in most part of the lumen. Score 2: Relatively wide root canal with organic remnant in the margins. Score 3: Absolutely clean root canal. H&E staining. Original magnification: 10×. * = organic remnant. d = dentin.

2.5. Statistical Analyses

In order to test the hypothesis explaining the effect of the variables under study (i.e., PUI vs. CI removal of organic remnant), statistical analyses were carried out as follows: (i) Epps-Singleton (ES) test for equal distributions to assess the effect of each diameter separately and Kruskal-Wallis test for equal medians to test the diameter effect as a whole, (ii) Mann-Whitney pairwise test to test the diameter of the instrument on the canal cleanness score observed after biomechanical instrumentation (BIns), and (iii) Principal Coordinate Analysis to assess the overall effect of PUI compared to CI, using a one-way Analysis of Similarities (ANOSIM) as a post-hoc test. The rationale behind using an ES test instead of the widely used Kolmogorov-Smirnov (KS) two-sample test lies in the greater statistical power of the first test when compared with the second [22]. Regarding the ANOSIM post-hoc test, it is the non-parametric version of the one-way ANOVA for ranked ordinal data [23]. All the analyses were run in PAST 4.06b statistical program [24].

3. Results

3.1. Effect of PUI on the Organic Remnant Removal Regarding the Instrumentation with Different Diameters

When the instrumentation procedures were analysed separately, only the instrumentation with #25 at 2 mm crosscut from the apex showed statistically significant differences between the PUI and CI samples (1A vs. 2A) (Figure 2 and Table 1). After pooling the #25 and #35 groups, regardless of the depth of the observation (crosscuts of 2 and 4 mm from the apex), the pair #25 + CI vs. #35 + PUI showed statistically significant differences (group 2A vs. group 1B) (Figure 2 and Table 1).

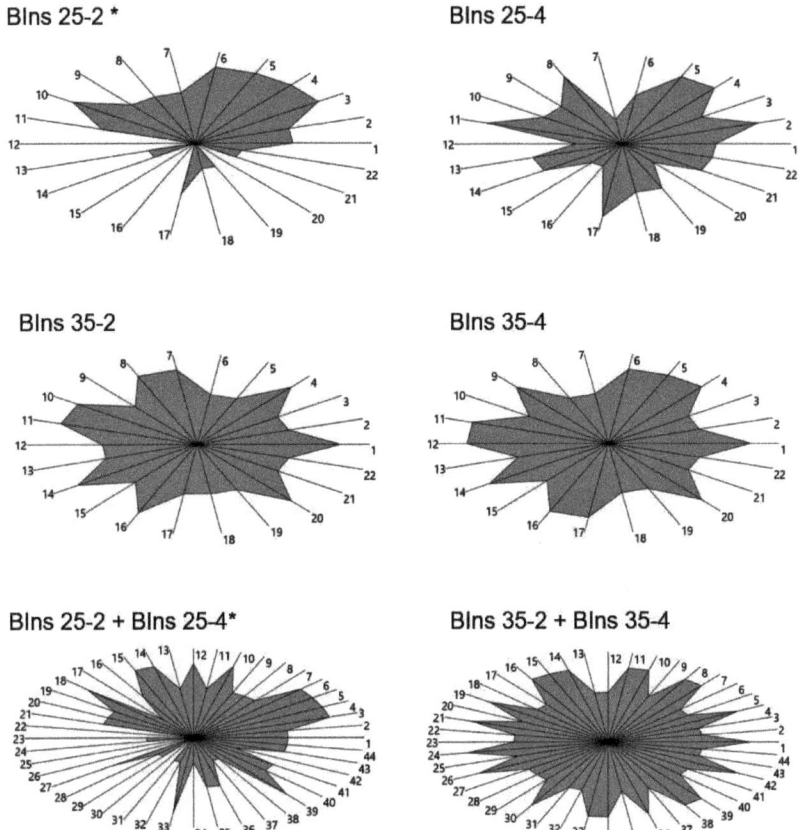

Figure 2. Frequency of cleanness scores registered after analysing the root transversal samples used in this study. In single diameter radar plots (first two rows) teeth 1–10 = PIU, and teeth 11–22 = CI. In pooled diameter radar plots (last row) teeth 1–20 = PIU, and teeth 21–44 = CI. * Statistically significant differences when comparing PIU and CI scores ($p < 0.001$, for details see Table 1). BIns = Biomechanical instrumentation (#-mm from apex).

Table 1. Effect of PUI on debris removal regarding the diameter of the instrument used during biomechanical instrumentation.

Instrument Size (#-mm from Apex)	Epps-Singleton W2	p Value (Same Distance)
25-2	43.58	7.84×10^{-9}
25-4	1.39	0.8460
35-2	0.40	0.9823
35-4	3.24×10^{-16}	1
25 (2, 4)	21.10	3×10^{-4}
35 (2, 4)	0.22	0.9944

A representative histological section, at 2 mm from the apex, is shown in Figure 3, with apical enlargement of #25 without PUI, where the presence of organic remnants is evident, (Figure 3A,B) vs. an apical histological section with enlargement of #25 with PUI, where the organic remnant is starkly reduced (Figure 3C,D).

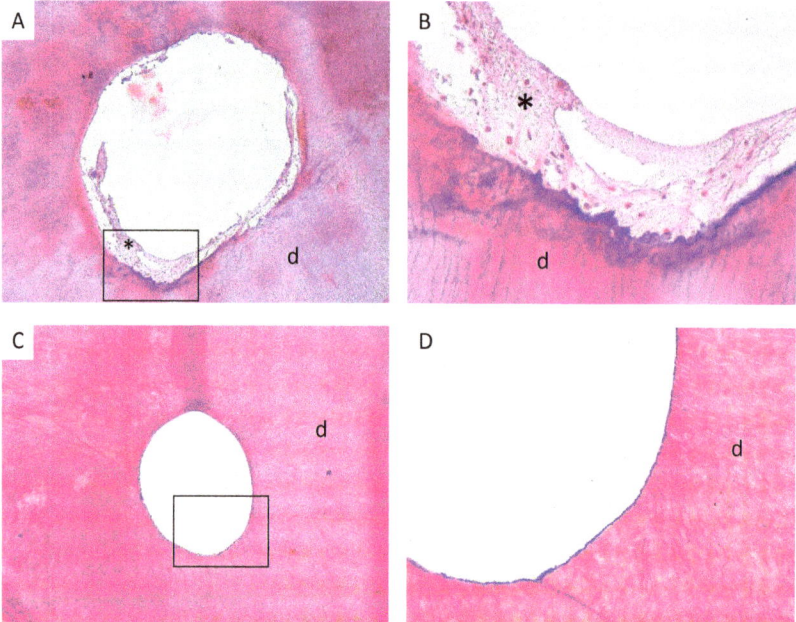

Figure 3. Representative images, at 2 mm from the apex, of root canals instrumented with RaCe system with and without PUI. (**A**,**B**): Root canals instrumented with RaCe system #25 without PUI. Organic remnant is observed adjacent to the walls of the apical canal. (**C**,**D**): Apical canals instrumented with RaCe system #25 with PUI. The walls of the apical canal are observed without organic remnants. H&E staining. Magnification: (**A**,**C**), 10× (**B**,**D**), 40× * = organic remnant. d = dentin.

3.2. Effect of PUI and the Diameter of Endodontic Instruments for Biomechanical Removal on Teeth Cleanness

Compared with the control samples, the cleanness of the teeth under the effect of PUI and endodontic instrumentation was significantly improved (Kruskal-Wallis test for equal medians: H (Chi^2) = 11.52, Hc (tie corrected) = 13.62, p (same) = 0.003474).

Regarding the endodontic instrumentation, the observed differences are mainly explained by the diameter of the operational device (#35 vs. #25), independently from the depth of the observation (2 vs. 4 mm from the apex) (Table 2). In addition, in the histological sections obtained from the samples of this study, we observed that none of the studied root canals were completely free from debris readily accumulated in the isthmus of mesial root canals (Figure 4).

Table 2. Effect of the diameter of the instrument on the canal cleanness score observed after biomechanical instrumentation (Mann-Whitney pairwise test, Bonferroni corrected p values). BIns = Biomechanical instrumentation (#-mm from apex).

	BIns 25-2	BIns 25-4
BIns 25-4	0.9076	
BIns 35-2	0.03814	0.5247
BIns 35-4	0.01547	0.1988

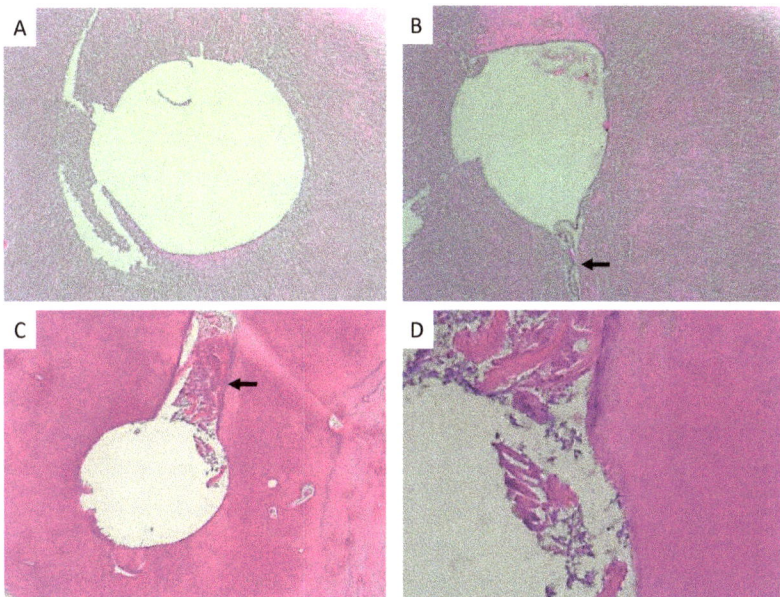

Figure 4. Representative images, at 2 mm from the apex, of roots canals prepared with different instrument diameters. (**A**): Root canal instrumented with #35 without PUI. Magnification 10×. (**B**): We can observe the remains of detritus in the isthmus after instrumentation (black arrow). Magnification 10×. (**C**): Root canal instrumented in a single pole with lime RaCe #25. We can observe the remains of detritus in the polar opposite (black arrow) Magnification 10×. (**D**): Approach of the previous case. Magnification 40×.

After applying a PCoA to the ordinal raw data obtained by the Langeland's ordinal scale for teeth cleanness, the effect of PUI explained 64.9% of the overall variance when compared with the control (conventional irrigation, CI). The percentage of PCo 1 expected by chance variance was below what was observed, implying a statistically significant difference between the PUI and CI samples (i.e., 52% vs. 64.9%, respectively, after a broken-stick model) (Figure 5). These results were corroborated by a one-way ANOSIM post-hoc test (R = 0.3383, p (same) = 0.0005, mean ranks = 95.7–134.8, using Manhattan similarity index after 9.999 permutations).

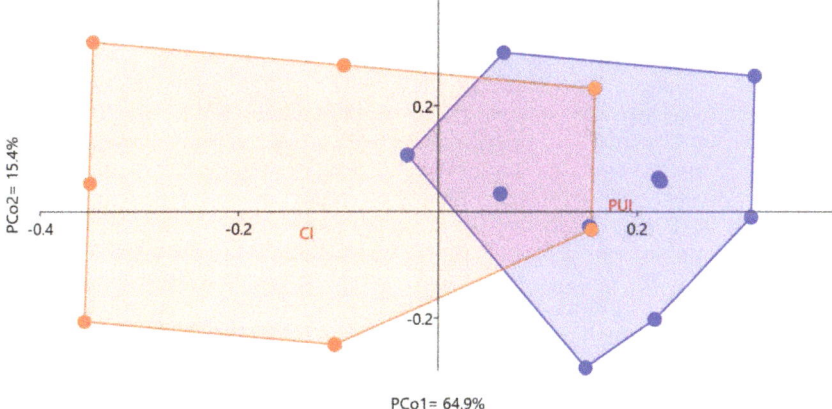

Figure 5. Principal Coordinate Analysis (PCoA) of the raw data. Visualization of the dissimilarities of the ordinal raw data

used in this study after assigning a location to each observation in a low-dimensional space represented by the Principal Coordinate axes, where PCo1 > PCo2 > ... > PCoZ.

Finally, Table 3 is a summary of our findings and it compares the elimination of organic material after the biomechanical rotary instrumentation of narrow, infected and curved root canals with or without PUI and apical enlargements of #25 and #35.

Table 3. Summary of the experimental design to assess the effect of three relevant variables on RCS cleanness: (1) Distance from the apex (depth); (2) Irrigation system (PUI vs. Conventional syringes); and (3) Diameter of the instrument used during biomechanical instrumentation (#25 vs. #35). A"+" sign indicates the presence of a significant effect of each of the analysed variables; its absence means that there are no differences between them. RCS = Root canal system; CI = Conventional irrigation.

Depth	Irrigation System		Diameter of the Instrument (RaCe 0.04 Taper)	
	PUI	CI	#25	#35
4 mm	+	−	−	+
2 mm	+	−	+	−

4. Discussion

We compared the effect of PUI on the efficacy of the elimination of organic material remaining into infected, narrow and moderated curved mandibular root canals after their instrumentation using the RaCe rotary files 0.04 taper with apical enlargements of #25 and #35, following an instrumentation protocol similar to the one we used in clinical practice.

Our results show that when PUI was combined with the RaCe rotary system instrumentation, there was no difference in the elimination of organic material between groups 1A and 1B (with apical enlargements of #25 and #35, respectively). Our results agree with the study of Lee et al. who compared different apical diameters with and without PUI [18]. They found that PUI reduces remnant pulp tissues in canals to small preparations. However, in the present study we performed an instrumentation and irrigation protocol which is closer to the real clinical practice than the one used by Lee et al., who used a single file protocol. In addition, we used infected and moderate curved root canals instead of vital pulp teeth. Regarding the latter, there is a consensus that PUI is more effective than traditional syringe irrigation, removing more efficiently the organic tissue, planktonic bacteria and dentine debris from the root canal. These phenomena could be explained because the ultrasound creates a higher speed and flow volume of the irrigant in the canal during irrigation, thereby eliminating more debris, producing less apical packing, allowing better access of the chemical product to accessory canals and even causing a flush effect to be produced by ultrasound but not manual irrigation [3,13].

On the other hand, in our study when the instrumentation was performed without PUI in apical enlargements of #25 and #35, the difference in the elimination of organic material was significant, with a pronounced reduction in the 2B group (with apical enlargement of #35) compared with 2A group (with apical enlargement of #25). This is in agreement with several studies regarding apical enlargement that establish a directly proportional relationship between the increase of last instrument diameter and the reduction of organic and bacterial remaining [5–7,10,15,21,25–28]. In fact, during canal preparation, apical size has been crucial in defining the successful debridement of the RCS because the penetration of the irrigant into the apical one-third of the canal and the removal of debris depend on the final size of the instrument used in the canals; so, an increase in the apical preparation size significantly enhances the root canal disinfection [10,25].

In addition, several studies have shown the relevance not only of the apical preparation but also of the taper in the instrumentation of the apical one-third of root canals. Regarding this, a previous study by Plotino et al. (2014) showed that the cleanliness of the apical canal walls was better when the apical preparation was performed after a basic preparation of a size #25/0.06 taper, irrespective of the technique used to perform the apical preparation [29]. Srikanth et al. (2015) showed that for proper penetration of irrigants, removal of debris and the smear layer from the apical third region, the enlargement to #30 file size is adequate when the suitable coronal taper is achieved. A more recent study by Xu et al. (2018) determined that when the apical size increased to #40, the remnant debris significantly decreased in the mesial roots of mandibular first molars [30].

In our study, we observed an important reduction of the organic remnant when using PUI during apical preparations up to #25 (1A vs. 2A groups). In addition, the amount of organic remnant in group 1A was comparable with what we observed in group 2B. In other words, using PUI instead of CI improves the #25-diameter efficiency as well as the #35-diameter with a CI protocol. This is particularly relevant when the clinician is instrumenting complex root canal morphology (e.g., mesiobuccal roots of upper molars), where it often becomes impossible to reach apical diameters of #35 or higher without transportation and/or perforation risk. Additionally, we found a cleaner area of the samples studied at 4 mm from the apex with and without PUI, compared to the area at 2 mm from the apex which had the highest content of detritus. This coincides with Paqué et al. (2005), who found an increase in the amount of debris towards the apical region using RaCe without PUI [31]. We believe that this may be explained by an increased flow, and therefore, greater solvent action of hypochlorite in this region, at 4 mm from the apex.

It is important to note that none of the root canals from the four groups analysed in this study was completely free from hard-tissue debris, with debris readily accumulated in the isthmus of mesial root canals (Figures 2 and 3). In this regard, we consider that all rotary instrumentations must be complemented by a thorough manual instrumentation in order to achieve optimal debridement, because those systems tend to keep a centred positioned inside the canal, failing to reach both internal and external pole of the canal. This, together with activation of sodium hypochlorite during instrumentation, could more effectively eliminate the presence of organic debris within the canals, especially from areas which are difficult to access or inaccessible by mechanized instrumentation.

One of the limitations of this study was the use of an ordinal scale to assess a change which is intrinsically infinitesimal, like the quantity of organic remnant found in RCS after instrumentation. This limitation can be overcome by calculating and comparing the surface occupied by debridement in the root canal of the control and experimental histological samples. A further development of this study will be to evaluate the debridement efficacy of infected root canals using EndoActivator (Dentsply Maillefer) or XP-Endo Finisher (FKG Dentaire) compared with PUI.

5. Conclusions

This work adds evidence regarding the clinical treatment of infected and curved root canals, showing that the use of PUI becomes fundamental when the augmentation up to #35 or #40 of apical diameter is difficult, if not impossible, because of the presence of curves or little amount of dentinal wall in the apical third of the root canal. Therefore, we consider that clinicians should incorporate PUI as part of their regular therapeutic strategy, since it helps to remove pulp tissue from isthmus and flattened root canals from vital teeth. Also, in cases of infected root canals, it might have an antibacterial effect by disorganizing biofilm into root canals, thus significantly improving the prognosis of these treatments.

Author Contributions: Conceptualization, M.A., G.M. and F.E.G.; Methodology, M.A., G.M. and F.E.G.; Validation, J.O., C.D., A.O.-P. and C.P.; Formal Analysis, G.M. and F.E.G.; Investigation, J.O., C.D., A.O.-P. and C.P.; Resources, M.A., J.O., C.D., A.O.-P., G.M. and F.E.G.; Data Curation, J.O., C.D. and A.O.-P.; Writing—Original Draft Preparation, M.A., J.O., C.D. and F.E.G.; Writing—Review & Editing, M.A., J.O., A.O.-P., C.P., J.C.R., D.S., G.M. and F.E.G.; Visualization, A.O.-P., G.M. and F.E.G.; Supervision, M.A. and F.E.G.; Project Administration, M.A. and F.E.G.; Funding Acquisition, M.A., G.M. and F.E.G. All authors have read and agreed to the published version of the manuscript.

Funding: This work was partially supported by CONICYT, Programa de Investigación Asociativa Anillos en Ciencia y Tecnología ACT N-096 grant (G.M.) and the Faculty of Dentistry, University of Chile, FIOUCH 17-007 grant (F.E.G.). The APC was funded by the Faculty of Dentistry, University of Chile.

Institutional Review Board Statement: The present study was performed in agreement with the guidelines of the Declaration of Helsinki and approved by the Ethical Committee of the Faculty of Dentistry, University of Chile (Pri-ODO 15479).

Informed Consent Statement: Written consent from patients was waived because the teeth used in the study were samples that had been discarded after extraction either in public dental services or in the Dental Clinic of the Faculty of Dentistry, University of Chile. However, all patients had given oral consent for further use of the discarded samples.

Data Availability Statement: Data obtained from this study is not available publicly. Information regarding these data should be requested to the corresponding authors.

Acknowledgments: The rotary instruments used in this study were donated by FKG Dentaire SA. We thank Juan Fernández from the Language and Translation services, Faculty of Dentistry, Universidad de Chile and Claudia Trajtemberg, MPhil University of Cambridge, UK, for kindly proofreading and checking the spelling and grammar of this manuscript.

Conflicts of Interest: The authors declare that there is no conflict of interest regarding the publication of this article.

References

1. Cesario, F.; Hungaro Duarte, M.A.; Duque, J.A.; Alcalde, M.P.; de Andrade, F.B.; Reis So, M.V.; De Vasconcelos, B.C.; Vivan, R.R. Comparisons by microcomputed tomography of the efficiency of different irrigation techniques for removing dentinal debris from artificial grooves. *J. Conserv. Dent.* **2018**, *21*, 383–387. [CrossRef]
2. Dioguardi, M.; Di Gioia, G.; Illuzzi, G.; Laneve, E.; Cocco, A.; Troiano, G. Endodontic irrigants: Different methods to improve efficacy and related problems. *Eur. J. Dent.* **2018**, *12*, 459–466. [CrossRef] [PubMed]
3. Mozo, S.; Llena, C.; Forner, L. Review of ultrasonic irrigation in endodontics: Increasing action of irrigating solutions. *Med. Oral Patol. Oral Cir. Bucal.* **2012**, *17*, e512–e516. [CrossRef]
4. Kumar, T.; Dhillon, J.S.; Gill, G.S.; Singla, R.; Rani, S.; Dhillon, M. An in vitro comparison of the antimicrobial efficacy of positive pressure and negative pressure irrigation techniques in root canals infected with Enterococcus faecalis. *J. Conserv. Dent.* **2018**, *21*, 438–442. [CrossRef]
5. Baugh, D.; Wallace, J. The role of apical instrumentation in root canal treatment: A review of the literature. *J. Endod.* **2005**, *31*, 333–340. [CrossRef] [PubMed]
6. Tan, B.T.; Messer, H.H. The effect of instrument type and preflaring on apical file size determination. *Int. Endod. J.* **2002**, *35*, 752–758. [CrossRef] [PubMed]
7. Siqueira, J.F., Jr.; Lima, K.C.; Magalhaes, F.A.; Lopes, H.P.; de Uzeda, M. Mechanical reduction of the bacterial population in the root canal by three instrumentation techniques. *J. Endod.* **1999**, *25*, 332–335. [CrossRef]
8. Waltimo, T.M.; Orstavik, D.; Siren, E.K.; Haapasalo, M.P. In vitro yeast infection of human dentin. *J. Endod.* **2000**, *26*, 207–209. [CrossRef]
9. Berkiten, M.; Okar, I.; Berkiten, R. In vitro study of the penetration of Streptococcus sanguis and Prevotella intermedia strains into human dentinal tubules. *J. Endod.* **2000**, *26*, 236–239. [CrossRef]
10. Srikanth, P.; Krishna, A.G.; Srinivas, S.; Reddy, E.S.; Battu, S.; Aravelli, S. Minimal Apical Enlargement for Penetration of Irrigants to the Apical Third of Root Canal System: A Scanning Electron Microscope Study. *J. Int. Oral Health* **2015**, *7*, 92–96.
11. Reddy, J.M.; Latha, P.; Gowda, B.; Manvikar, V.; Vijayalaxmi, D.B.; Ponangi, K.C. Smear layer and debris removal using manual Ni-Ti files compared with rotary Protaper Ni-Ti files—An In-Vitro SEM study. *J. Int. Oral Health* **2014**, *6*, 89–94. [PubMed]
12. Brunson, M.; Heilborn, C.; Johnson, D.J.; Cohenca, N. Effect of apical preparation size and preparation taper on irrigant volume delivered by using negative pressure irrigation system. *J. Endod.* **2010**, *36*, 721–724. [CrossRef] [PubMed]
13. van der Sluis, L.W.; Versluis, M.; Wu, M.K.; Wesselink, P.R. Passive ultrasonic irrigation of the root canal: A review of the literature. *Int. Endod. J.* **2007**, *40*, 415–426. [CrossRef] [PubMed]
14. van der Sluis, L.W.; Shemesh, H.; Wu, M.K.; Wesselink, P.R. An evaluation of the influence of passive ultrasonic irrigation on the seal of root canal fillings. *Int. Endod. J.* **2007**, *40*, 356–361. [CrossRef] [PubMed]
15. Harrison, A.J.; Chivatxaranukul, P.; Parashos, P.; Messer, H.H. The effect of ultrasonically activated irrigation on reduction of Enterococcus faecalis in experimentally infected root canals. *Int. Endod. J.* **2010**, *43*, 968–977. [CrossRef] [PubMed]
16. Freire, L.G.; Iglecias, E.F.; Cunha, R.S.; Dos Santos, M.; Gavini, G. Micro-Computed Tomographic Evaluation of Hard Tissue Debris Removal after Different Irrigation Methods and Its Influence on the Filling of Curved Canals. *J. Endod.* **2015**, *41*, 1660–1666. [CrossRef] [PubMed]

17. Leoni, G.B.; Versiani, M.A.; Silva-Sousa, Y.T.; Bruniera, J.F.; Pecora, J.D.; Sousa-Neto, M.D. Ex vivo evaluation of four final irrigation protocols on the removal of hard-tissue debris from the mesial root canal system of mandibular first molars. *Int. Endod. J.* **2017**, *50*, 398–406. [CrossRef] [PubMed]
18. Lee, O.Y.S.; Khan, K.; Li, K.Y.; Shetty, H.; Abiad, R.S.; Cheung, G.S.P.; Neelakantan, P. Influence of apical preparation size and irrigation technique on root canal debridement: A histological analysis of round and oval root canals. *Int. Endod. J.* **2019**, *52*, 1366–1376. [CrossRef] [PubMed]
19. Schneider, S.W. A comparison of canal preparations in straight and curved root canals. *Oral Surg. Oral Med. Oral Pathol.* **1971**, *32*, 271–275. [CrossRef]
20. Langeland, K.; Liao, K.; Pascon, E.A. Work-saving devices in endodontics: Efficacy of sonic and ultrasonic techniques. *J. Endod.* **1985**, *11*, 499–510. [CrossRef]
21. Siqueira, J.F., Jr.; Araujo, M.C.; Garcia, P.F.; Fraga, R.C.; Dantas, C.J. Histological evaluation of the effectiveness of five instrumentation techniques for cleaning the apical third of root canals. *J. Endod.* **1997**, *23*, 499–502. [CrossRef]
22. Goerg, S.J.; Kaiser, J. Nonparametric Testing of Distributions—The Epps—Singleton Two-Sample Test using the Empirical Characteristic Function. *Stata. J.* **2009**, *3*, 454–465. [CrossRef]
23. Clarke, K.R. Nonparametric Multivariate Analyses of Changes in Community Structure. *Austral Ecol.* **1993**, *18*, 117–143. [CrossRef]
24. Hammer, O.; Harper, D.A.T.; Ryan, P.D. PAST: Paleontological Statistics Software Package for Education and Data Analysis. *Palaeontol. Electron.* **2001**, *4*, e9.
25. Rodrigues, R.C.V.; Zandi, H.; Kristoffersen, A.K.; Enersen, M.; Mdala, I.; Orstavik, D.; Rocas, I.N.; Siqueira, J.F., Jr. Influence of the Apical Preparation Size and the Irrigant Type on Bacterial Reduction in Root Canal-treated Teeth with Apical Periodontitis. *J. Endod.* **2017**, *43*, 1058–1063. [CrossRef]
26. Usman, N.; Baumgartner, J.C.; Marshall, J.G. Influence of instrument size on root canal debridement. *J. Endod.* **2004**, *30*, 110–112. [CrossRef] [PubMed]
27. Albrecht, L.J.; Baumgartner, J.C.; Marshall, J.G. Evaluation of apical debris removal using various sizes and tapers of ProFile GT files. *J. Endod.* **2004**, *30*, 425–428. [CrossRef] [PubMed]
28. Dalton, B.C.; Orstavik, D.; Phillips, C.; Pettiette, M.; Trope, M. Bacterial reduction with nickel-titanium rotary instrumentation. *J. Endod.* **1998**, *24*, 763–767. [CrossRef]
29. Plotino, G.; Grande, N.M.; Tocci, L.; Testarelli, L.; Gambarini, G. Influence of Different Apical Preparations on Root Canal Cleanliness in Human Molars: A SEM Study. *J. Oral Maxillofac. Res.* **2014**, *5*, e4. [CrossRef]
30. Xu, K.; Wang, J.; Wang, K.; Gen, N.; Li, J. Micro-computed tomographic evaluation of the effect of the final apical size prepared by rotary nickel-titanium files on the removal efficacy of hard-tissue debris. *J. Int. Med. Res.* **2018**, *46*, 2219–2229. [CrossRef] [PubMed]
31. Paque, F.; Musch, U.; Hulsmann, M. Comparison of root canal preparation using RaCe and ProTaper rotary Ni-Ti instruments. *Int. Endod. J.* **2005**, *38*, 8–16. [CrossRef]

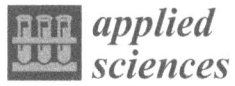

Article

Advantages of Dynamic Navigation in Prosthetic Implant Treatment in Terms of the Clinical Evaluation and Salivary Pro-Inflammatory Biomarkers: A Clinical Study

Kacper Wachol [1,*], Tadeusz Morawiec [1], Agnieszka Szurko [2], Domenico Baldi [3], Anna Nowak-Wachol [4], Joanna Śmieszek-Wilczewska [1] and Anna Mertas [5]

[1] Department of Dental Surgery, Faculty of Medical Sciences in Zabrze, Medical University of Silesia, 15 Poniatowskiego Street, 40-055 Katowice, Poland
[2] Faculty of Science and Technology, University of Silesia, 75 Pułku Piechoty 1A Street, 41-500 Chorzów, Poland
[3] Department of Surgical and Integrated Diagnostics Sciences, University of Genoa, Via Balbi 5, 16126 Genoa, Italy
[4] Doctoral School, Department of Dental Propedeutics, Faculty of Medical Sciences in Zabrze, Medical University of Silesia in Katowice, 15 Poniatowskiego Street, 40-055 Katowice, Poland
[5] Department of Microbiology and Immunology, Faculty of Medical Sciences in Zabrze, Medical University of Silesia in Katowice, 19 Jordana Str., 41-808 Zabrze, Poland
* Correspondence: kacper.wachol@sum.edu.pl

Citation: Wachol, K.; Morawiec, T.; Szurko, A.; Baldi, D.; Nowak-Wachol, A.; Śmieszek-Wilczewska, J.; Mertas, A. Advantages of Dynamic Navigation in Prosthetic Implant Treatment in Terms of the Clinical Evaluation and Salivary Pro-Inflammatory Biomarkers: A Clinical Study. *Appl. Sci.* **2023**, *13*, 9866. https://doi.org/10.3390/app13179866

Academic Editor: Bruno Chrcanovic

Received: 4 July 2023
Revised: 30 August 2023
Accepted: 30 August 2023
Published: 31 August 2023

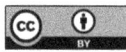

Copyright: © 2023 by the authors. Licensee MDPI, Basel, Switzerland. This article is an open access article distributed under the terms and conditions of the Creative Commons Attribution (CC BY) license (https://creativecommons.org/licenses/by/4.0/).

Abstract: Successful implantation in augmented areas relies on adequate bone density and quality, along with thorough planning. The minimisation of the risks involved in the surgery and recovery phases is also of tremendous relevance. The aims of the present research were to clinically and biochemically evaluate the healing process after implant surgery (dental implants) using dynamic surgical navigation following prior bone augmentation. Thirty healthy patients who had implant treatment were analysed. The study participants (30 patients) were randomised between two groups. The 15 patients in the study group were treated with Navident dynamic navigation by using a flapless technique. The control group included 15 subjects in whom the implantation procedure was performed classically using the elevation flap full-thickness method. In all cases, the patient's clinical condition, the patient's subjective visual assessment of post-operative pain using the Visual Analogue Scale (VAS), and the levels of the salivary biomarkers interleukin 6 (IL 6) and C-reactive protein (CRP) immediately before surgery on the first post-operative day and on the seventh post-operative day were assessed. The healing process was shown to be faster in patients in the study group due to the low invasiveness of the treatment, which was confirmed by lower levels of pro-inflammatory cytokines in the study group versus the control group. The statistical analysis used Student's t-test and Mann–Whitney test. The implementation of dynamic navigation and the application of the flapless technique reduced post-operative trauma, leading to a reduced risk of infection, reduced patient discomfort, and faster recovery.

Keywords: dentistry; implantology; cytokine; saliva; biomarkers; flapless implantology; dynamic navigation; minimally invasive implantology

1. Introduction

Conventional implant surgery involves incisions of the alveolar mucosa and elevation of the mucoperiosteal flap to visualise and access the bone. This approach ensures the identification and protection of the underlying vital anatomical structures: vessels, nerves, or the maxillary sinus [1,2]. Insufficient bone in the regions to be treated with implants requires prior bone regeneration. The materials involved in bone augmentation can be classified as autogenous (grafts taken directly from the patient's tissues), allogenic (human bone material), xenogenic (derived from animals), or alloplastic (synthetic or natural provenance) [3]. Recently, an autogenous bone substitute extracted from the appropriately processed dentin of retained teeth has been successfully used to meet biological and physical criteria [4,5].

In the case of reduced alveolar bone, elevation of the full-thickness or partial-thickness flap results in loss of bone mass and increased osteoclast activity [6], which further aggravates the local anatomical conditions [7,8]. In extreme cases, it can lead to complications, such as injury to the inferior alveolar nerve or nasopalatine nerve and the perforation of the nasal cavity or the maxillary sinus, including accidental migration of a dental implant into the sinus [9,10].

Recently, surgical navigation techniques have been developed that provide safety, aesthetics, and comfort with a minimally invasive surgical method and are well accepted among both doctors and patients [11]. Navigation can be divided into static (using templates) and dynamic surgical navigation. The use of dynamic navigation techniques does not require the use of preprepared templates. Digital planning helps to optimise the position of the implant, taking into account the requirements for future prosthetic restoration. The accurate tracking of the position of each instrument in the surgical field by the navigation system allows for high precision in restricted anatomical conditions, shorter duration, and better outcomes regarding the procedure performed, along with less patient exposure to the procedure-related risks of infection, pain, and stress [12,13].

Researchers are attempting to objectively assess the body's response to a range of conditions, not only systemic, such as systemic lupus erythematosus (SLE), tuberculosis, or malignant processes [14,15], but also oral conditions, including periodontitis [16], caries [17,18], lichen planus [19], or peri-implantitis [20]. To this end, the levels of various cytokines, such as IL-1β, IL-2, IL-4, IL-5, IL-6, IL-7, IL-8, IL-10, IL-12, IFN-γ, TNF-α, and CRP, are monitored for diagnostic and prognostic purposes, and their fluctuations are reflected in the patient's clinical condition or to assess the severity of the disease [21,22].

Cytokine concentrations can be assessed in body fluids, tissues, and cells [23], and recently, human saliva has been more widely used [24]. In comparison to blood, saliva collection is a non-invasive procedure, does not involve nursing personnel, and does not evoke negative associations. Therefore, saliva sampling is especially suitable in cases where blood sampling is difficult, e.g., in very small children, the elderly, or anxious individuals [25,26]. Inflammatory mediators can affect leukocyte, osteoblast, and osteoclast activity and promote systemic and local tissue remodelling [27,28]. The frequently assessed biomarkers of inflammation are CRP and IL-6, and clinical use has been confirmed in studies [29,30].

Interleukin-6 (IL-6) is a pleiotropic cytokine involved in multiple inflammatory responses, with roles in immune regulation [31] and pathological conditions, including both acute and chronic inflammatory diseases [32]. IL-6 initiates and up-regulates inflammation, triggers the release of acute phase proteins, regulates the inflammatory response, attracts immune cells to sites of injury or infection, and stimulates coagulation [33]. IL-6 levels in saliva have different correlations with serum levels based on the conditions studied, e.g., Behçet's disease [34] or oral lichen planus treated with photo-biomodulation [35].

C-reactive protein (CRP) operates mostly in the innate immune defence, with increased values in reaction to infection, inflammation, tissue injury, necrosis, malignant tumours, and allergic reactions [36]. CRP has a clinical diagnosis benefit as a marker of systemic inflammation and as an independent risk factor for cardiovascular disease in both adults and paediatric patients [37,38].

The main purpose of this study was to compare values of IL-6, CRP, and VAS between two surgery techniques and the evaluation of the potential benefits of dynamic navigation (compared to the classical method) by assessing the salivary levels of soluble inflammatory mediators (CRP, IL-6) and VAS pain intensity.

2. Materials and Methods
2.1. Patients

Implant treatment was performed on 30 patients enrolled from July 2019 to December 2020 for the rehabilitation of extracted dentition. An extraoral and intraoral examination and a CBCT scan (Carestream Dental CS 8100 3d, Carestream Dental LLC, Atlanta, GA, USA) were conducted. Patients were eligible for the study according to the criteria outlined in Table 1. Out of a total of 87 patients, 30 participants (12 men and 18 women) were finally qualified.

Table 1. Patient eligibility criteria.

Inclusion Criteria	Exclusion Criteria
aged 18–65 years	critical systemic disease (ASA III-IV)
absence of systemic disease comorbidities	generalised immunodeficiency
adequate oral hygiene (API < 15%)	autoimmune disease
	clinically and radiologically diagnosed inflammatory conditions (active caries, gingivitis and periodontitis, mucosal diseases, e.g., leukoplakia, lichen planus)
	active nicotinism
	use of antibiotics in the past 2 weeks

All participants were informed about the purpose and methodology of this study and gave written informed consent. The approval of the Bioethics Committee of the Silesian Medical Chamber in Katowice was obtained (Resolution No. 24/2019 on 25 June 2019).

The patients were then randomly divided into two groups of 15 patients: a study group and a control group. In the study group, implants were carried out using Navident dynamic navigation (Navident, ClaroNav, Toronto, ON, Canada) which allows for surgery using a flapless technique—Figure 1.

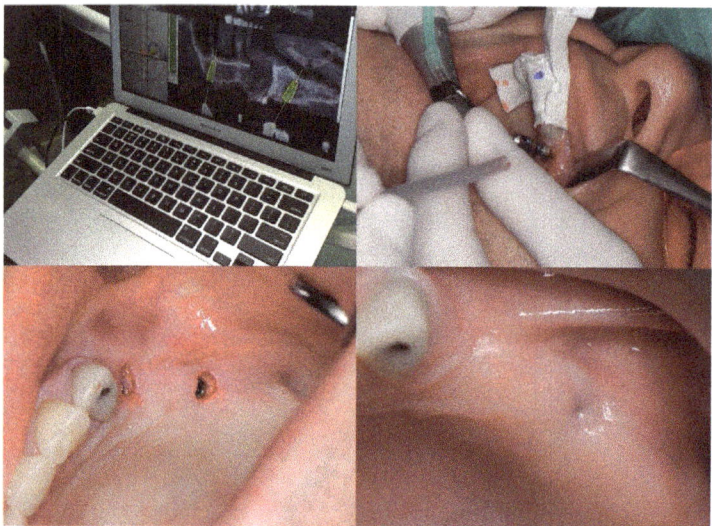

Figure 1. Dynamic navigation system in use with status immediately after surgery and clinical appearance after 7 days.

In the control group, implant treatment was carried out in a classic manner with the elevation of the mucoperiosteal flap—Figure 2. Due to the study methodology, surgery and follow-up visits were performed in the morning.

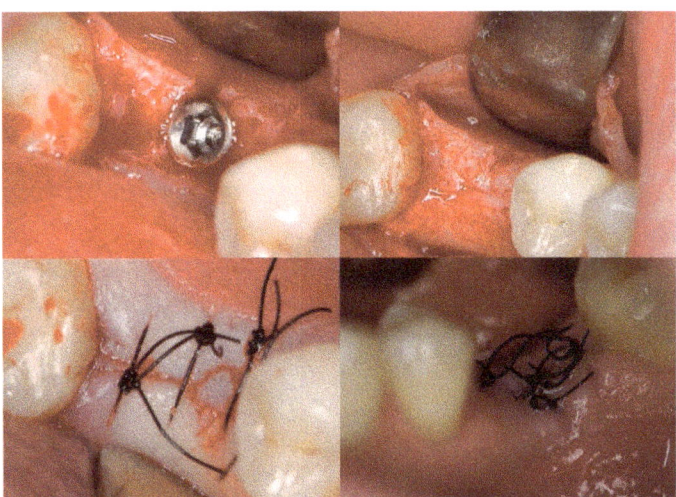

Figure 2. Implantation in the control group. Visible sutures immediately after the procedure and after 7 days. All patients were carefully examined immediately before surgery, on the first post-operative day, and on the seventh post-operative day and were asked to rate their pain on a 10-degree VAS (Visual Analogue Scale) [38].

2.2. Saliva Samples

The samples of unstimulated whole saliva were collected in the morning, after a minimum hunger period of two hours (between 9 and 11 a.m.), using the Salivette® system (Sarstedt, Nümbrecht, Germany). Briefly, the patient removed the swab from Salivette® and placed the swab in the mouth. Then, the patient chewed the swab for about 1 min to stimulate salivation. Next, the patient returned the swab with the absorbed saliva to the Salivette®. The obtained saliva samples were then centrifuged for 2 min at $1000\times g$, and the obtained supernatants were pipetted into Eppendorf tubes which were stored at $-80\,°C$ until the day of the CRP and IL-6 assay. Then, these saliva samples were completely thawed, vortexed, and centrifuged at $1500\times g$ for 15 min to remove mucins and other particulate matter which may interfere with antibody binding and affect the CRP or IL-6 test results.

2.3. Determination of Saliva CRP Concentration

The concentration of CRP in the saliva samples was determined by using the Salivary C-Reactive Protein ELISA Kit Generation II (Salimetrics, State College, PA, USA), which is an enzyme-linked immunoassay (ELISA) for the quantitative measurement of human CRP in oral fluid. This is an indirect sandwich ELISA kit wherein a "sandwich" is formed when the precoated captured anti-CRP antibody present on the plate binds CRP from the standard (Salimetrics' High and Low CRP Generation II Controls) and tested samples. After each incubation, the unbound components were washed away. Bound anti-CRP antibody enzyme conjugate was then added, and the levels of detected CRP were measured by the reaction of the horseradish peroxidase enzyme to the substrate tetramethylbenzidine. The effect of this reaction is a blue colour in the solutions in the plate wells. Next, a yellow colour was formed after stopping the reaction with an acidic solution, and then the optical density was measured at 450 nm using a microplate reader EonTM Microplate Spectrophotometer (BioTek, Winooski, VT, USA). The corresponding concentration of CRP in pg/mL was determined from the standard curve (nonlinear regression curve fit) using the average optical density values of the controls and saliva samples. The functional sensitivity of the Salivary C-Reactive Protein ELISA Kit Generation II is 19.44 pg/mL.

2.4. Determination of Saliva IL-6 Concentration

The concentration of IL-6 in the saliva samples was determined using the Salivary IL-6 ELISA Kit (Salimetrics, State College, PA, USA), which is a sandwich immunoassay for the quantitative measurement of salivary IL-6. This is a sandwich ELISA kit wherein the IL-6 standard (Salimetrics' High and Low IL-6 Controls) and tested samples bind to the antibody binding sites on a microtiter plate. After incubation, the unbound components were washed away. Next, biotin conjugated to goat antibodies and to human IL-6 was added and attached to the bound IL-6. After incubation, the unbound components were washed away, and streptavidin (conjugated to horseradish peroxidase) was added (and binds to the biotin conjugated and the goat antibodies), and the levels of detected IL-6 were measured by the reaction of the horseradish peroxidase enzyme to the substrate tetramethylbenzidine. The effect of this reaction is a blue colour in the solutions in the plate wells. Next, a yellow colour was formed after stopping the reaction with an acidic solution, and then the optical density was measured at 450 nm using a microplate reader (EonTM Microplate Spectrophotometer; BioTek, Winooski, VT, USA). The corresponding concentration of IL-6 in pg/mL was determined from a standard curve (four-parameter nonlinear regression curve fit) using the average optical density values of the controls and saliva samples. The functional sensitivity of the Salivary IL-6 ELISA Kit is 2.08 pg/mL.

2.5. Statistical Analysis

The results obtained were then collected, and statistical analyses were performed using the STATISTICA 10 program (StatSoft Polska, Kraków, Poland). For each analysis, the Shapiro–Wilk test was performed to check the type of distribution of measurable features. We checked whether the distribution of the variables was normal and if the variances were homogeneous. On the basis of those positive results, it was decided that parametric tests (including Student's *t*-test for independent groups in the case of, for example, the analysis of different parameters (CRP, Il-6, and VAS) would be performed to observe changes over time between the groups of patients treated with the standard procedure and the patients free-lobe treated. When the essential assumptions for the parametric tests were not met, nonparametric tests were used (including the Mann–Whitney test). Data are expressed as the mean and median values ± standard deviation (SD) and standard error (SE). The level of significance was $p < 0.05$. The results are presented in box graphs.

3. Results

Comparison of CRP concentration ratio at 1st day after surgery (Day 1) and before treatment (Day 0) obtained for study group treated by flapless method was 3.74 and control group treated with standard procedure was 2.5.

Comparison of CRP concentration ratio at 7th day after surgery (Day 7) and before treatment (Day 0) obtained for study group treated by flapless method was 1.2 and control group treated with standard procedure was 1.7.

Comparison of VAS scale ratio (Day 1/Day 0) at 1st day after surgery (Day 1) and before treatment (Day 0) obtained for study group treated by flapless method was 1.04 and control group treated with standard procedure was 1.5.

Comparison of VAS scale ratio (Day 7/Day 0) at 7th day after surgery (Day 7) and before treatment (Day 0) obtained for study group treated by flapless method was 0.51 and control group treated with standard procedure was 0.52.

The presented box graphs in Figures 3 and 4 show the differences between the CRP concentration ratio from day 1 after surgery and before treatment, as well as the CRP concentration ratio measured on day 7 after surgery and before treatment, obtained for the study group treated with the free-lobe method and the control group treated with the standard procedure, respectively.

Despite the fact that there were no significant differences between the mean values for the CRP concentration ratio on Day 1/Day 0 as well as on Day 7/Day 0 when comparing the study group treated with the flapless method and the control group treated with the standard procedure, there are some observable tendencies that may show completely different characters. First of all, the concentration of CRP decreases with time after surgery in both studied groups. However, the ratio coefficient calculated on day 1 after surgery seems to be higher for the study group and on day 7 after the tendency is opposed. This may suggest that the inflammatory state in the study group treated with the flapless method decreased faster over time than in the control group. Moreover, on day 7 after the procedure, the concentration drop is deeper for the study group. Such results are not statistically significant, so they may show some tendencies that can only be confirmed by using a larger group of patients.

The next analyses are presented as box graphs in Figures 5 and 6, which show the differences in the VAS scale ratios on day 1 after surgery and before treatment as well as the VAS scale ratio calculated on day 7 after surgery and before treatment, obtained for the study group treated with the flapless method and the control group treated with the standard procedure, respectively.

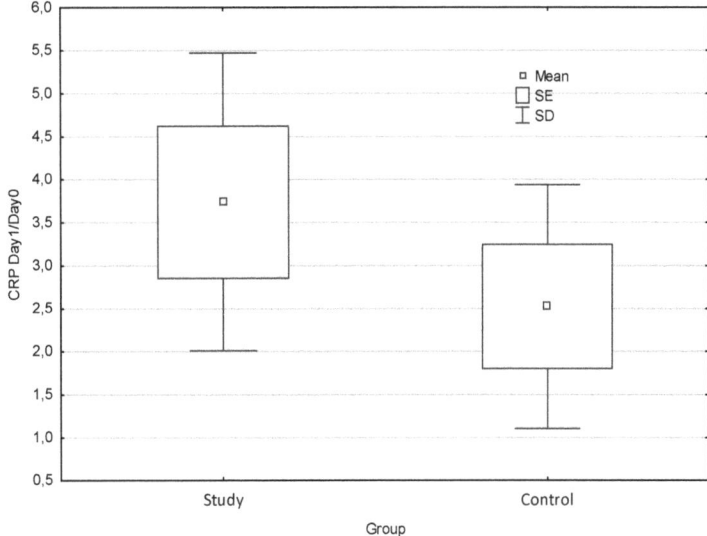

Figure 3. Comparison of CRP concentration ratio on day 1 after surgery (Day 1) and before treatment (Day 0), obtained for the study group treated with the flapless method and the control group treated with the standard procedure.

The obtained results show statistically significant ($p = 0.005$) differences between the VAS scale ratio (Day1/Day0) on day 1 after surgery and before treatment, obtained for the study group treated with the flapless method and the control group treated with the standard procedure; the significantly higher value was obtained for the control group (VAS = 1.5), and for the study group, it was nearly 0.5 lower. Such results prove that the flapless method leads to less pain reported by patients just after surgery than does the standard method. Further measurements showed that the pain felt and described by patients from both groups is similar and much lower than before the surgery.

Figure 7 presents a box graph that shows the differences between the saliva Il-6 concentration ratios on day 1 after surgery and before treatment as well as the ratio calculated on day 7 after surgery and before treatment, obtained for the study group treated with the flapless method and the control group treated with the standard procedure.

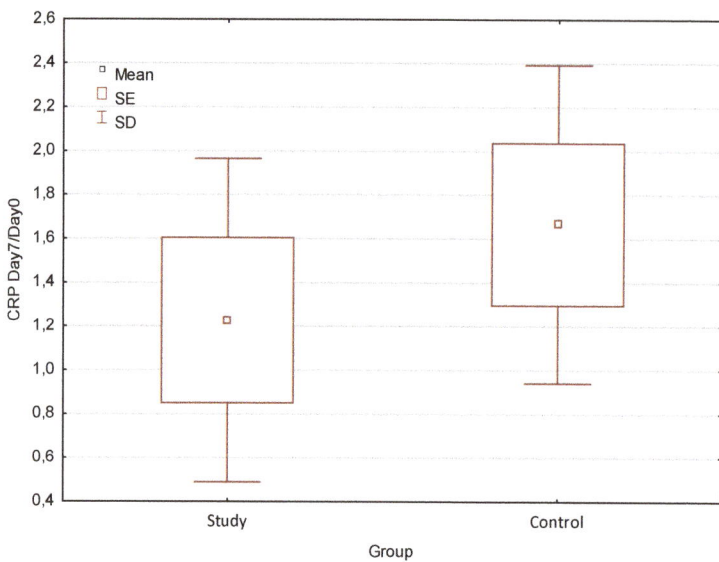

Figure 4. Comparison of CRP concentration ratio on day 7 after surgery (Day 7) and before treatment (Day 0), obtained for the study group treated with the flapless method and the control group treated with the standard procedure.

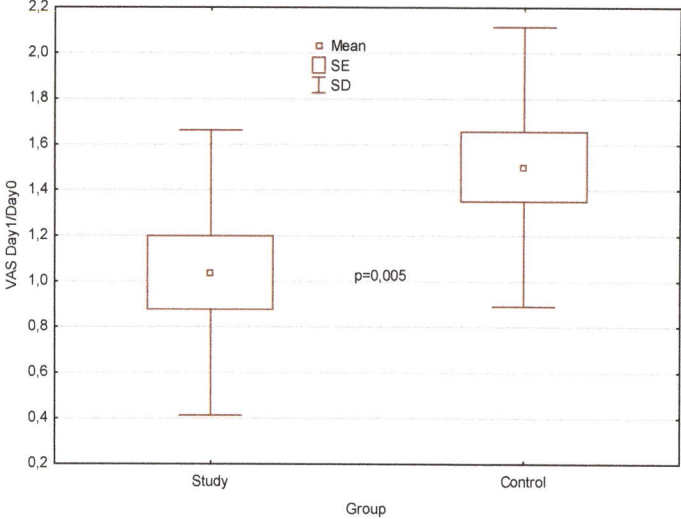

Figure 5. Comparison of VAS scale ratio (Day 1/Day 0) on day 1 after surgery (Day 1) and before treatment (Day 0), obtained for the study group treated with the flapless method and the control group treated with the standard procedure.

It should be noted that there were no significant differences between the studied groups. However, some tendencies can be seen, such as a significantly higher mean increase in the salivary Il-6 concentration in the control group on the first post-operative day. On the other hand, the Il-6 concentration ratio on day 7 after treatment seems to be similar and significantly lower in comparison to the ratios calculated after the first day for both groups.

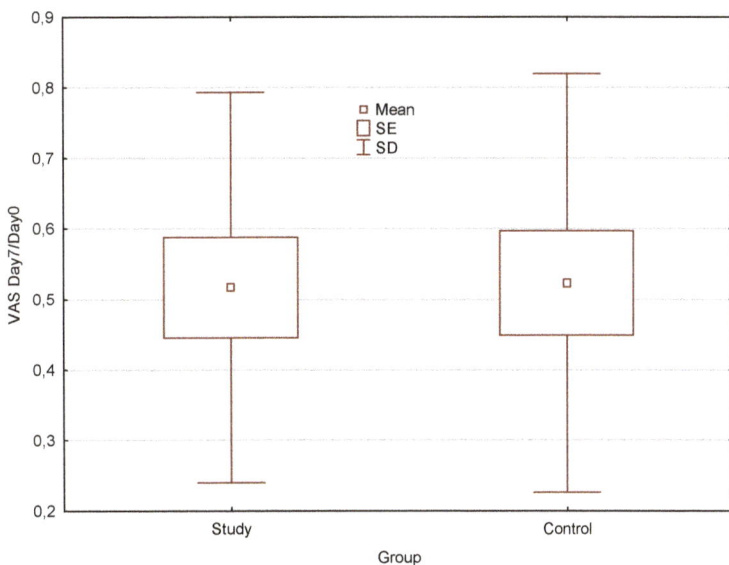

Figure 6. Comparison of VAS scale ratio (Day 7/Day 0) on day 7 after surgery (Day 7) and before treatment (Day 0), obtained for the study group treated with the flapless method and the control group treated with the standard procedure.

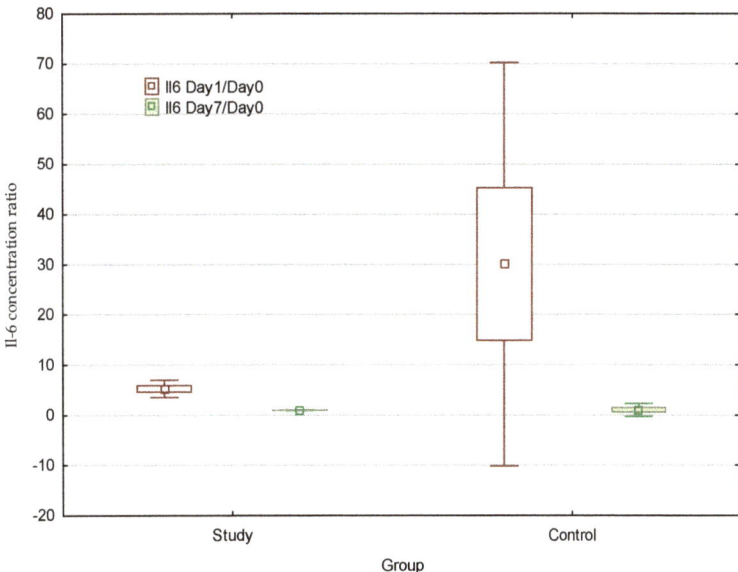

Figure 7. Box graph presenting the differences between saliva Il-6 concentration ratios on day 1 after surgery and before treatment (brown), as well as the ratios calculated on day 7 after surgery and before treatment (green), obtained for the study group treated with the flapless method and the control group treated with the standard procedure.

Generally, the saliva concentration with the pro-inflammatory factors considered (CRP, Il-6) and the VAS pain scale are lower after flapless surgery compared to the standard procedure. However, conclusions must be drawn cautiously due to the small size of the study groups and the observed trends. Only in some cases was a statistically significant

(p = 0.005) higher VAS scale ratio (Day1/Day0) confirmed on day 1 after surgery when compared to the pretreatment ratio obtained for the treated control group.

4. Discussion

Saliva is one of the most important body fluids. It performs a number of vital functions, including ensuring a humid environment in the mouth, participating in water regulation, pre-digestion, protecting oral cavity structures from damage, acting as an antimicrobial agent, remineralising enamel, and participating in the perception of taste or pronunciation. Its composition and properties determine systemic homeostasis, and fluctuations in certain parameters enable it to be useful as a diagnostic marker for a number of pathologies and as a screening and treatment tool for oral squamous cell carcinoma, for instance [39].

It is very important to be able to test inflammatory markers in a non-invasive way by testing a saliva sample. Until now, the most common way to test inflammatory biomarker levels has been from a blood serum sample, which involves venipuncture and trauma, which is an invasive procedure and involves qualified personnel, laboratory equipment, and significant financial resources. In contrast, saliva collection is non-invasive, stress-free, and painless and provides an effective alternative diagnostic method [40].

A range of scientific papers that have recently been published discusses the potential use of IL-6 and CRP in the monitoring and early diagnosis of oral diseases. A study by Dineshkumar et al. [41] evaluated IL-6 among a large group of 100 patients with potentially malignant lesions (PML) in the oral cavity, 100 diagnosed oral squamous cell carcinoma (OSCC) cases, and 100 controls. Among other things, it showed a twofold to threefold higher level of inflammatory markers in saliva than in serum in those patients with diagnosed OSCC when compared with PML and a group of healthy subjects, demonstrating 96% specificity and 99% sensitivity for IL-6 in saliva in distinguishing PML from OSCC.

A study by Fonseca et al. [19] assessed the levels of a variety of pro-inflammatory cytokines in 22 edentulous patients who presented with clinical mucositis or peri-implantitis. Assessing a broad panel of markers, including, as in our study, IL-6, showed that the total IL-6 levels tended to be higher in patients with peri-implantitis in relation to a comparison group that only manifested mucositis around the implants. This demonstrated that the level of severity of the inflammatory reaction developing around the implant is reflected in IL-6 levels.

A pilot study by Draft et al. [42] on seven patients with implants, compared to three patients in the control group, assessed the levels of total antioxidant status (TAS), amounts of IL-6, IL-8, and TNF-α (tumour necrosis factor), and salivary lactate dehydrogenase (LDH) levels in correlation with bone loss around the implant over one year. Two patients in the study group had the lowest TAS levels, the highest IL-6 and IL-8 levels, and by far the highest marginal bone loss (1.0 and 0.85 mm at one year in relation to results in the range of 0.02–0.08 mm in the other implant patients). Admittedly, no strong assumptions can be drawn on such a small group; however, the authors did give consideration to screening implant patients using saliva biomarkers. Those with low TAS values or elevated levels of pro-inflammatory cytokines should undergo more frequent follow-up visits for close monitoring and the prevention of more severe complications.

A study by Cennamo et al. [43] published in May of 2023 highlights the role of point-of-care tests for the detection of salivary levels of cytokines (including IL-6) as an important tool for early diagnosis and timely treatment of inflammatory-based diseases such as periodontitis. The SPR-POF biosensor solution was presented, which allows for detecting IL-6 levels from 40 pM to 2 nM, while the GNG biosensor was designed to detect IL-6 range from 680 aM to 25 fM. The devices have applications in the diagnosis of plasma and salivary concentrations, which appears to be crucial for monitoring an individual response to a specific therapy for a particular disease.

Systemic C-reactive protein (CRP) is a sensitive marker of systemic inflammation and an independent risk factor for CVD (cardiovascular disease) [36,37].

A pilot study by Azar and Richard [43] conducted on 45 young Canadians (mean age: 18.89 years, SD = 2.62) determined the CRP levels from a saliva sample in active smokers, passive smokers, and nonsmokers. The CRP levels were highest in active smokers, lower in passive smokers, and lowest in nonsmokers. Passive smokers had significantly higher CRP levels than nonsmokers. Interestingly, the difference in CRP levels in the passive and active smokers did not reach significance. In addition, the investigators stated that salivary CRP levels appear to have a similar relationship with tobacco smoke exposure (TSE) as it is a widely used serum biomarker counterpart [44].

A cohort study [19] on 30 patients with oral lichen planus and 30 healthy patients showed that the levels of TNF-α, G-GSF, IL-1α, IL-1β, and IL-8 were statistically significantly higher in OLP patients than in the healthy group. Spearman's rank correlation analysis showed that levels of TNF-α, GM-CSF, MIP-1α, MIP-1β, IL-1β, and IL-6 in saliva were positively correlated with the severity of the OLP lesion, meaning they have great potential as biomarkers for diagnosing and predicting the prognosis of OLP.

In implant manufacturing, several concepts have been developed for coating the implant surface and local delivery of agents regarding antimicrobial, bioactive, or therapeutic effects. For example, a coating of bioactive materials (calcium phosphates and hydroxyapatite (HA)) increases the bioactivity of the surface, improving osteointegration. Bisphosphonate coatings are designed to stimulate osteoblasts and inhibit osteoclast activity and bone resorption, and implants coated with gentamicin and polylactic acid have antimicrobial effects [45].

However, bone loss with implants progresses independently of the coatings applied to the implant surface. In the case of reduced alveolar bone, the dehiscence of the full as well as partial-thickness flap consequently leads to a loss of bone mass and increased osteoclast activity [6], which further aggravates the local anatomical conditions [7,8]. Hence, the innovative approach is complimentary implantation, which reduces the invasiveness of the procedure, improves and accelerates the healing process, and reduces the pain sensation of patients, as confirmed in our study.

The complementary technique may also lead to less bone loss compared to the traditional technique, as confirmed by a meta-analysis [46].

According to the analysis by Carosi et al. [47], computer-assisted flapless implant placement by means of mucosa-supported templates in complete arch restorations can be considered a reliable and predictable treatment choice despite the potential effects that the flapless approach can bring to the overall treatment.

Furthermore, on the basis of a comparative analysis of the planning and execution of freehand implant treatment using navigation, it has been shown that dynamic navigation may improve the quality and safety of surgical procedures and reduce the risk of complications compared to freehand implant placement [48].

Dynamic surgical navigation is also used during zygomatic implant placement procedures for the reconstruction of edentulous maxilla among patients whose osseous conditions do not allow for the placing of implants into the alveolar bone of the maxilla. A study by Bhalerao et al. confirmed that free zygomatic implant placement under dynamic navigation guidance represents a technique with minimal surgical complications [49].

Research confirms that surgery with the flapless technique provides a lower temperature for the operated area and bone bed, which contributes to improved healing and reduced likelihood of perioperative complications; this is confirmed by thermographic studies in patients operated on with flapless and classical techniques [50,51].

Equally important is the pre-operative and post-operative care of the surgical patient. Clinical studies have shown satisfactory efficacy in eliminating pathological oral flora with therapeutic preparations of natural origin, such as tea tree oil and ethanolic propolis extract [52,53], and preparation for surgery by rinsing with antiseptics before surgery, i.e., chlorhexidine, may reduce the risk of post-operative complications [54,55].

Our clinical study reveals an innovative approach to the issue of the biochemical and clinical assessment of healing in implant patients. The currently available literature has not previously explored a similar topic, indicating that there is potential space for further in-depth study of this issue. It should also be taken into account that the analysis of saliva samples and their testing requires a certain research and analytical background and an appropriate selection of patients for comparative methods. In the future, as the availability of diagnostic methods increases and their cost decreases, monitoring the clinical status of patients with objective results will allow for individual modifications to the therapy conducted.

In addition, complex surgical treatment requires the monitoring of many clinical parameters, and patient saliva may be only one of them. This also implies the limitations of the treatment method presented in this paper, which may include the patient's general health, old age, or significant general obstructions that would disqualify the patient from surgical treatment.

In these cases, alternatives for the reconstruction of the lost dentition with implants may be proposed. In this case, "classic" prosthetic solutions such as bridges or removable denture or telescopic prosthetic devices supported by the current residual dentition may be used.

5. Conclusions

The results of this study confirm the advantages of dynamic navigation in implant treatment, supplementing previous knowledge in this aspect with observations of changes in CRP and IL-6 levels and pain intensity in the first week after surgery.

Objectively, pain is lower in the free methods than in the conventional methods and a lower level of inflammation was observed on the basis of lower biomarker parameters in the study group.

Dynamic navigation may reduce patient discomfort and facilitate faster recovery, as could be indicated by lower levels of pro-inflammatory cytokines compared to the control group.

Author Contributions: Conceptualization, K.W., T.M. and A.M.; methodology, K.W., T.M. and A.M.; software, K.W. and A.S.; validation, K.W. and T.M.; formal analysis K.W. and D.B.; investigation, K.W., A.M. and A.N.-W.; resources, K.W., T.M., A.M. and J.Ś.-W.; data curation, K.W., A.M. and J.Ś.-W.; writing—original draft preparation, K.W. and A.N.-W.; writing—review and editing, K.W., T.M. and D.B.; visualization, A.S.; supervision, K.W., T.M. and A.M.; project administration, K.W. and T.M.; funding acquisition, K.W. and T.M. All authors have read and agreed to the published version of the manuscript.

Funding: This research was funded by the Medical University of Silesia in Katowice with research numbers PCN-2-032/N/0/K and PCN-1-066/N/0/O.

Institutional Review Board Statement: This study was conducted according to the guidelines of the Declaration of Helsinki and approved by the Bioethics Committees of the Silesian Medical Chamber in Katowice (Resolution no. 24/2019, as of 25 June 2019).

Informed Consent Statement: Informed consent was obtained from all subjects involved in this study.

Data Availability Statement: The data presented in this study are available from the corresponding authors.

Conflicts of Interest: The authors declare no conflict of interest.

References

1. Kageyama, I.; Maeda, S.; Takezawa, K. Importance of anatomy in dental implant surgery. *J. Oral Biosci.* **2021**, *63*, 142–152. [CrossRef]
2. Greenstein, G.; Cavallaro, J.; Tarnow, D. Practical Application of Anatomy for the Dental Implant Surgeon. *J. Periodontol.* **2008**, *79*, 1833–1846. [CrossRef] [PubMed]
3. Sheikh, Z.; Sima, C.; Glogauer, M. Bone Replacement Materials and Techniques Used for Achieving Vertical Alveolar Bone Augmentation. *Materials* **2015**, *8*, 2953–2993. [CrossRef]
4. Gual-Vaques, P.; Polis-Yanes, C.; Estrugo-Devesa, A.; Ayuso-Montero, R.; Mari-Roig, A.; Lopez-Lopez, J. Autogenous teeth used for bone grafting: A systematic review. *Med. Oral. Patol. Oral. Cir. Bucal.* **2018**, *23*, e112–e119. [CrossRef] [PubMed]

5. Kubaszek, B.; Morawiec, T.; Mertas, A.; Wachol, K.; Nowak-Wachol, A.; Śmieszek-Wilczewska, J.; Łopaciński, M.; Cholewka, A. Radiological and Microbiological Evaluation of the Efficacy of Alveolar Bone Repair Using Autogenous Dentin Matrix—Preliminary Study. *Coatings* **2022**, *12*, 909. [CrossRef]
6. Fickl, S.; Kebschull, M.; Schupbach, P.; Zuhr, O.; Schlagenhauf, U.; Hürzeler, M.B. Bone loss after full-thickness and partial-thickness flap elevation. *J. Clin. Periodontol.* **2011**, *38*, 157–162. [CrossRef]
7. Araujo, M.G.; Lindhe, J. Dimensional ridge alterations following tooth extraction. An experimental study in the dog. *J. Clin. Periodontol.* **2005**, *32*, 212–218. [CrossRef]
8. Araújo, M.G.; Lindhe, J. Ridge alterations following tooth extraction with and without flap elevation: An experimental study in the dog. *Clin. Oral Implant. Res.* **2009**, *20*, 545–549. [CrossRef]
9. Volberg, R.; Mordanov, O. Canalis Sinuosus Damage after Immediate Dental Implant Placement in the Esthetic Zone. *Case Rep. Dent.* **2019**, *2019*, 3462794. [CrossRef]
10. An, J.-H.; Park, S.-H.; Han, J.J.; Jung, S.; Kook, M.-S.; Park, H.-J.; Oh, H.-K. Treatment of dental implant displacement into the maxillary sinus. *Maxillofac. Plast. Reconstr. Surg.* **2017**, *39*, 35. [CrossRef]
11. Pellegrino, G.; Bellini, P.; Cavallini, P.F.; Ferri, A.; Zacchino, A.; Taraschi, V.; Marchetti, C.; Consolo, U. Dynamic Navigation in Dental Implantology: The Influence of Surgical Experience on Implant Placement Accuracy and Operating Time. An in Vitro Study. *Int. J. Environ. Res. Public Health* **2020**, *17*, 2153. [CrossRef] [PubMed]
12. Vercruyssen, M.; Laleman, I.; Jacobs, R.; Quirynen, M. Computer-supported implant planning and guided surgery: A narrative review. *Clin. Oral Implant. Res.* **2015**, *26* (Suppl. S11), 69–76. [CrossRef] [PubMed]
13. Bover-Ramos, F.; Viña-Almunia, J.; Cervera-Ballester, J.; Peñarrocha-Diago, M.; García-Mira, B. Accuracy of Implant Placement with Computer-Guided Surgery: A Systematic Review and Meta-Analysis Comparing Cadaver, Clinical, and In Vitro Studies. *Int. J. Oral Maxillofac. Implant.* **2018**, *33*, 101–115. [CrossRef] [PubMed]
14. Zian, Z.; Bouhoudan, A.; Mourabit, N.; Azizi, G.; Mechita, M.B. Salivary Cytokines as Potential Diagnostic Biomarkers for Systemic Lupus Erythematosus Disease. *Mediat. Inflamm.* **2021**, *2021*, 8847557. [CrossRef]
15. Diesch, T.; Filippi, C.; Fritschi, N.; Filippi, A.; Ritz, N. Cytokines in saliva as biomarkers of oral and systemic oncological or infectious diseases: A systematic review. *Cytokine* **2021**, *143*, 155506. [CrossRef]
16. Teles, R.P.; Likhari, V.; Socransky, S.S.; Haffajee, A.D. Salivary cytokine levels in subjects with chronic periodontitis and in periodontally healthy individuals: A cross-sectional study. *J. Periodontal Res.* **2009**, *44*, 411–417. [CrossRef]
17. Gornowicz, A.; Bielawska, A.; Bielawski, K.; Grabowska, S.Z.; Wójcicka, A.; Zalewska, M.; Maciorkowska, E. Pro-inflammatory cytokines in saliva of adolescents with dental caries disease. *Ann. Agric. Environ. Med.* **2012**, *19*, 711–716.
18. Ribeiro, C.C.C.; Pachêco, C.d.J.B.; Costa, E.L.; Ladeira, L.L.C.; Costa, J.F.; da Silva, R.A.; Carmo, C.D.S. Proinflammatory cytokines in early childhood caries: Salivary analysis in the mother/children pair. *Cytokine* **2018**, *107*, 113–117. [CrossRef]
19. Zhu, Z.-D.; Ren, X.-M.; Zhou, M.-M.; Chen, Q.-M.; Hua, H.; Li, C.-L. Salivary cytokine profile in patients with oral lichen planus. *J. Dent. Sci.* **2022**, *17*, 100–105. [CrossRef]
20. Fonseca, F.J.P.O.; Junior, M.M.; Lourenço, E.J.V.; Teles, D.d.M.; Figueredo, C.M. Cytokines expression in saliva and peri-implant crevicular fluid of patients with peri-implant disease. *Clin. Oral Implant. Res.* **2014**, *25*, e68–e72. [CrossRef]
21. Vohra, F.; Alkhudhairy, F.; Al-Kheraif, A.A.; Akram, Z.; Javed, F. Peri-implant parameters and C-reactive protein levels among patients with different obesity levels. *Clin. Implant. Dent. Relat. Res.* **2018**, *20*, 130–136. [CrossRef] [PubMed]
22. Melguizo-Rodríguez, L.; Costela-Ruiz, V.J.; Manzano-Moreno, F.J.; Ruiz, C.; Illescas-Montes, R. Salivary Biomarkers and Their Application in the Diagnosis and Monitoring of the Most Common Oral Pathologies. *Int. J. Mol. Sci.* **2020**, *21*, 5173. [CrossRef] [PubMed]
23. Decker, M.-L.; Gotta, V.; Wellmann, S.; Ritz, N. Cytokine profiling in healthy children shows association of age with cytokine concentrations. *Sci. Rep.* **2017**, *7*, 17842. [CrossRef] [PubMed]
24. Chauhan, A.; Yadav, S.S.; Dwivedi, P.; Lal, N.; Usman, K.; Khattri, S. Correlation of Serum and Salivary Cytokines Level with Clinical Parameters in Metabolic Syndrome With Periodontitis. *J. Clin. Lab. Anal.* **2016**, *30*, 649–655. [CrossRef] [PubMed]
25. Szabo, Y.Z.; Slavish, D.C. Measuring salivary markers of inflammation in health research: A review of methodological considerations and best practices. *Psychoneuroendocrinology* **2021**, *124*, 105069. [CrossRef]
26. Cazalis, J.; Tanabe, S.; Gagnon, G.; Sorsa, T.; Grenier, D. Tetracyclines and chemically modified tetracycline-3 (CMT-3) modulate cytokine secretion by lipopolysaccharide-stimulated whole blood. *Inflammation* **2009**, *32*, 130–137. [CrossRef]
27. Sorsa, T.; Tjäderhane, L.; Konttinen, Y.T.; Lauhio, A.; Salo, T.; Lee, H.M.; Golub, L.M.; Brown, D.L.; Mäntylä, P. Matrix metalloproteinases: Contribution to pathogenesis, diagnosis and treatment of periodontal inflammation. *Ann. Med.* **2006**, *38*, 306–321. [CrossRef]
28. Shahidi, M.; Jafari, S.; Barati, M.; Mahdipour, M.; Gholami, M.S. Predictive value of salivary microRNA-320a, vascular en-dothelial growth factor receptor 2, CRP and IL-6 in Oral lichen planus progression. *Inflammopharmacology* **2017**, *25*, 577–583. [CrossRef]
29. Shiva, A.; Arab, S.; Mousavi, S.J.; Zamanian, A.; Maboudi, A. Serum and Salivary Level of Nitric Oxide (NOx) and CRP in Oral Lichen Planus (OLP) Patients. *J. Dent.* **2020**, *21*, 6–11.
30. Rose-John, S. Interleukin-6 Family Cytokines. *Cold Spring Harb. Perspect. Biol.* **2017**, *10*, a028415. [CrossRef]
31. Tanaka, T.; Narazaki, M.; Kishimoto, T. IL-6 in Inflammation, Immunity, and Disease. *Cold Spring Harb. Perspect. Biol.* **2014**, *6*, a016295. [CrossRef] [PubMed]

32. Vilotić, A.; Nacka-Aleksić, M.; Pirković, A.; Bojić-Trbojević, Z.; Dekanski, D.; Krivokuća, M.J. IL-6 and IL-8: An Overview of Their Roles in Healthy and Pathological Pregnancies. *Int. J. Mol. Sci.* **2022**, *23*, 14574. [CrossRef] [PubMed]
33. Novak, T.; Hamedi, M.; Bergmeier, L.A.; Fortune, F.; Hagi-Pavli, E. Saliva and Serum Cytokine Profiles During Oral Ulceration in Behçet's Disease. *Front. Immunol.* **2021**, *12*, 724900. [CrossRef] [PubMed]
34. Abboud, C.S.; Brandão, E.H.d.S.; Cunha, K.R.L.; Brito, K.d.S.; Gallo, C.d.B.; Molon, A.C.; Horliana, A.C.R.T.; Franco, A.S.L.; Thongprasom, K.; Rodrigues, M.F.S.D. Serum and salivary cytokines in patients with oral lichen planus treated with Photobiomodulation. *Oral Dis.* **2021**, *29*, 1250–1258. [CrossRef]
35. Markanday, A. Acute Phase Reactants in Infections: Evidence-Based Review and a Guide for Clinicians. *Open Forum Infect. Dis.* **2015**, *2*, ofv098. [CrossRef]
36. Broyles, S.T.; Staiano, A.E.; Drazba, K.T.; Gupta, A.K.; Sothern, M.; Katzmarzyk, P.T. Elevated C-Reactive Protein in Children from Risky Neighborhoods: Evidence for a Stress Pathway Linking Neighborhoods and Inflammation in Children. *PLoS ONE* **2012**, *7*, e45419. [CrossRef]
37. Kuppa, A.; Tripathi, H.; Al-Darraji, A.; Tarhuni, W.M.; Abdel-Latif, A. C-Reactive Protein Levels and Risk of Cardiovascular Diseases: A Two-Sample Bidirectional Mendelian Randomization Study. *Int. J. Mol. Sci.* **2023**, *24*, 9129. [CrossRef]
38. Klimek, L.; Bergmann, K.-C.; Biedermann, T.; Bousquet, J.; Hellings, P.; Jung, K.; Merk, H.; Olze, H.; Schlenter, W.; Stock, P.; et al. Visual analogue scales (VAS): Measuring instruments for the documentation of symptoms and therapy monitoring in cases of allergic rhinitis in everyday health care: Position Paper of the German Society of Allergology (AeDA) and the German Society of Allergy and Clinical Immunology (DGAKI), ENT Section, in collaboration with the working group on Clinical Immunology, Allergology and Environmental Medicine of the German Society of Otorhinolaryngology, Head and Neck Surgery (DGHNOKHC). *Allergo J. Int.* **2017**, *26*, 16–24. [CrossRef]
39. Sahibzada, H.A.; Khurshid, Z.; Khan, R.S.; Naseem, M.; Siddique, K.M.; Mali, M.; Zafar, M.S. Salivary IL-8, IL-6 and TNF-α as Potential Diagnostic Biomarkers for Oral Cancer. *Diagnostics* **2017**, *7*, 21. [CrossRef]
40. Ouellet-Morin, I.; Danese, A.; Williams, B.; Arseneault, L. Validation of a high-sensitivity assay for C-reactive protein in human saliva. *Brain, Behav. Immun.* **2011**, *25*, 640–646. [CrossRef]
41. Dineshkumar, T.; Ashwini, B.K.; Rameshkumar, A.; Rajashree, P.; Ramya, R.; Rajkumar, K. Salivary and Serum Interleukin-6 Levels in Oral Premalignant Disorders and Squamous Cell Carcinoma: Diagnostic Value and Clinicopathologic Correlations. *Asian Pac. J. Cancer Prev.* **2016**, *17*, 4899–4906. [CrossRef]
42. Azar, R.; Richard, A. Elevated salivary C-reactive protein levels are associated with active and passive smoking in healthy youth: A pilot study. *J. Inflamm.* **2011**, *8*, 37. [CrossRef] [PubMed]
43. Cennamo, N.; Piccirillo, A.; Bencivenga, D.; Arcadio, F.; Annunziata, M.; Della Ragione, F.; Guida, L.; Zeni, L.; Borriello, A. Towards a point-of-care test to cover atto-femto and pico-nano molar concentration ranges in interleukin 6 detection exploiting PMMA-based plasmonic biosensor chips. *Talanta* **2023**, *256*, 124284. [CrossRef] [PubMed]
44. O'Loughlin, J.; Lambert, M.; Karp, I.; McGrath, J.; Gray-Donald, K.; Barnett, T.A.; Delvin, E.E.; Levy, E.; Paradis, G. Association between cigarette smoking and C-reactive protein in a representative, population-based sample of adolescents. *Nicotine Tob. Res.* **2008**, *10*, 525–532. [CrossRef] [PubMed]
45. Zafar, M.S.; Fareed, M.A.; Riaz, S.; Latif, M.; Habib, S.R.; Khurshid, Z. Customized Therapeutic Surface Coatings for Dental Implants. *Coatings* **2020**, *10*, 568. [CrossRef]
46. Lahoti, K.; Dandekar, S.; Gade, J.; Agrawal, M. Comparative evaluation of crestal bone level by flapless and flap techniques for implant placement: Systematic review and meta-analysis. *J. Indian Prosthodont. Soc.* **2021**, *21*, 328–338. [CrossRef]
47. Carosi, P.; Lorenzi, C.; Lio, F.; Cardelli, P.; Pinto, A.; Laureti, A.; Pozzi, A. Accuracy of Computer-Assisted Flapless Implant Placement by Means of Mucosa-Supported Templates in Complete-Arch Restorations: A Systematic Review. *Materials* **2022**, *15*, 1462. [CrossRef]
48. Wachol, K.; Morawiec, T.; Nowak-Wachol, A.; Kubaszek, B.; Kasprzyk-Kucewicz, T.; Baldi, D.; Machorowska-Pieniążek, A.; Skucha-Nowak, M.; Cholewka, A. Comparative Analysis of Implant Prosthesis Treatment Planning and Execution Following Bone Repair Procedures Using Dynamic Surgical Navigation in Augmented Areas. *Coatings* **2022**, *12*, 1099. [CrossRef]
49. Bhalerao, A.; Marimuthu, M.; Wahab, A.; Ayoub, A. Flapless placement of zygomatic implants using dynamic navigation: An innovative technical note. *Br. J. Oral Maxillofac. Surg.* **2022**, *61*, 136–140. [CrossRef]
50. Kasprzyk-Kucewicz, T.; Cholewka, A.; Bałamut, K.; Kownacki, P.; Kaszuba, N.; Kaszuba, M.; Stanek, A.; Sieroń, K.; Stransky, J.; Pasz, A.; et al. The applications of infrared thermography in surgical removal of retained teeth effects assessment. *J. Therm. Anal. Calorim.* **2020**, *144*, 139–144. [CrossRef]
51. Kaszuba, N.; Kasprzyk-Kucewicz, T.; Szurko, A.; Wziatek-Kuczmik, D.; Stanek, A.; Morawiec, T.; Cholewka, A. How to use thermal imaging in selected surgical dental procedures? *Thermol. Int.* **2021**, *31*, 172–181.
52. Morawiec, T.; Dziedzic, A.; Niedzielska, I.; Mertas, A.; Tanasiewicz, M.; Skaba, D.; Kasperski, J.; Machorowska-Pieniążek, A.; Kucharzewski, M.; Szaniawska, K.; et al. The Biological Activity of Propolis-Containing Toothpaste on Oral Health Environment in Patients Who Underwent Implant-Supported Prosthodontic Rehabilitation. *Evidence-Based Complement. Altern. Med.* **2013**, *2013*, 1–12. [CrossRef] [PubMed]
53. Wiatrak, K.; Morawiec, T.; Rój, R.; Kownacki, P.; Nitecka-Buchta, A.; Niedzielski, D.; Wychowański, P.; Machorowska-Pieniążek, A.; Cholewka, A.; Baldi, D.; et al. Evaluation of Effectiveness of a Toothpaste Containing Tea Tree Oil and Ethanolic Extract of

Propolis on the Improvement of Oral Health in Patients Using Removable Partial Dentures. *Molecules* **2021**, *26*, 4071. [CrossRef] [PubMed]
54. Hassan, S.; Dhadse, P.; Bajaj, P.; Sethiya, K.; Subhadarsanee, C. Pre-procedural Antimicrobial Mouth Rinse: A Concise Review. *Cureus* **2022**, *14*, e30629. [CrossRef]
55. Pałka, Ł.; Nowakowska-Toporowska, A.; Dalewski, B. Is Chlorhexidine in Dentistry an Ally or a Foe? A Narrative Review. *Healthcare* **2022**, *10*, 764. [CrossRef]

Disclaimer/Publisher's Note: The statements, opinions and data contained in all publications are solely those of the individual author(s) and contributor(s) and not of MDPI and/or the editor(s). MDPI and/or the editor(s) disclaim responsibility for any injury to people or property resulting from any ideas, methods, instructions or products referred to in the content.

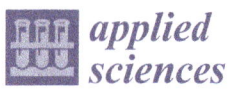

Article

Reliability and Agreement of Three Devices for Measuring Implant Stability Quotient in the Animal Ex Vivo Model

Monica Blazquez-Hinarejos [1], Constanza Saka-Herrán [1], Victor Diez-Alonso [1], Raul Ayuso-Montero [2,3,*], Eugenio Velasco-Ortega [4] and Jose Lopez-Lopez [3,5]

[1] Faculty of Medicine and Health Sciences (Dentistry), University of Barcelona, 08007 Barcelona, Spain; mblazquezhinarejos@gmail.com (M.B.-H.); constanzasakah@gmail.com (C.S.-H.); victor.diez.a@gmail.com (V.D.-A.)
[2] Department of Odontostomatology, Faculty of Medicine and Health Sciences (Dentistry), University of Barcelona, 08007 Barcelona, Spain
[3] Oral Health and Masticatory System Group, Bellvitge Biomedical Research Institute, IDIBELL, University of Barcelona, 08007 Barcelona, Spain; 18575jll@gmail.com
[4] Department of Stomatology, Faculty of Dentistry, University of Seville, 41009 Seville, Spain; evelasco@us.es
[5] Department of Odontostomatology, Faculty of Medicine and Health Sciences (Dentistry), Barcelona University Dental Hospital, University of Barcelona, 08007 Barcelona, Spain
* Correspondence: raulayuso@ub.edu

Abstract: Resonance frequency analysis (RFA) is the most extended method for measuring implant stability. The implant stability quotient (ISQ) is the measure obtained by different RFA devices; however, inter- and intra-rater reliability and agreement of these instruments remain unknown. Thirty implants were placed in three different pig mandibles. ISQ was measured parallel and perpendicular (lingual) to the peg axis with Osstell® Beacon, Penguin® and MegaISQ® by two different investigators and furthermore, one performed a test-retest. Intraclass correlation coefficient was calculated to assess the intra- and inter-rater reliability. Pearson correlation coefficient was used to assess the agreement. Intraclass correlation coefficients ranged from 0.20 to 0.65 for the Osstell® Beacon; 0.57 to 0.86 for the Penguin®; and −0.01 to 0.60 for the MegaISQ®. The highest ISQ values were obtained using Penguin® (66.3) in a parallel measurement; the lowest, using the MegaISQ® (60.1) in a parallel measurement. The highest correlation values with the other devices were obtained by MegaISQ® in a parallel measurement. Osstell® Beacon and MegaISQ® showed lower reliability than Penguin®. Osstell® had good agreement for measuring ISQ both in parallel and perpendicular, and MegaISQ® had the best agreement for measuring ISQ in parallel.

Keywords: resonance frequency analysis; implant stability quotient; reliability; agreement

Citation: Blazquez-Hinarejos, M.; Saka-Herrán, C.; Diez-Alonso, V.; Ayuso-Montero, R.; Velasco-Ortega, E.; Lopez-Lopez, J. Reliability and Agreement of Three Devices for Measuring Implant Stability Quotient in the Animal Ex Vivo Model. *Appl. Sci.* **2021**, *11*, 3453. https://doi.org/10.3390/app11083453

Academic Editors: Ricardo Castro Alves, José João Mendes and Ana Cristina Mano Azul

Received: 15 March 2021
Accepted: 9 April 2021
Published: 12 April 2021

Publisher's Note: MDPI stays neutral with regard to jurisdictional claims in published maps and institutional affiliations.

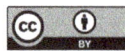

Copyright: © 2021 by the authors. Licensee MDPI, Basel, Switzerland. This article is an open access article distributed under the terms and conditions of the Creative Commons Attribution (CC BY) license (https://creativecommons.org/licenses/by/4.0/).

1. Introduction

Implant stability is critical in implant therapy and varies during the osseointegration process, reflecting bone/implant interface changes [1,2]. Low levels of implant micromotion are necessary to avoid implant failure and to achieve successful osseointegration [3–5].

Several existing methods have addressed measuring implant stability, including theoretical [6] and experimental modal analysis [7]. Among these, Periotest, insertion torque value (ITV), and implant stability quotient (ISQ) using resonance frequency analysis [8] are the ones widely used clinically. Periotest is a damping method that requires to strike the implant abutment [9], ITV measures the newton centimeters used to screw the implant into the bone [5], and ISQ sensors register the response of the electromagnetic stimulation of an abutment fixed to the implant called transducer peg, measuring the implant stability [10]. Periotest and ISQ are considered modal analysis methods based on the displacement signal secondary to an external impulse force [7]. Successfully integrated implants involve low implant micromotion levels, which usually correspond to low Periotest values and high ITV and ISQ values. These ITV and ISQ values are inversely correlated with low implant micromotion. However, the relationship between ITV and implant micromotion becomes exponential for higher ITV values [5]. Besides, ITV only measures implant stability at the moment of the insertion [8]. For these reasons, ISQ is usually the preferred method to measure implant stability.

Devices used to measure ISQ return a quotient value ranged from 0 to 100 corresponding to minimum and maximum vibration, respectively [11]. According to existing literature, a minimum ISQ value of 57 corresponds to a maximum implant micromotion of 150 µm. Clinically, this micromotion represents implant stability and it is required to maintain osseointegration [2,5].

There are several studies analyzing the reliability of existing devices for measuring the ISQ. These analyses have focused on two devices: Osstell® (W&H, Göteborg, Sweden) and Penguin® (Integration Diagnostics Sweden AB, Göteborg, Sweden) [12–14]. For instance, Buyukguclu et al. [12] reported better reliability for Osstell®, while Romanos et al. [13] reported that both devices were sensitive and reliable. Bural et al. reported excellent reliability for Penguin®, but they did not report the reliability of Osstell® [14]. Norton et al. [15] reported the agreement between the measurements obtained by two different Osstell® versions and Penguin®, and the authors considered these differences not clinically relevant. Therefore, reliability results reported so far are contradictory.

Osstell® Beacon is the wireless version of Osstell® that can be connected online to the Osstell® database for statistical analysis. The smartpegs for Ostell® are not autoclavable. On the other hand, the multipegs for Penguin® are autoclavable and the device is wireless. MegaISQ® (Megagen Implant CO, Daegu, Korea) is a portable, but not wireless device that uses the Osstell® smartpegs. To the best of our knowledge, inter- and intra-rater reliability and agreement among Osstell® Beacon, Penguin® and MegaISQ® have not yet been investigated.

The goal of this study was to determine and compare the inter- and intra-rater reliability of Osstell® Beacon and MegaISQ® versus Penguin® as control. This study also aimed to explore the agreement between these devices for ISQ measurement. This study was conducted in vitro by two investigators to obtain the inter- and intra-rater reliability and the agreement level among these three devices.

2. Materials and Methods

In this in vitro study, 30 BioHorizons® Internal implants (BioHorizons, Birmingham, AL, USA) were inserted in fresh pig mandibles (Figure 1). The manufacturer drilling protocol was used to place 10 implants (4.6 mm diameter, 12 mm height) in 10 different positions of 3 different mandibles (Figure 1). Considering an alpha error of 0.05 and a beta error of 0.2, in a two-sided test, a minimum of 20 samples were necessary from each group to identify a statistically significant difference greater than or equal to two units. Based on a recent study [16], standard deviation was assumed to be 5 and the correlation coefficient measurement was 0.9.

ISQ was measured using three different devices: Osstell® Beacon (W&H, Göteborg, Sweden), Penguin® (Integration Diagnostics Sweden AB, Göteborg, Sweden) and MegaISQ® (Megagen Implant CO, Daegu, Korea). The transducer peg for each device (smartpeg for Osstell and MegaISQ and multipeg for Penguin) was inserted on each implant according to the manufacturer's instructions, and two measurements were recorded parallel and perpendicular (lingual) to the longitudinal axis of the peg. Due to the reliability provided by previous studies [12–15], Penguin® was used as the control.

The smartpeg for Osstell®, the multipeg for Penguin® and the smartpeg for MegaISQ® were removed between each measurement, and the stability of the 30 implants placed in the three different mandibles was evaluated with the three devices.

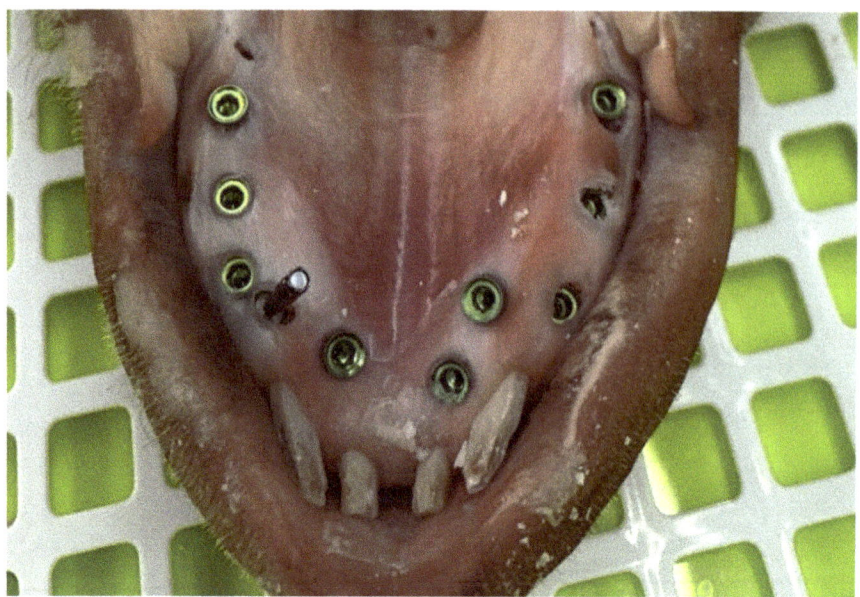

Figure 1. Implant locations in a representative mandible with a Penguin® multipeg inserted in one of the implants.

All procedures were repeated by two different experienced and calibrated investigators (MB and RA) after the implant insertion, in order to assess the inter-rater reliability, and one operator (RA) repeated the procedures 5 min later in order to perform a test-retest check for measuring the intra-rater reliability in the same conditions. While it was not possible to blind the device used, the order in which implants were measured and which device was used was randomized. The measurements were coded by these two operators in order to blind the statistical analysis.

Statistical Analysis

Shapiro–Wilks and Levene tests were respectively used for assessing criteria of normality and homogeneity of variances (Supplementary Table S1). Test-retest was used to calculate the intraclass correlation coefficient (ICC) using a mixed model with a random effect on the individual in order to assess the intra- and inter-rater reliability. ICC values were classified as poor-moderate-good according to Koo et al. criteria. [17]. Absolute ISQ values obtained using each method were reported as mean (95%CI). The agreement between the devices was assessed by means of the Pearson correlation coefficient. To establish the level of agreement and the correlation between the different devices a mean value from the two operators was calculated. All analyses were performed using the IBM Statistics for Windows v24.0 software package (IBM Corp., New York, NY, USA) ($p < 0.05$).

3. Results

Table 1 shows the implant stability measurements obtained by each device. As shown, using Penguin in parallel measurement yields the highest ISQ values; in contrast, using the MegaISQ® in a perpendicular measurement results in the lowest values.

Table 1. Mean values (95% CI) of implant stability quotient (ISQ) according to the device and the orientation.

Device	Technique	ISQ	Difference with Mean ISQ Values 62.1 (59.2 to 65)
OSSTELL® Beacon	parallel	62.2 (59.5 to 64.9)	0.1 (−0.1 to 0.1)
	perpendicular	60.6 (58.0 to 63.3)	−1.5 (−1.7 to −1.15)
PENGUIN®	parallel	66.3 (62.4 to 70.1)	4.2 (3.25 to 5.1)
	perpendicular	63.1 (60.0 to 66.3)	1 (0.85 to 1.3)
MEGAISQ®	parallel	60.1 (57.5 to 62.6)	−2 (−2.4 to −1.65)
	perpendicular	60.2 (57.5 to 62.8)	−1.9 (−2.2 to −1.65)

ISQ—implant stability quotient. 95% CI—95% confidence interval.

The difference between the values obtained with each device and technique and the mean ISQ values is shown in Figure 2. The mean of these differences was 0.13 (95% CI: −5.79 to 6.05) for the Osstell® Beacon in a parallel measurement; −1.45 (95% CI: −7.78 to 4.88) for the Osstell® Beacon in a perpendicular measurement; 4.2 (95% CI: −6.20 to 14.60) for the Penguin® in a parallel measurement; 1.03 (95% CI: −7.40 to 9.47) for the Penguin® in a perpendicular measurement; −2.02 (95% CI: −7.30 to 3.27) for the MegaISQ® in a parallel measurement and −1.09 (95% CI: −13.03 to 9.23) for MegaISQ® in a perpendicular measurement.

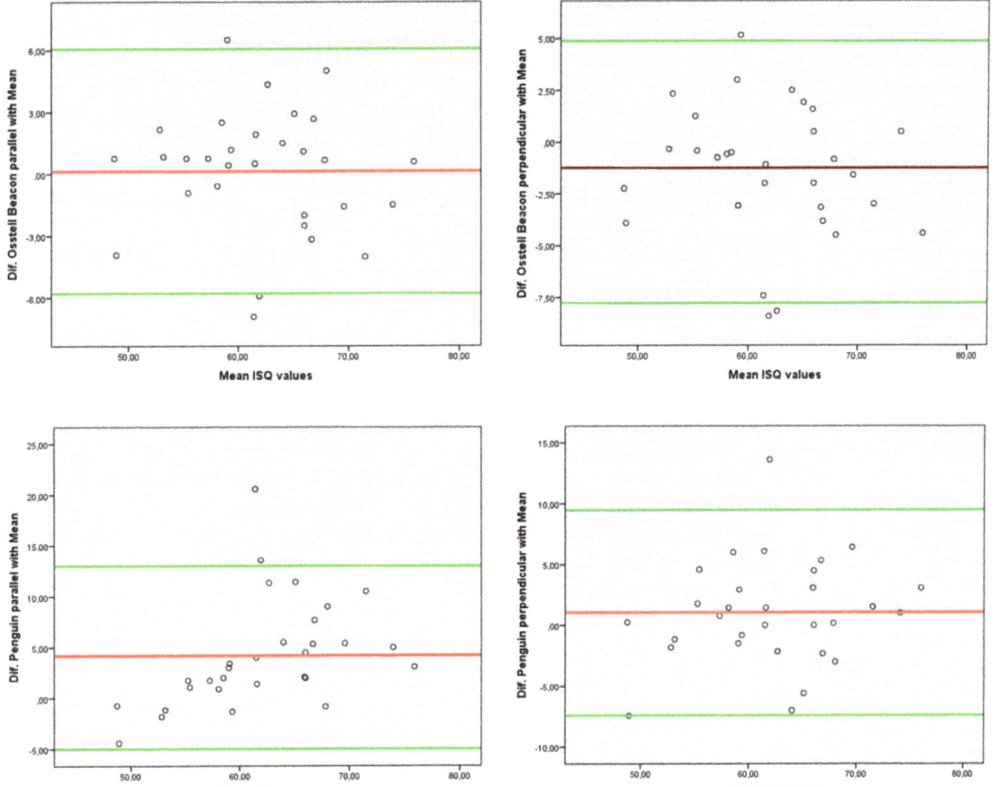

Figure 2. Cont.

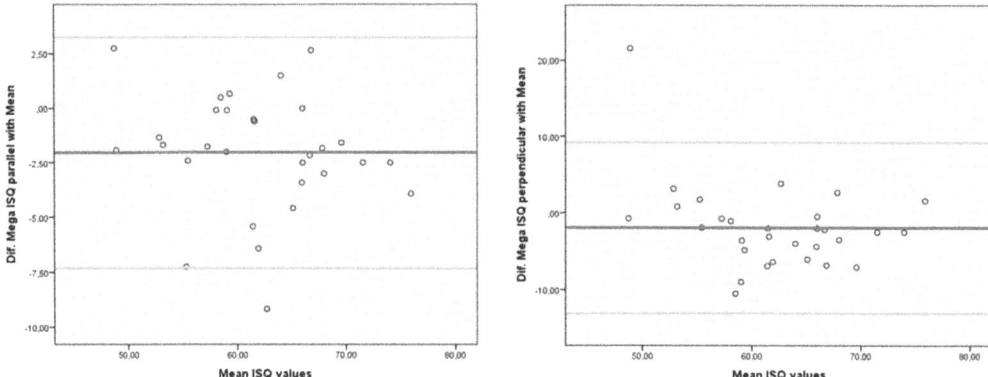

Figure 2. Bland–Altman plot with the difference between the measurements of each device and technique and the mean ISQ values.

Table 2 shows the reliability scores for the three devices. The highest inter- and intra-rater reliability was obtained by Penguin® when measuring in parallel. The lowest inter-rater reliability was obtained by MegaISQ® measuring perpendicularly, Osstell® Beacon measuring perpendicularly, and MegaISQ® measuring in parallel. The lowest intra-rater reliability was obtained by Osstell® Beacon.

Table 2. Reliability (ICC; 95% CI) of the three devices used to measure ISQ.

Reliability		ICC Classification		
INTER-RATER			INTRA-RATER	
METHOD	ICC (95% CI)		ICC (95% CI)	
OSSTELL®B parallel	0.37 (0.40 to 0.64)	poor	0.65 (0.38 to 0.81)	moderate
OSSTELL®B perpendicular	0.20 (−0.17 to 0.52)	poor	0.47 (0.13 to 0.71)	poor
PENGUIN® parallel	0.86 (0.72 to 0.93)	good	0.85 (0.70 to 0.92)	good
PENGUIN® perpendicular	0.57 (0.26 to 0.77)	moderate	0.78 (0.56 to 0.89)	good
MEGAISQ® parallel	0.26 (−0.11 to 0.57)	poor	0.60 (0.26 to 0.79)	moderate
MEGAISQ® perpendicular	−0.01 (−0.38 to 0.36)	poor	0.57 (0.27 to 0.77)	moderate

ICC—intraclass correlation coefficient, two-way random, absolute agreement for single measurement; OSSTELL®B—Osstell® Beacon.

A matrix with the Pearson correlation coefficients is shown in Table 3. The highest correlation value with the other devices was obtained by MegaISQ® measuring parallel; however, this device obtained the lowest correlation value when measuring perpendicular. Osstell® Beacon obtained high correlation values with the other devices measuring either in parallel or perpendicular. Penguin® obtained correlation values lower than Osstell® Beacon, both measuring parallel and perpendicular, but higher than MegaISQ® when measuring perpendicular.

Table 3. Matrix of Pearson correlation coefficients for the different devices used to measure ISQ.

	Osstell® Beacon Parallel	Osstell® Beacon Perpend.	PENGUIN® Parallel	PENGUIN® Perpend.	MEGAISQ® Parallel	MEGAISQ® Perpend.	TOTAL
OSSTELL® Beacon parallel	1	0.723 **	0.667 **	0.555 **	0.766 **	0.405 **	4.12
OSSTELL® Beacon perpend.	0.723 **	1	0.575 **	0.652 **	0.653 **	0.525 **	4.13
PENGUIN® parallel	0.667 **	0.575 **	1	0.760 **	0.691 **	0.298 *	3.99
PENGUIN® perpend.	0.555 **	0.652 **	0.760 **	1	0.675 **	0.404 **	4.05
MEGAISQ® parallel	0.766 **	0.653 **	0.691 **	0.675 **	1	0.449 **	4.23
MEGAISQ® perpend.	0.405 **	0.525 **	0.298 *	0.404 **	0.449 **	1	3.08

* $p < 0.01$; ** $p < 0.001$; perpend.—perpendicular.

4. Discussion

Based on the ICC scores, our results suggest that Osstell® Beacon and MegaISQ® exhibited lower reliability than Penguin®. The reliability of Penguin® was good in parallel measurements, and between moderate to good when measuring perpendicularly. Osstell® Beacon presented a poor to moderate reliability when measuring parallel and poor when measuring perpendicular, and MegaISQ® obtained poor to moderate reliability when measuring both parallel and perpendicular. The lower reliability obtained by Osstell® Beacon and MegaISQ® compared to Penguin® can be attributed to differences in the electromagnetic functioning, since these devices use the same smartpeg from Osstell®, and Penguin® uses a magnetized multipeg. From these results, Penguin® should be used to monitor the implant micromotion and the evolution of osseointegration.

Our ICC scores were lower than a recent study [14]; however, in this study, the mean of the perpendicular and parallel ISQ values was considered as the final ISQ of each implant, then the differences of each device measuring parallel or perpendicular could be not detected. High ICC scores were also reported for both Penguin® and Osstell®, but only when the implant surrounding material was stiff [12]. The differences in bone density between studies could explain the different results obtained.

The inter-rater ICC values obtained in our study were mostly lower than the intra-rater ICC values for the majority of devices and techniques. This observation suggests that the values obtained from these devices can be operator dependent. All three devices presented higher ICC values when measuring parallel than perpendicular. One study reported increased variability and reduced reliability when measuring buccolingual [14]. These results suggest that the clinical evaluation of implant micromotion by means of parallel ISQ could be recommended.

Osstell® Beacon showed lower values than previous studies using different types of Osstell® (Osstell® ISQ and Osstell® IDX) [14,18]. These differences can be attributed to the bone density and the device version. In our study, the highest ISQ values were obtained using Penguin® and the lowest values were obtained using MegaISQ®. This observation can lead the clinician to overestimate the implant stability with Penguin®. The MegaISQ® values were the lowest, suggesting that MegaISQ® tends to underestimate the implant stability. However, the difference between the MegaISQ® values and the mean was twice as low as with Penguin, then the underestimation of MegaISQ® has not reached the magnitude of the Penguin® overestimation. These differences could be clinically relevant when the ISQ measure is around 57 corresponding to the minimum threshold of osseointegration. This value can be interpreted as a correct osseointegration of a failed implant with Penguin® or as a failed implant with a correct osseointegration with MegaISQ®.

Comparing the correlation between each instrument, MegaISQ® measuring parallel had the higher correlation to the others (considering every instrument and technique). However, the same instrument obtained the lowest correlation when measuring perpendicular (lowest Pearson correlation coefficient and widest difference of agreement with the mean ISQ values in the Bland–Altman plot). On the other hand, Osstell® Beacon obtained good correlation for measuring both parallel and perpendicular (and the narrowest difference of agreement with the mean ISQ values), and Penguin® had similar correlation values with the other methods measuring parallel and perpendicular.

This study has some limitations. The bone density can affect ISQ values [19] and no previous evaluation of the different bone locations where implants were placed was done. However, some aspects that could affect ISQ values, such as implant length and diameter were controlled using the same implant size for all measurements. Another limitation was the manual tightening of the transducers, but this technique was previously reported to be objective and reliable [20]. Finally, it was not possible to blind the investigators within the instrument used, and the study was performed in an animal model. Therefore, further research is needed to clinically assess in vivo the behavior of these devices.

5. Conclusions

Within the limitations of this study, Osstell® Beacon and MegaISQ® showed a larger deviation in the measurements than Penguin®; Penguin® exhibited moderate to good inter-rater reliability and good intra-rater reliability for measuring the implant micromotion; Osstell® Beacon had good agreement for measuring ISQ both parallel and perpendicular and MegaISQ® had the best agreement for measuring ISQ parallel, but not for measuring perpendicular.

Supplementary Materials: The following are available online at https://www.mdpi.com/article/10.3390/app11083453/s1, Table S1. Normality and homogeneity of variances.

Author Contributions: Conceptualization, J.L.-L., R.A.-M. and E.V.-O.; Methodology, R.A.-M., J.L.-L., C.S.-H. and E.V.-O.; Software, R.A.-M. and C.S.-H.; Validation, M.B.-H., C.S.-H., V.D.-A., J.L.-L., R.A.-M. and E.V.-O.; Formal Analysis, R.A.-M. and C.S.-H.; Investigation, V.D.-A., M.B.-H., J.L.-L. and R.A.-M.; Resources, R.A.-M. and J.L.-L.; Data Curation, V.D.-A., M.B.-H. and R.A.-M.; Writing—Original Draft Preparation, R.A.-M. and J.L.-L.; Writing—Review and Editing, M.B.-H., R.A.-M. and E.V.-O.; Visualization, R.A.-M., J.L.-L.; Supervision, J.L.-L., R.A.-M. and E.V.-O.; Project Administration, M.B.-H., R.A.-M. and J.L.-L. All authors have read and agreed to the published version of the manuscript.

Funding: This research received funding from Biohorizons-Camlog® Ibérica with the grant number 018582/2019, and from the Faculty of Medicine and Health Sciences, University of Barcelona.

Data Availability Statement: Data of obtained from this study is not available publicly. Information regarding these data should be requested to the corresponding author.

Acknowledgments: The authors gratefully acknowledge Jordi Martinez-Gomis for the statistical analysis support.

Conflicts of Interest: The authors declare no conflict of interest.

References

1. Turkyilmaz, I.; Sennerby, L.; Tumer, C.; Yenigul, M.; Avci, M. Stability and marginal bone level measurements of unsplinted implants used for mandibular overdentures: A 1-year randomized prospective clinical study comparing early and conventional loading protocols. *Clin. Oral Implant. Res.* **2006**, *17*, 501–505. [CrossRef] [PubMed]
2. Huwiler, M.; Pjeturson, B.E.; Bosshardt, D.D.; Salvi, G.E.; Lang, N.P. Resonance Frequency Analysis (RFA) in relation to jaw bone characteristics during early healing. *Clin. Oral Implant. Res.* **2007**, *18*, 275–280. [CrossRef] [PubMed]
3. Trisi, P.; Perfetti, G.; Baldoni, E.; Berardi, D.; Colagiovanni, M.; Scogna, G. Implant micromotion is related to peak insertion torque and bone density. *Clin. Oral Implant. Res.* **2009**, *20*, 467–471. [CrossRef] [PubMed]

4. Winter, W.; Klein, D.; Karl, M. Micromotion of dental implants: Basic mechanical considerations. *J. Med. Eng.* **2013**, *2013*, 1. [CrossRef] [PubMed]
5. Brizuela-Velasco, A.; Alvarez-Arenal, A.; Gil-Mur, F.J.; Herrero-Climent, M.; Chávarri-Prado, D.; Chento-Valiente, Y.; Dieguez-Pereira, M. Relationship between torque and resonance frequency measurements, performed by resonance frequency analysis, in micromobility of dental implants: An in vitro study. *Implant Dent.* **2015**, *24*, 607–611. [CrossRef] [PubMed]
6. Zanetti, E.M.; Ciaramella, S.; Calì, M.; Pascoletti, G.; Martorelli, M.; Asero, R.; Watts, D.C. Modal analysis for implant stability assessment: Sensitivity of this methodology for different implant designs. *Dent. Mater.* **2018**, *34*, 1235–1245. [CrossRef] [PubMed]
7. Atsumi, M.; Park, S.H.; Wang, H.L. Methods used to assess implant stability: Current status. *Int. J. Oral Maxillofac. Implant.* **2007**, *22*, 743–754.
8. Aparicio, C.; Lang, N.P.; Rangert, B. Validity and clinical significance of biomechanical testing of implant/bone interface. *Clin. Oral Implant. Res.* **2006**, *17* (Suppl. S2), 2–7. [CrossRef] [PubMed]
9. Lee, D.H.; Shin, Y.H.; Park, J.H.; Shim, J.H.; Shin, S.W.; Lee, J.Y. The reliability of anycheck device related to healing abutment diameter. *J. Adv. Prosthodont.* **2020**, *12*, 83–88. [CrossRef] [PubMed]
10. Brizuela-Velasco, A.; Chávarri-Prado, D. The functional loading of implants increases their stability: A retrospective clinical study. *Clin. Implant. Dent. Relat. Res.* **2019**, *21*, 122–129. [CrossRef] [PubMed]
11. Santamaría-Arrieta, G.; Brizuela-Velasco, A.; Fernández-González, F.J.; Chávarri-Prado, D.; Chento-Valiente, Y.; Solaberrieta, E.; Chávarri-Prado, D.; Chento-Valiente, Y.; Solaberrieta, E. Biomechanical evaluation of oversized drilling technique on primary implant stability measured by insertion torque and resonance frequency analysis. *J. Clin. Exp. Dent.* **2016**, *1*, 307–311. [CrossRef]
12. Buyukguclu, G.; Ozkurt-Kayahan, Z.; Kazazoglu, E. Reliability of the Osstell implant stability quotient and Penguin resonance frequency analysis to evaluate implant stability. *Implant Dent.* **2018**, *27*, 429–433. [CrossRef] [PubMed]
13. Romanos, G.E.; Bastardi, D.J.; Kakar, A.; Moore, R.; Delgado-Ruiz, R.A.; Javed, F. In vitro comparison of resonance frequency analysis devices to evaluate implant stability of narrow diameter implants at varying drilling speeds in dense artificial bone blocks. *Clin. Implant Dent. Relat. Res.* **2019**, *21*, 1023–1027. [CrossRef] [PubMed]
14. Bural, C.; Dayan, C.; Geçkili, O. Initial stability measurements of implants using a new magnetic resonance frequency analyzer with titanium transducers: An ex vivo study. *J. Oral Implantol.* **2020**, *46*, 35–40. [CrossRef] [PubMed]
15. Norton, M.R. Resonance Frequency Analysis: Agreement and correlation of implant stability quotients between three commercially available instruments. *Int. J. Oral Maxillofac. Implant.* **2018**. [CrossRef] [PubMed]
16. Lee, J.; Pyo, S.W.; Cho, H.J.; An, J.S.; Lee, J.H.; Koo, K.T.; Lee, Y.M. Comparison of implant stability measurements between a resonance frequency analysis device and a modified damping capacity analysis device: An in vitro study. *J. Periodontal. Implant Sci.* **2020**, *50*, 56–66. [CrossRef] [PubMed]
17. Koo, T.K.; Li, M. A Guideline of Selecting and Reporting Intraclass Correlation Coefficients for Reliability Research. *J. Chiropr. Med.* **2016**, *15*, 155–163. [CrossRef] [PubMed]
18. Becker, W.; Hujoel, P.; Becker, B.E. Resonance frequency analysis: Comparing two clinical instruments. *Clin. Implant Dent. Relat. Res.* **2018**, *20*, 308–312. [CrossRef] [PubMed]
19. Sim, C.P.; Lang, N.P. Factors influencing resonance frequency analysis assessed by Osstell mentor during implant tissue integration: I. Instrument positioning, bone structure, implant length. *Clin. Oral Implant. Res.* **2010**, *21*, 598–604. [CrossRef] [PubMed]
20. Kästel, I.; de Quincey, G.; Neugebauer, J.; Sader, R.; Gehrke, P. Does the Manual Insertion Torque of Smartpegs Affect the Outcome of Implant Stability Quotients (ISQ) During Resonance Frequency Analysis (RFA)? *Int. J. Implant Dent.* **2019**, *5*, 42. [CrossRef] [PubMed]

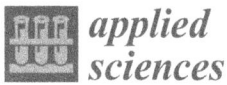

Review

Bisphosphonates and Their Influence on the Implant Failure: A Systematic Review

Cristiana Gomes Rebelo [1], Juliana Campos Hasse Fernandes [2], Nuno Bernardo [1], Patrícia Couto [1] and Gustavo Vicentis Oliveira Fernandes [1,3,*]

[1] Center for Interdisciplinary Research in Health (CIIS), Universidade Católica Portuguesa—Faculty of Dental Medicine (FMD-UCP), 3504-505 Viseu, Portugal
[2] Private Practice, Ann Arbor, MI 48109, USA
[3] Periodontics and Oral Medicine Department, University of Michigan School of Dentistry, Ann Arbor, MI 48109, USA
* Correspondence: gustfernandes@gmail.com

Abstract: Objective: The goal of this systematic review was to study the relationship between the use of bisphosphonates (oral or intravenous) and its effect on implant osseointegration. Methods: The focused question was "In patients medicated with bisphosphonates and who underwent surgery to place dental implants, what is the influence of that medication (of different generations) on the failure of dental implants (O)?" Following specific eligibility criteria, four databases (PubMed/MEDLINE, Scopus, Web of Science, DOAJ) were electronically screened to search the articles. Specific MeSH terms were used in combinations with Boolean Operators "AND" and "OR" for the research. In addition, a manual search was done. The data extracted were the (i) author, (ii) year of publication, (iii) country, (iv) research question, (v) study design, (vi) patient information, (vii) the number of patients included, (viii) patient/implant status, (ix) the number of implants evaluated, (x) type of implant, (xi) risk factors, and (xii) findings obtained. Moreover, the following were also registered: the (i) type, generation, duration, and route for BP administrated; (ii) the presence of any systemic condition and drug treatment; (iii) follow-up (months); and (iv) implant failure rate (%). The quality assessment of the included studies was carried out using the Modified Newcastle–Ottawa scale. Results: A total of 491 articles were found (183 in PubMed/MEDLINE, 171 in Scopus, 65 in Web of Science, and 72 articles in DOAJ), and 17 articles were considered for full-text reading. After the exclusion of 3 articles, 14 were included in this systematic review (11 case reports, 2 retrospective, and 1 prospective study). The reasons for the bisphosphonates intaking included osteoporosis, multiple myeloma, breast cancer, knee cancer, and osteogenesis imperfecta. The oral administration involved Alendronato (eight studies), Risedronate (three studies), and Ibandronate (three studies); whereas the intravenous administrations were Zoledronate (seven studies), Clodronato (one study), and Pamidronato (three studies). The duration of use of bisphosphonates at the time of implant placement was diverse; it ranged from no interruption of bisphosphonate intaking up to its discontinuation for 2, 3, or 6 months before surgery, with respective use being resumed 1, 3, or 8 months after surgery. Antibiotic treatment (amoxicillin + clavulanic acid) was performed before the intervention in two cases and after the intervention in three cases. Finally, the percent of implant failure rate when intaking BPs had an average of 49.96%. Conclusions: Within the limitation of this systematic review, it was possible to conclude that a high mean failure rate of implant osseointegration (49.96%) was found, regardless of the generation of bisphosphonates used. Moreover, the failure rate was lower in patients using second generation bisphosphonates (Alendronate and Pamidronato) and was higher with the IV administration compared to the oral administration of bisphosphonates.

Keywords: bisphosphonates; dental implants; osseointegration; medication-related osteonecrosis of the jaw

Citation: Rebelo, C.G.; Fernandes, J.C.H.; Bernardo, N.; Couto, P.; Fernandes, G.V.O. Bisphosphonates and Their Influence on the Implant Failure: A Systematic Review. *Appl. Sci.* **2023**, *13*, 3496. https://doi.org/10.3390/app13063496

Academic Editors: Ricardo Castro Alves, José João Mendes and Ana Cristina Mano Azul

Received: 24 February 2023
Revised: 6 March 2023
Accepted: 7 March 2023
Published: 9 March 2023

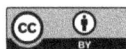

Copyright: © 2023 by the authors. Licensee MDPI, Basel, Switzerland. This article is an open access article distributed under the terms and conditions of the Creative Commons Attribution (CC BY) license (https://creativecommons.org/licenses/by/4.0/).

1. Introduction

Osseointegration is defined as a connection between the living bone and the implant surface in a stable and functional way. This involves anchoring the implant by forming bone tissue around the implant without fibrous tissue growth at the bone–implant interface [1]. This direct contact between the implant surface and the bone is decisive for the success of the implant, since it decreases the risk of failure, improves stability, and promotes implant longevity. In order to enhance osseointegration, it is possible to change the roughness of the implant surface [2].

Over the years, studies have been carried out to find the most suitable material for the composition of the implants and the consequent success or failure of their osseointegration [3–5]. The most scientifically studied implants are titanium implants, and more recently, investigations and comparisons with zirconia material have emerged [3–5]. According to Hanawa (2020) [6], titanium has shown excellent biocompatibility, corrosion-resistance, and high fracture toughness based on high strength and elongation. Compared to titanium, zirconia reported a significantly reduced bacterial biofilm formation and increased microcirculation in the peri-implant soft tissues [3]. Regarding peri-implant soft tissues, both materials have similar integration properties. However, titanium appears to have a faster initial osseointegration process when compared to zirconia. Survival rates of more than 96% for titanium implants with microrough surfaces have been reported after being followed for 10 years [3]. On the other hand, Sivaraman et al. (2018) [7] reported higher success rates (95.8%) for titanium and zirconia implants (90.9%) in the mandible compared to the maxilla, at 71.9% and 55%, respectively.

Nevertheless, the use of bisphosphonate (BP) may impair the osseointegration. It is a class of drugs that are frequently selected when there is an alteration in the bone metabolism, which are utilized to prevent bone loss [8]. It can be administered orally (e.g., daily, weekly, or monthly) for treatment of osteoporosis and Paget's disease, or intravenously (every 3 months or annually) to treat malignant skeletal oncological diseases [9]. BPs can also be classified according to generations, with the first generation being non-nitrogenous and including drugs such as Clodronate, Etidronate, and Tiludronate. The second and third generation, on the other hand, contain nitrogen. Regarding the second generation, it includes drugs such as Alendronate, Neridronate, and Pamidronate and the third generation includes drugs such as Risedronate, Minodronate, Zoledronate, and Ibandronate [9].

Despite the fact that they increase the quality of life of the patients, there is an elevated risk that BPs can cause osteonecrosis of the jaw. This is characterized by an exposure of necrotic bone in the mandibular region that normally persists for 8 or more weeks [10]. Patients who have been treated with BPs intravenously have shown a greater chance of developing medication-related osteonecrosis of the jaw (MRONJ) or implant loss compared to oral-intaking therapy [11].

In a study developed by Gelazius et al. [10], patients taking BPs who were treated intravenously lost 6 implants out of 68, which yielded an 8.82% for failure rate; patients treated with intraoral therapy had a failure of 5 implants in 423 (1.18%), which was more than 7-fold less. They considered the dental implant a failure if the implant had mobility, active inflammation for more than 8 weeks without healing with antibiotic therapy, drainage of purulent secretion near the implant, the presence of necrotic bone or unhealed soft tissue, or implant loss [10].

A study by Chen et al. [12] showed that Zoledronate (the third generation of BPs) and Alendronate (the second-generation BPs) improved titanium implant osseointegration in ovariectomized rats. In this case, a single dose injection of Zoledronate (0.1 mg/kg) was shown to be able to increase bone implant contact (BIC), osseointegration, more than the oral administration of Alendronate (7 mg/kg/week) [12]. However, in oral mucosa cells, which provide the first physical and immunological barrier to prevent bacterial invasion, these BPs have been shown to have a difficult adhesion and metabolism [13]. In addition, the potential risk of medication-related osteonecrosis of the jaw (MRONJ) or loss of the implant associated with BP therapy cannot be disregarded, and more standardized studies are needed to provide more accurate information on this subject.

Therefore, the aim of this review was to systematically study, in the literature, the association of bisphosphonates (oral or intravenous) and its effect on implant osseointegration. The null hypothesis was that there is an impairment of the bone formation/osseointegration around implants when the patient is intaking bisphosphonates (BPs).

2. Material and Methods

2.1. Focused Question

A focused question was constructed according to the Preferred Reporting Items for Systematic Reviews and Meta-Analyses (PRISMA) guidelines and Participants Intervention Control Outcomes (PICO) protocol. The focused question presented in this systematic review was "In patients medicated with bisphosphonates (P) and who underwent surgery to place dental implants (I), what is the influence of that medication (of different generations) (C) on the failure of dental implants (O)?" (Table 1).

Table 1. PICO characterization.

Participants (P)	Patients using bisphosphonates
Intervention (I)	Placement of one or more dental implants
Control (C)	Different generations and administration routes of BFs
Outcomes (O)	Dental implant failure rate

2.2. Eligibility Criteria

Inclusion criteria were (i) patients undergoing therapy with BPs (oral or intravenous), (ii) patients undergoing a dental implant placement procedure, (iii) using different generations and routes of BPs, (iv) that studied the influence of BPs intake on implant failure, (v) random controlled trials, case-control, case series, retrospective studies, prospective studies, (vi) trials conducted between 2000–2021, and (vii) in English language. The exclusion criteria included the following: (i) patients undergoing drug therapy other than BPs, (ii) patients whose surgical procedure was not the placement of dental implants, (iii) studies that did not refer to the type of BP used, (iv) studies that did not assess the relationship between dental implants and local/systemic therapy with BPs, (v) reviews, meta-analysis, commentaries, editorial, in vitro or preclinical studies, letters to the editor, duplicated articles, and (vi) other languages.

2.3. Literature Search and Screening

Four databases (PubMed/MEDLINE, Scopus, Web of Science, DOAJ) were used to electronically search for the articles. The following MeSH (Medical Subject Headings) terms were used: "Diphosphonates", "Bisphosphonates", "Clodronate", "Etidronate", "Alendronate", "Pamidronate", "Risedronate", "Ibandronate", "Dental Implants", "Bisphosphonate-Associated Osteonecrosis of the Jaw" and their related entry terms were used in different combinations using the Boolean Operators "AND" and "OR" for the research and specific related-terms with the theme of this study. In addition, a manual search was made by each one of the researchers with the terms: "Osseointegration", "Tiludronate", "Neridronate", "Minodronate", "Zolendronate" (Table 2).

2.4. Data Extraction

The data collected from the included articles were inserted in an Excel spreadsheet (Microsoft Excel® for Mac, v. 16, Redmond, WA, USA, USA). They were the following: (i) author, (ii) year of publication, (iii) country, (iv) research question, (v) study design, (vi) patient information, (vii) number of patients included, (viii) patient/implant status, (ix) number of implants evaluated, (x) type of implant, (xi) risk factors, and (xii) findings obtained. Moreover, the following were also registered: the (i) type, generation, duration, and route for BP administrated; (ii) the presence of any systemic condition and drug treatment; (iii) follow-up (months); and (iv) implant failure rate (%).

Table 2. Search strategy.

Database	Equation Implemented	Filters
Pubmed/MEDLINE	((((((((((((diphosphonates [MeSH Terms]) OR bisphosphonates [MeSH Terms]) OR clodronate [MeSH Terms]) OR etidronate [MeSH Terms]) OR alendronate [MeSH Terms]) OR pamidronate [MeSH Terms]) OR risedronate [MeSH Terms]) OR ibandronate [MeSH Terms]) OR "bisphosphonate- associated osteonecrosis of the jaw" [MeSH Terms]) OR tiludronate) OR neridronate) OR minodronate) OR zoledronate AND (osseointegration OR dental implants [MeSH Terms])	In English, from January 2000 to December 2021, humans
Scopus	ALL ((diphosphonates OR bisphosphonates OR clodronate alendronate OR risedronate OR bisphosphonate-associated AND osteonecrosis AND jaw) OR tiludronate OR neridronate OR etidronate OR pamidronate OR ibandronate OR (minodronate OR zoledronate) AND (osseointegration OR dental AND implants) AND (failure AND rate)) AND PUBYEAR > 1999 AND PUBYEAR < 2022 AND (LIMIT-TO (PUBSTAGE, "final")) AND (LIMIT-TO (DOCTYPE, "ar")) AND (LIMIT-TO (EXACTKEYWORD, "Humans")) AND (LIMIT-TO (LANGUAGE, "English")) AND (LIMIT-TO (SRCTYPE, "j"))	In English, from January 2000 to December 2021, humans, final stage
Web of Science	(diphosphonates OR bisphosphonates OR clodronate OR etidronate OR alendronate OR pamidronate OR risedronate OR ibandronate OR (bisphosphonate-associated AND osteonecrosis AND of AND the AND jaw) OR tiludronate OR neridronate OR minodronate OR zoledronate) AND (osseointegration OR dental implants) AND failure (All Fields)	In English, from January 2000 to December 2021
DOAJ	(diphosphonates OR bisphosphonates OR clodronate OR etidronate OR alendronate OR pamidronate OR risedronate OR ibandronate OR (bisphosphonate-associated AND osteonecrosis AND of AND the AND jaw) OR tiludronate OR neridronate OR minodronate OR zoledronate) AND (osseointegration OR dental implants) AND failure (All Fields)	In English, from January 2000 to December 2021, humans

2.5. Quality Assessment

After the selection of articles, an assessment of their quality was carried out. For this, we used the Modified Newcastle–Ottawa scale, in which the following parameters were evaluated: representativeness, selection, comparability, blinding and, finally, the follow up. All parameters had a maximum score of 1 value, except for comparability, which can be evaluated up to a score of 2 values, totaling 7 points. From 0 to 3 points, the study was considered to have a low level of quality; between 4–6 was considered a moderate level; and a 7 score was considered a high level of quality.

3. Results

After carrying out the search, 491 articles were found. Of these, 183 articles were identified in PubMed/MEDLINE, 171 in Scopus, 65 in Web of Science, and 72 articles in DOAJ. Then, the articles that were duplicated (n = 214) were eliminated, which resulted in 277 studies. After analyzing the title and abstract, another 260 articles were excluded. Then, a total of 17 articles remained for full-text reading. After performing the full reading, four more articles were excluded due to lack of information and detail on the patient follow up. Thus, 13 articles were included in this systematic review (10 case reports, 2 retrospective studies, and 1 prospective study). The agreements between reviewers were, for initial assessment, k = 0.97 and, for assessment of the final inclusion, k = 0.91 (Figure 1).

The demographic data for the patients/implants and studies included are summarized in Tables 3 and 4. A total of 67 patients were analyzed and 163 dental implants were placed in the studies included. All of them were Caucasian, with a mean age of 62 years old (58 female and 9 male). The mean follow-up period was 28.9 months (ranging from 12 months to 48 months). The risk factors reported were hypertension, tobacco, poor oral hygiene, and diabetes, and all of these factors were respectively linked to higher implant failure rates of 8%, 19%, 2%, and 7%. Most of the diseases for which BPs were taken were osteoporosis, multiple myeloma, breast cancer, lung cancer, prostate cancer, knee cancer, and osteogenesis imperfecta.

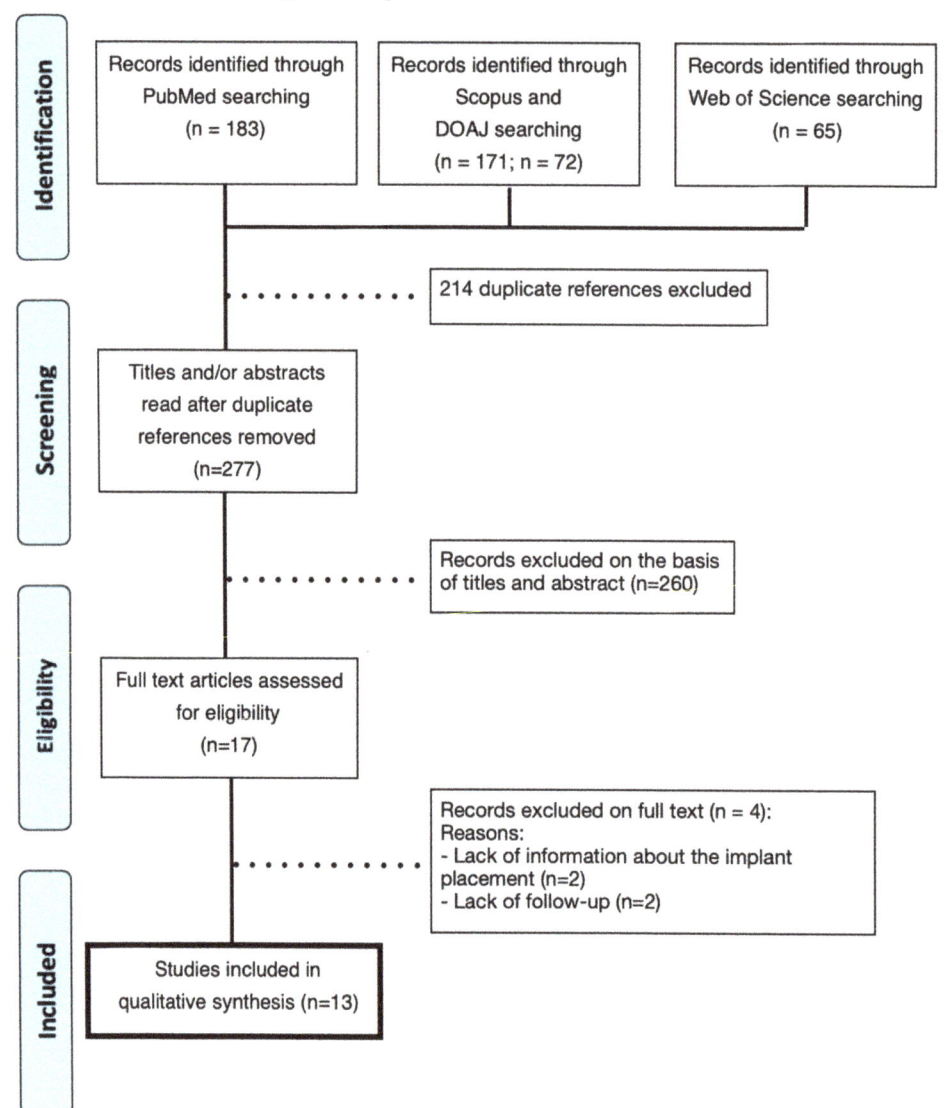

Figure 1. Article selection strategy, according to the PRISMA Flowchart (Preferred Reporting Items for Systematic Reviews and Meta-Analyses).

The routes of BP administration were oral and intravenous. A total of 42 patients (63%) were on therapy with BPs administered orally, and 25 patients (37%) received BPs through IV. For oral administration, the drugs were Alendronate [14–21], Risedronate [16,17,21], and Ibandronate [14,17,19], whereas those administered intravenously were Zoledronate [14,17,19,22–26], Clodronate [27], and Pamidronate [14,19,26]. The duration of the use of BPs at the time of implant placement was diverse. It varied from no interruption of BP intake to its discontinuation from 2, 3, or for 6 months before surgery, with respective resumption 1, 3, or 8 months after surgery. Antibiotic treatment (amoxicillin + clavulanic acid) was performed before the intervention in two cases and before and after surgical treatment in three cases. Use only after intervention was not found. Antibiotic treatment proved to be effective in cases where it was used as a pre- and post-surgical therapy. Finally, a percentage of implant survival in the group taking BPs had an average failure rate of 42.27%. Four studies did not have any implant failure [15,16,22,24].

The most prevalent BPs corresponded to the second generation (Alendronate and Pamidronate), which were used in 61% of the cases, followed by the third generation (Zoledronate, Ibandronate, and Risedronate), which were found in 38% of the cases; only one case utilized first generation BPs (Clodronate). Regarding this variable, a lower failure rate was noted when patients used the second-generation BPs (37%), followed by third generation (38%) and first generation (100%). Moreover, when patients discontinued BP therapy (45% of the cases), lower failure rates were obtained than patients with continuous use (55%). The quality assessment of the study was considered to be of low/moderate level, with all studies excepting Yajima et al. presenting values between 2 and 5 (Figure 2).

Study ID	SELECTION			COMPARABILITY	OUTCOME		Total score (out of 7)
	Representativeness of exposed sample (Maximum: *)	Selection of non-exposed sample (Maximum: *)	Ascertainment of exposure (Maximum: *)	Comparability on the basis of the design or analysis (Maximum: **)	Assessment of outcome (Maximum: *)	Adequacy of follow-up (Maximum: *)	
Flieger (2019)			*		*	*	3
Bayani et al. (2019)			*		*	*	3
Holzinger et al. (2014)	*		*	*	*	*	5
Tripodakis et al. (2012)			*		*	*	3
Caicedo-Rubio et al. (2017)			*		*	*	3
Favia et al. (2015)			*		*	*	3
Junquera et al. (2011)			*		*	*	3
Kwon et al. (2014)	*		*	*	*	*	5
Shirota et al. (2009)			*		*		2
Yajima et al. (2017)	*	*	*	**	*	*	7
Favia et al. (2011)			*		*	*	3
Jacobsen et al. (2013)	*		*	*	*	*	5
Storelli et al. (2019)			*		*	*	3

Figure 2. Qualitative assessment of the studies by the Modified Newcastle-Ottawa Quality Assessment scale for Cohort and Case-Control Studies (m-NOS). (Flieger (2019) [15]; Bayani et al. (2019) [21]; Holzinger et al. (2014) [14]; Tripodakis et al. (2012) [16]; Caicedo-Rubio et al. (2017) [23]; Favia et al. (2015) [22]; Junquera et al. (2011) [24]; Kwon et al. (2014) [17]; Shirota et al. (2009) [25]; Yajima et al. (2017) [18]; Favia et al. (2011) [26]; Jacobsen et al. (2013) [19]; Storelli et al. (2019) [20]). * 1 point for the score; ** 2 points for the score.

Table 3. Characteristics of the patients and implants studied.

	Authors (Year)	Country	Research Question	Patient Information	Design (n)	Pacient Status/Implant	N. of Implants Assessed (Site)	Risk Factors	Results
1	Flieger (2019) [15]	Poland	Placement of two missing teeth with insertion of immediate implants in a patient medicated with BPs	F, 56 yo	n = 1; case report	Absence of bone loss in both implants; normal peri-implant soft tissue condition (no signs of inflammation)	2 (15, 24)	Hypertension	implant survival
2	Bayani et al. (2019) [21]	Iran	Report of implant placement in a patient with MRONJ	M, 54 yo	n = 1; case report	Minimal bone loss	1 (14)	Non-smoking, good oral hygiene	implant survival
3	Holzinger et al. (2014) [14]	Austria	Development of MRONJ in patients treated with BPs who received implants.	F; average of 65.7 ± 8.5 yo	n = 13; retrospective study	NR	1 (47)	7 former smokers; and 5 smokers	Implant failure (MRONJ)
4	Tripodakis et al. (2012) [16]	Greece	Care in the placement of implants and prevention of MRONJ in patients with BP therapy	F, 70 and 65 yo	n = 2; case report	No observed complications	3 (14, 15, 17) 14 (13, 14, 16, 17, 25, 26, 27, 28, 36, 37, 38, 46, 47, 48)	1 with hypertension and hyperlipidemia	implant survival
5	Caicedo-Rubio et al. (2017) [23]	Spain	Insertion of implants in a patient treated with IV bisphosphonates	M, 61 yo	n = 1; case report	Generalized gingival inflammation; peri-implant tissues without inflammation; loss of 1.25 mm of crestal bone in the implant area 36	3 (36, 37, 46)	Smoker (20 cigarettes/day); Stroke prior to 2007; poor oral hygiene	implant survival
6	Favia et al. (2015) [22]	Italy	Patient with breast cancer affected by MRONJ	F, 66 yo	n = 1; case report	Pain; purulent secretion; right-sided inferior alveolar nerve paresthesia	7 (16, 31, 35, 36, 41, 44, 46)	Poor oral hygiene	Implant failure (MRONJ)
7	Junquera et al. (2011) [24]	Spain	Mandibular dental implant placement in a patient with MRONJ	M, 59 yo	n = 1; case report	Left lower lip paresthesia; purulent discharge; necrotic bone	2	NR	Implant failure (MRONJ)
8	Kwon et al. (2014) [17]	Korea	Analysis of MRONJ characteristics around dental implants	2 M, 17 F; 42 to 85 yo	n = 19; prospective study	Necrotic bone exposure, purulent discharge; fistula; swelling for more than 8 weeks	23	Hypertension; and Diabetes	Implant failure (MRONJ)

Table 3. *Cont.*

	Authors (Year)	Country	Research Question	Patient Information	Design (n)	Pacient Status/Implant	N. of Implants Assessed (Site)	Risk Factors	Results
9	Shirota et al. (2009) [25]	Japan	MRONJ around implants in maxillary molars	F, 54 yo	n = 1; case report	Pain; bone exposure; redness; swelling	3 (15, 25, 27)	NR	Implant failure (MRONJ)
10	Yajima et al. (2017) [18]	Japan	BMD and influence of the use of BP's on early implant failure	F, >60 yo	n = 11; retrospective study	NR	25	Diabetes, smoking, steroid, poor oral hygiene were excluded	Implant survival and failure cases
11	Favia et al. (2011) [26]	Italy	Occurrence of MRONJ after implant insertion	F, 65 yo	n = 1; case report	non-loading	2 (35, 36)	No pre-existing bone lesions	Implant failure (MRONJ)
12	Jacobsen et al. (2013) [19]	Switzerland	Report of 14 patients with mandibular osteopathology associated with BP therapy and dental implant insertion	11 F and 3 M	n = 14; case series	purulent; periapical radiolucency surrounding the implants	23	NR	Implant failure (MRONJ)
13	Storelli et al. (2019) [20]	Italy	MRONJ after implant placement in a patient undergoing oral BF therapy	F, 77 years old	n = 1; case report	Necrotic bone; pain; abscess; nerve paresthesia; fistula; exposed bone; lack of healing	8	Non-smoking, hypothyroidism, hypercholesterolemia, hypertension, arterial fibrillation	Implant failure (MRONJ)

BMD = bone mineral density; BP = bisphosphonates; F = female; M = male; wk = weeks; y = years; yo = years old; NR = not reported.

Table 4. Comparison of the characteristics of the variables studied.

	Authors (Year)	BP Type	BP Generation	Route of Administration	Antibiotic Treatment	Duration	Patient/Implant Status	Type of the Dental Implant	Risk Factors	Implant Failure Rate (%)
1	Flieger (2019) [15]	Alendronate	2nd	Oral 70 mg/week for 24 months	Before surgery amoxicillin + clavulanic acid. 1000 mg day/7 days	No discontinuation	Absence of bone loss; normal condition of peri-implant soft tissue (no signs of inflammation)	ICX-plus (3.45 × 10 mm) at bone level	Hypertension	0%
2	Bayani et al. (2019) [21]	Zoledronate	3rd	IV 3.5 mg/month for 22 months	Before surgery 2 g amoxicillin/clavulanic acid. After: 1000 mg 2×/day/7 days	Discontinued 6 months before surgery and resumed 8 months after	Minimal bone loss	Superline; Dentium (3.6 × 10 mm)	Non-smoking, good oral hygiene	0%
3	Holzinger et al. (2014) [14]	Zolendronate (n = 7) Alendronate (n = 3) Pamidronate (n = 2) Ibandronate (n = 1)	3rd (n = 8) 2nd (n = 5)	7—IV 4 mg/month 3—Oral 70 mg/week 2—Oral 90 mg/month 1—IV 3 mg each 3 months	NR	3—BPs after implant placement 3—BPs before implant placement 7—BPs before and after implant placement	NR	NR	7 former smokers; and 5 smokers	63.8%
4	Tripodakis et al. (2012) [16]	Risedronate Alendronate	2nd 3rd	1—Oral for 2 months 1—Oral for 4 years	24 h before surgery 500 mg of amoxicillin up to 10 days after surgery	Discontinued 3 months before surgery and resumed 3 months after surgery	No complications observed	Branemark System Mk III Groovy a 13 mm; SPI, Alpha Bio 16 mm	1 with hypertension and hyperlipidemia	0%
5	Caicedo-Rubio et al. (2017) [23]	Zoledronate	3rd	IV 5 mg each 6 months for 4 years	Before surgery, amoxicillin 500 mg every 8 h until 6 days after surgery	Discontinued 2 months before surgery and resumed 1 month after	Generalized gingival inflamation; peri-implants good health; 1.25 mm loss of of crestal bone in the implant area 36	MIS Implants Technologies LTD 7.5 × 10 mm and 75 × 11.5 mm subcrestal	Smoker (20 cigarettes/day); Stroke prior to 2007; poor oral hygiene	0%
6	Favia et al. (2015) [22]	Zoledronate	3rd	IV 4 mg monthly for 33 months	NR	6 months after implant placement	Pain; pus secretion; right inferior alveolar nerve paresthesia	NR	Poor oral hygiene	57.1%
7	Junquera et al. (2011) [24]	Zoledronate	3rd	IV 4 mg monthly	NR	9 months after implant placement	Lower left labial paraesthesia; purulent secretion; necrotic bone	Endosseous dental implants	NR	50%

Table 4. Cont.

	Authors (Year)	BP Type	BP Generation	Route of Administration	Antibiotic Treatment	Duration	Patient/Implant Status	Type of the Dental Implant	Risk Factors	Implant Failure Rate (%)
8	Kwon et al. (2014) [17]	Zolendronate Alendronate Ibandronate Risedronate	3rd 2nd	Oral ou IV	NR	Started before surgery (n = 16) and after (n = 3)	Necrotic bone exposure, pus secretion; fistula; swelling for more than 8 weeks	NR	Hypertension; and Diabetes	15.8%
9	Shirota et al. (2009) [25]	Pamidronate Zolendronate	2nd 3rd	IV (P 17 times and Zolendronate 9 times) in 16 months	NR	4 years after implant placement	Pain; bone exposure; redness; swelling	NR	NR	66.7%
10	Yajima et al. (2017) [18]	Alendronate	2nd	Oral	NR	No discontinuation. Using BF: 3.8 + 2.1 years	NR	NR	Diabetes, smoking, steroid, poor oral hygiene were excluded	12%
11	Favia et al. (2011) [26]	Clodronate	1st	IV 300 mg twice a month	NR	Discontinuation 3 months before surgery	Purulent secretion; periapical radiolucency surrounding the implants	NR	No pre-existing bone lesions	100%
12	Jacobsen et al. (2013) [19]	9— Zoledronate 2— Alendronate 1— Ibandronate 2— Pamidronate	2nd 3rd	IV e Oral in 3 months	NR	NR	Necrotic bone; ache; abscess; nerve paraesthesia; fistula; exposed bone; no healing	NR	NR	100%
13	Storelli et al. (2019) [20]	Alendronate	2nd	Oral 70 mg once a week	NR	No discontinuation. Use started 3 years before surgery	Inflamed peri-implant tissues; bleeding on probing; bone resorption < 2 mm around implants; purulent secretions; exposure of necrotic bone; mobility	NR	Non-smoking, hypothyroidism, hypercholesterolemia, hypertension, arterial fibrillation	100%

BP, bisphosphonate; BRONJ, bisphosphonate-related osteonecrosis of the jaw; IV, intravenous.

4. Discussion

The objective of the present systematic review was to analyze the negative influence of BPs on dental implant osseointegration. Of the 67 Caucasian patients who were included, there was a predominance of females (58 patients) most of whom were in an age for menopause, over 50 years old, and had an elevated risk for osteoporosis [27]. On the other hand, male patients constituted the minority (9 individuals). That pathology can be diagnosed in other age groups and also in men. Worldwide, this pathology affects a total of 200 million women, with a growing trend in North America and Europe [28].

4.1. BP Use and Dental Implants

BPs are prescribed in several pathologies, whether they affect the bone (osteoporosis, OI, Paget's disease) or in malignant pathologies (malignant hypercalcemia, bone metastases, lung and breast cancer, and MM), because they prevent bone resorption. Of the studies included in this systematic review, 44 patients had osteoporosis, 8 had MM, 10 had breast cancer, 2 had lung cancer, 1 had prostate cancer, 1 had Langerhans cell histiocytosis, and 1 had OI. The administration of BPs is more prevalent in patients with osteoporosis, since, as reported in the literature, this is one of the most common bone pathologies in developed countries and one which has the most indication for the prescription of these drugs due to the risk of occurrence of bone fractures [29].

Of all the studies included, the presence of patients undergoing therapy with second generation (Alendronate, Pamidronate) [14–20,25] and third generation BPs (Risedronate, Zoledronate and Ibandronate) [14,16,17,19,21–25] were greater than the use of first generation (Clodronate) [26]. The first generation seems to show a decreasing trend in use nowadays. On the other hand, the failure rate for osseointegration proved to be lower in patients who used therapy with second generation of BPs (about 37%) compared to patients who had therapy with first and third generations. Second generation BPs have been shown to be a well-tolerated drug, with low side effects. This fact has been shown through their growing use in recent years [30].

The interruption of therapy with BPs was a parameter with varied results in this systematic review, from patients who did not discontinue to patients who discontinued for 2, 3, or 6 months before surgery, with respective resumption for 1, 3, or 8 months after surgery. Tripodakis et al. [16] reported the case of two female patients, both in their seventh decade of life, who requested rehabilitation with implant placement. The patients were medicated with second and third generation BPs (Alendronate and Risedronate). After consultation with the attending physician, the patients discontinued BPs 3 months before and resumed 3 months after implant placement. They received antibiotic therapy after surgical interventions, and the treatment plan was completed uneventfully and without complications during a 2-year follow up. In another study, Flieger [15] reported the case of a female patient (56 years old), who intended to carry out the prosthetic reconstruction of the crown of two molars lost in the maxilla with the placement of two implants. She was medicated with Alendronate (a second-generation BP) for osteoporosis. There was no bone loss around both implants, and it was observed that the peri-implant soft tissue did not show any signs of inflammation. Bayani et al. [21] reported that the placement of dental implants in patients with MM undergoing therapy with third generation BPs (Zoledronate) can be performed. Therefore, a meticulous selection of cases, an adequate medical consultation, and a minimally invasive surgery should be considered.

Flieger [15], Yajima et al. [18], and Storelli et al. [20] recommended that patients (n = 13) not interrupt their therapy with BPs during implant placement surgery. Fliger [15] and Yajima et al. [18] obtained a low failure rate in the implant placement procedure of 0% and 12% respectively. On the contrary, Storelli et al. [20] had a complete failure rate (100%). Similarly, in the study carried out by Kwon et al. [17], a complete failure of implant placement was observed in patients who started therapy with BPs before implant placement surgery.

Otherwise, Bayani et al. [21] reported the discontinuation of BP therapy for 6 months before surgery that was resumed therapy 8 months after surgery. The failure rate was 0%, and no complications were observed. The same happened with Tripodakis et al. [16] who interrupted therapy 3 months before the surgery and resumed it for 3 months after. After 17 implants were placed, none of them failed. Caicedo-Rubio et al. [23] discontinued the therapy 2 months before the surgery and resumed it 1 month later, and they also obtained 0% for implant failure rate. This fact suggests an association between discontinuing BP therapy with a low rate of dental implant failure (around 45%) than for non-interruption therapy (around 55%). These data may still be different depending on the involvement of risk factors. Moreover, the cumulative dose and duration of drug exposure, medical comorbidities (corticosteroids, diabetes, immunosuppressive conditions), and dental co-morbidities (extractions, implant placement, invasive procedures, periodontal disease, trauma, infection) must be verified. In this way, all the most invasive dental procedures constitute a risk when we are facing patients who use BPs.

According to Holzinger et al. [14], the occurrence of complications seems to be delayed when dental implants are inserted before starting BP therapy. However, the incidence of complications seems to be higher when implants are placed after BP treatment or during its therapy. Thus, it is suggested as ideal to proceed with implant placement before initiating BPs therapy; once therapy is started, the risk becomes higher.

Specifically, for four studies without implant failure [15,16,21,23], all cases reported types of study that must be carefully interpreted, due to the low level of scientific weight, Bayani et al. [21] found excellent results after a 1-year follow up in a 54-year-old man patient with multiple myeloma (MM) who complained of difficulty in mastication and esthetical concern for his upper anterior teeth. He received a monthly infusion of 3.5 mg of the IV BP drug Zoledronate for a period of 22 months, which is considered a long period and a high-risk treatment. The other two studies, Flieger [15] and Tripodakis et al. [16], had 2-year follow up periods without complications and bone loss. Similar results were obtained by Caicedo-Rubio et al. [23], after 4-year follow up, which showed no evidence of pathology in the peri-implant tissues.

4.2. Dental Implants Characteristics

Flieger [15] performed a surgical procedure using two implants with widths of 3.45 mm and lengths of 10 mm at the tissue level. Bayani et al. [21] opted for the placement of a bone-level implant that was 3.6 mm in diameter and 10 mm in length. Tripodakis et al. [16] placed a total of 17 implants that were 13 mm long at the bone level. Caicedo-Rubio et al. [23] placed three implants of 3.75 × 10 mm and 3.75 × 11.5 mm at the subcrestal level; Junquera et al. [24] placed two subcrestal implants. All these implants showed a significantly acceptable success rate, except for the implants placed by Junquera et al. [24], which resulted in severe complications and implant failure due to the MRONJ. The literature showed in the Hammerle et al.'s study [31] that the placement of implants at the subcrestal level was not recommended for these types of patients, who can achieve greater marginal bone loss [32].

4.3. Implants Associated with Risk Factors

Implant placement can also be influenced by risk factors, local or systemic, which can lead to complications. This includes cases of smoker patients, patients with pathologies (diabetes), with poor oral hygiene, and with a history of recent stroke (first 6 months after the episode) [33]. According to several authors, the risk of implant failure is greater with the increase in the number of cigarettes smoked per day; therefore, this factor is considered a real risk factor for implant placement [14]. On the other hand, Caicedo-Rubio et al. [23] reported that smoker patients and those with poor oral hygiene had favorable results for the implants. These data must be carefully analyzed due to the reduced sample size present in the study. This fact has led researchers to exclude from their studies all smoker patients,

patients with diabetes, those using steroids, or those with poor oral hygiene, precisely because of the higher implant failure risk [18].

In our study, we found a somewhat significant failure rate in the case of smoker patients (19%), patients who had diabetes (7%), hypertensive patients (8%), and those who had poor oral hygiene (2%). However, even though the patients did not present any risk factor, they had very similar failure rates to those with risk factors. In the case of diabetes mellitus, this was closely related to oral health. From the data available to date, it increases the susceptibility to infection and impairs the tissue healing. In addition, there is evidence that patients with diabetes are more likely to develop complications than patients without this pathology [17].

4.4. MRONJ and Route of Administration

Several studies have focused on the risk factors for MRONJ development with the treatment of IV BPs (nitrogenated) and performing tooth extractions (identified as important risk factors) [10]. There is scientific evidence showing that drugs (Pamidronate and Zolendronate) whose route of administration is exclusively IV have been strongly associated with cases of MRONJ [19]. This can be explained because these drugs are more potent and have greater bioavailability due to the type of administration (IV).

For this purpose, Shirota et al. [25] described a case of a 54-year-old woman with gum ulceration, bone exposure, and intense spontaneous pain around implants. The patient in question had undergone IV therapy with BPs (Pamidronate and Zolendronate) for 2 years to treat bone metastases from breast cancer. The authors reported MRONJ related to BPs, with symptoms of necrotic bone for more than 8 weeks; the patient did not undergo radiotherapy in the maxillofacial area.

Drugs, such as Alendronate and Risedronate, are administered exclusively orally. It has been reported that these drugs are safer and have a lower risk of MRONJ [16]. This was observed in the Flieger's study [15] of a a 56-year-old woman who underwent rehabilitation of two missing molars in the maxilla. She was taking oral Alendronate and, during the time of osteoporosis treatment with Alendronate, there were no episodes of MRONJ.

Upon analyzing the studies included in this systematic review, it was not possible to be precise in presenting the failure rates for both routes of administration, due to the lack of data provided by the studies. Nevertheless, there was a consensus among authors that the IV route of administration results in a high number of failure cases. Thus, the oral route of administration still seems to be the safest route.

4.5. MRONJ and Implant Failure

MRONJ can be manifested through several signs and symptoms. Its development may present clinical manifestations such as the presence of pain, necrotic bone, bone exposure, the presence of purulent secretion, redness, abscess, swelling, paresthesia of the right inferior alveolar nerve, an ill-defined radiolucent area, bleeding upon probing, bone resorption around the implants, and the presence of mobility. These symptoms can persist for more than 8 weeks. It is a problem with a multifactorial origin; it is difficult to predict its occurrence.

Favia et al. [22] showed failure in four of the seven implants placed in the same patient that were related to the occurrence of MRONJ. In this case, the reported symptoms were essentially pain, the presence of purulent secretion, and paresthesia of the inferior alveolar nerve on the right side associated with an ill-defined radiolucent area that extended from the right posterior mandible to the opposite region of the premolar. These data were attributed to the patient's poor oral hygiene. As for the remaining implants that still showed acceptable osseointegration, it was not possible to conclude what would be the long-term prognosis, since the follow-up only occurred after 18 months.

Similar results happened with Junquera et al. [24]. The patient had two implants presenting features compatible with MRONJ (necrotic bone, left lower lip paresthesia, and purulent secretion in only one of the implants). Also, Shirota et al. [25] reported a case with three implants placed; two of them presented pain, bone exposure, redness, and swelling.

On the other hand, we had cases, in this study, where there was complete failure of the implants, and all patients developed MRONJ. Kwon et al. [17] and Jacobsen et al. [19] obtained the same results from evaluating a total of 23 implants, which all failed with reports of necrotic bone exposure, purulent secretion, pain, abscess, paresthesia, fistula, and swelling for more than 8 weeks.

Storelli et al. [20] reported a case of MRONJ in a 77-year-old female patient. After receiving oral implant rehabilitation and an immediate-load fixed prosthesis in the maxilla, she began to report pain and purulent secretions, which were neglected by the responsible professional. She returned to see the same professional after another episode of acute pain. The fixed prosthesis was removed and exposure of necrotic bone around the implants was observed. In this case, all implants failed. The patient was submitted to surgery to remove necrotic bone blocks. This was the most severe case analyzed in this systematic review.

4.6. Study Limitations

One of the main limitations of this study was the non-inclusion of randomized clinical trials. This occurred because there is scarce and limited literature. It was confirmed by the analysis of the quality of the included studies, in which the majority were classified as low and moderate quality. Several variables were studied that likely caused bias in analyzing the influence of BPs on implant placement. However, we presented the most clinically relevant results that can be interpreted from a trend perspective. Some of the studies included in this systematic review did not include all information regarding the influence of the route of administration on the implant failure rate. This situation made a statistical treatment of the variable under analysis impossible. Thus, it is suggested that, in a future investigation, the exploration of this theme be continued and that a longitudinal cohort study be developed.

5. Conclusions

Within the limitation of this systematic review, it was possible to conclude that a high mean for failure rate of implant osseointegration (49.96%) was found, regardless of the generation of BPs used. Moreover, the failure rate was lower in patients using second generation BPs (Alendronate and Pamidronate) and when there was an interruption of the BP therapy when placing implants when compared, respectively, with third generation and the continuous administration. Otherwise, it was higher with the IV administration compared to the oral administration of BPs. Furthermore, if the patients were smokers, diabetic, had hypertension, or poor oral hygiene, they were more prone to failure of the implants placed. However, more studies must be conducted to better understand the clinical findings associated with BPs and implant therapy.

Funding: This research received no external funding.

Conflicts of Interest: The authors declare no conflict of interest.

References

1. Jayesh, R.S.; Dhinakarsamy, V. Osseointegration. *J. Pharm. Bioallied Sci.* **2015**, *7*, 226–229.
2. Albrektsson, T.; Wennerberg, A. On osseointegration in relation to implant surfaces. *Clin. Implant Dent. Relat. Res.* **2019**, *21*, 4–7. [CrossRef]
3. Borges, H.; Correia, A.R.M.; Castilho, R.M.; Fernandes, G.V.O. Zirconia Implants and Marginal Bone Loss: A Systematic Review and Meta-Analysis of Clinical Studies. *Int. J. Oral Maxillofac. Implants* **2020**, *35*, 707–720. [CrossRef]
4. Fernandes, G.V.O.; Costa, B.M.G.N.; Trindade, H.F.; Castilho, R.M.; Fernandes, J.C.H. Comparative analysis between extra-short implants (≤6 mm) and 6 mm-longer implants: A meta-analysis of randomized controlled trial. *Aust. Dent. J.* **2022**, *67*, 194–211. [CrossRef]
5. Fernandes, P.R.E.; Otero, A.I.P.; Fernandes, J.C.H.; Nassani, L.M.; Castilho, R.M.; Fernandes, G.V.O. Clinical Performance Comparing Titanium and Titanium-Zirconium or Zirconia Dental Implants: A Systematic Review of Randomized Controlled Trials. *Dent. J.* **2022**, *10*, 83. [CrossRef]
6. Hanawa, T. Zirconia versus titanium in dentistry: A review. *Dent. Mater. J.* **2020**, *39*, 24–36. [CrossRef]

7. Sivaraman, K.; Chopra, A.; Narayan, A.I.; Balakrishnan, D. Is zirconia a viable alternative to titanium for oral implant? A critical review. *J. Prosthodont. Res.* **2018**, *62*, 121–133. [CrossRef]
8. Cremers, S.; Drake, M.T.; Ebetino, F.H.; Bilezikian, J.P.; Russell, R.G.G. Pharmacology of bisphosphonates. *Br. J. Clin. Pharmacol.* **2019**, *85*, 1052–1062. [CrossRef]
9. Nayak, S. Application of bisphosphonates in dentistry: A review of literature. *Indian J. Public Health Res. Dev.* **2019**, *10*, 299–303. [CrossRef]
10. Gelazius, R.; Poskevicius, L.; Sakavicius, D.; Grimuta, V.; Juodzbalys, G. Dental Implant Placement in Patients on Bisphosphonate Therapy: A Systematic Review. *J. Oral Maxillofac. Res.* **2018**, *9*, e2. [CrossRef]
11. Freitas, N.R.; Lima, L.B.; Moura, M.B.; Veloso-Guedes, C.C.F.; Simamoto-Júnior, P.C.; Magalhães, D. Bisphosphonate treatment and dental implants: A systematic review. *Med. Oral Patol. Oral Cir. Bucal* **2016**, *21*, e644–e651.
12. Chen, B.; Li, Y.; Yang, X.; Xu, H.; Xie, D. Zoledronic acid enhances bone-implant osseointegration more than alendronate and strontium ranelate in ovariectomized rats. *Osteoporos Int.* **2013**, *24*, 2115–2121. [CrossRef]
13. Basso, F.G.; Pansani, T.N.; Soares, D.G.; Cardoso, L.M.; Hebling, J.; de Souza Costa, C.A. Influence of bisphosphonates on the adherence and metabolism of epithelial cells and gingival fibroblasts to titanium surfaces. *Clin. Oral Investig.* **2018**, *22*, 893–900. [CrossRef]
14. Holzinger, D.; Seemann, R.; Matoni, N.; Ewers, R.; Millesi, W.; Wutzl, A. Effect of dental implants on bisphosphonate-related osteonecrosis of the jaws. *J. Oral Maxillofac. Surg.* **2014**, *72*, e1–e8. [CrossRef]
15. Flieger, R. Bilateral bone ridge splitting in maxilla with immediate implant placement in a patient with osteoporosis: A clinical report with 2-year follow-up. *Case Rep. Dent.* **2019**, *6*, 1458571. [CrossRef]
16. Tripodakis, A.P.; Kamperos, G.; Nikitakis, N.; Sklavounou-Andrikopoulou, A. Implant therapy on patients treated with oral bisphosphonates. *J. Osseointegration* **2012**, *4*, 9–14.
17. Kwon, T.G.; Lee, C.O.; Park, J.W.; Choi, S.Y.; Rijal, G.; Shin, H.I. Osteonecrosis associated with dental implants in patients undergoing bisphosphonate treatment. *Clin. Oral Implants Res.* **2014**, *25*, 632–640. [CrossRef]
18. Yajima, N.; Munakata, M.; Fuchigami, K.; Sanda, M.; Kasugai, S. Influence of bisphosphonates on implant failure rates and characteristics of postmenopausal woman mandibular jawbone. *J. Oral Implantol.* **2017**, *43*, 345–349. [CrossRef]
19. Jacobsen, C.; Metzler, P.; Rössle, M.; Obwegeser, J.; Zemann, W.; Grätz, K.W. Osteopathology induced by bisphosphonates and dental implants: Clinical observations. *Clin. Oral Investig.* **2013**, *17*, 167–175. [CrossRef]
20. Storelli, S.; Storelli, S.; Palandrani, G.; Dondi, C.; Tagliatesta, L.; Rossi, A. Severe case of Osteonecrosis following implant placement in a patient in therapy with bisphosphonates: A case report. *J. Oral Implantol.* **2019**, *45*, 139–144. [CrossRef]
21. Bayani, M.; Anooshirvani, A.A.; Keivan, M.; Mohammad-Rabei, E. Dental implant in a multiple myeloma patient undergoing bisphosphonate therapy: A case report. *Clin. Case Rep.* **2019**, *7*, 1043–1048. [CrossRef]
22. Favia, G.; Tempesta, A.; Limongelli, L.; Crincoli, V.; Piattelli, A.; Maiorano, E. Metastatic breast cancer in medication-related osteonecrosis around mandibular implants. *Am. J. Case Rep.* **2015**, *16*, 621–626. [CrossRef]
23. Caicedo-Rubio, M.; Ferrés-Amat, E.; Ferrés-Padró, E. Implant-supported fixed prostheses in a Patient with Osteogenesis Imperfecta: A 4-year follow-up. *J. Clin. Exp. Dent.* **2017**, *9*, e1482–e1486. [CrossRef]
24. Junquera, L.; Gallego, L.; Pelaz, A. Multiple Myeloma and Bisphosphonate-Related Osteonecrosis of the Mandible Associated with Dental Implants. *Case Rep. Dent.* **2011**, *2011*, 568246. [CrossRef]
25. Shirota, T.; Nakamura, A.; Matsui, Y.; Hatori, M.; Nakamura, M.; Shintani, S. Bisphosphonate-related osteonecrosis of the jaw around dental implants in the maxilla: Report of a case: Case Report. *Clin. Oral Implants Res.* **2009**, *20*, 1402–1408. [CrossRef]
26. Favia, G.; Piattelli, A.; Sportelli, P.; Capodiferro, S.; Iezzi, G. Osteonecrosis of the Posterior Mandible after Implant Insertion: A Clinical and Histological Case Report. *Clin. Implant Dent. Relat. Res.* **2011**, *13*, 58–63. [CrossRef]
27. Kanis, J.A.; Cooper, C.; Rizzoli, R.; Reginster, J.Y. Correction to: European guidance for the diagnosis and management of osteoporosis in postmenopausal women. *Osteoporos Int.* **2020**, *31*, 209. [CrossRef]
28. Lane, N.E. Epidemiology, etiology, and diagnosis of osteoporosis. *Am. J. Obstet. Gynecol.* **2006**, *194*, S3–S11. [CrossRef]
29. Serrano, A.J.; Begoña, L.; Anitua, E.; Cobos, R.; Orive, G. Systematic review and meta-analysis of the efficacy and safety of alendronate and zoledronate for the treatment of postmenopausal osteoporosis. *Gynecol. Endocrinol.* **2013**, *29*, 1005–1014. [CrossRef]
30. Aghaloo, T.; Pi-Anfruns, J.; Moshaverinia, A.; Sim, D.; Grogan, T.; Hadaya, D. The Effects of Systemic Diseases and Medications on Implant Osseointegration: A Systematic Review. *Int. J. Oral Maxillofac. Implants* **2019**, *34*, s35–s49. [CrossRef]
31. Hämmerle, C.H.; Brägger, U.; Bürgin, W.; Lang, N.P. The effect of subcrestal placement of the polished surface of ITI implants on marginal soft and hard tissues. *Clin. Oral Implants Res.* **1996**, *7*, 11–119. [CrossRef]
32. Pellicer-Chover, H.; Peñarrocha-Diago, M.; Peñarrocha-Oltra, D.; Gomar-Vercher, S.; Agustín-Panadero, R.; Peñarrocha-Diago, M. Impact of crestal and subcrestal implant placement in peri-implant bone: A prospective comparative study. *Med. Oral Patol. Oral Cir. Bucal* **2016**, *21*, e103–e110. [CrossRef]
33. Hwang, D.; Wang, H.L. Medical contraindications to implant therapy: Part I: Absolute contraindications. *Implant Dent.* **2006**, *15*, 353–360. [CrossRef]

Disclaimer/Publisher's Note: The statements, opinions and data contained in all publications are solely those of the individual author(s) and contributor(s) and not of MDPI and/or the editor(s). MDPI and/or the editor(s) disclaim responsibility for any injury to people or property resulting from any ideas, methods, instructions or products referred to in the content.

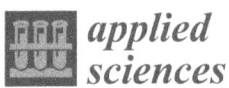

Article

Evaluation of the Trueness of Digital Implant Impressions According to the Implant Scan Body Orientation and Scanning Method

Bora Lee [1], Na-Eun Nam [2], Seung-Ho Shin [2], Jung-Hwa Lim [2], June-Sung Shim [3] and Jong-Eun Kim [3,*]

1 Department of Dental Education, Yonsei University College of Dentistry, Yonsei-ro 50-1, Seodaemun-gu, Seoul 03722, Korea; breezelee7@yuhs.ac
2 BK21 FOUR Project, Department of Prosthodontics, Yonsei University College of Dentistry, Yonsei-ro 50-1, Seodaemun-gu, Seoul 03722, Korea; jennynam5703@prostholabs.com (N.-E.N.); shin506@prostholabs.com (S.-H.S.); erin0313@prostholabs.com (J.-H.L.)
3 Department of Prosthodontics, Yonsei University College of Dentistry, Yonsei-ro 50-1, Seodaemun-gu, Seoul 03722, Korea; jfshim@yuhs.ac
* Correspondence: gomyou@yuhs.ac; Tel.: +82-2-2228-3160

Featured Application: This study presents a strategy for operators to acquire more accurate digital impressions in single implant cases in terms of the orientation of the scan body and the scanning method.

Abstract: This study investigated the trueness of a digital implant impression according to the orientation of the implant scan body (ISB) and the scanning method. With the flat surface of the ISB facing either the buccal or proximal direction, the ISB was scanned using one tabletop scanner (T500) and three types of intraoral scanner (TRIOS 3, CS3600, and i500). The effects of differences in the scanning method and ISB orientation were assessed. Postalignment data were subsequently obtained with the abutments generated using a digital library, and superimposed with reference data using a best-fit algorithm, followed by root-mean-square error (RMSE) analysis. The RMSE was lower in the buccal groups (28.15 ± 8.87 μm, mean ± SD) than in the proximal groups (31.94 ± 8.95 μm, $p = 0.031$), and lower in the full-scan groups (27.92 ± 10.80 μm) than in the partial-scan groups (32.16 ± 6.35 μm, $p = 0.016$). When using the tabletop scanner, the trueness was higher when the ISB was connected buccally (14.34 ± 0.89 μm) than when it was connected proximally (29.35 ± 1.15 μm, $p < 0.001$). From the findings of this study it can be concluded that the operator should connect the ISB so that its flat surface faces the buccal direction, and attempt to scan all areas. Additionally, it is advantageous to connect an ISB buccally when using a tabletop scanner.

Keywords: dental implant; digital impression; scan body; trueness; CAD/CAM

Citation: Lee, B.; Nam, N.-E.; Shin, S.-H.; Lim, J.-H.; Shim, J.-S.; Kim, J.-E. Evaluation of the Trueness of Digital Implant Impressions According to the Implant Scan Body Orientation and Scanning Method. *Appl. Sci.* **2021**, *11*, 3027. https://doi.org/10.3390/app11073027

Academic Editor: Bruno Chrcanovic

Received: 25 February 2021
Accepted: 24 March 2021
Published: 29 March 2021

Publisher's Note: MDPI stays neutral with regard to jurisdictional claims in published maps and institutional affiliations.

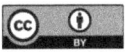

Copyright: © 2021 by the authors. Licensee MDPI, Basel, Switzerland. This article is an open access article distributed under the terms and conditions of the Creative Commons Attribution (CC BY) license (https://creativecommons.org/licenses/by/4.0/).

1. Introduction

Manufacturing an accurate dental prosthesis requires an accurate impression to be obtained. Precision impression materials, such as polyether and polyvinyl siloxane, have traditionally been used to fabricate fixed prostheses, and these have been selected by many clinicians for decades due to their excellent volume stability and precision [1]. However, the traditional method has inherent errors due to the shrinkage of the impression material during polymerization and expansion of the gypsum. The dimensional stability of the impression materials is also affected by the temperature, the time taken to make a model after taking the impression, the surface wettability of the gypsum, and the disinfection process [2–6].

Taking an impression for an implant prosthesis requires accurately transferring the position and orientation of the implant fixture, as well as the relationship with surrounding structures, such as the adjacent teeth, onto the master cast. An inaccurate impression procedure may result in a poor fit of the prosthesis and biological and mechanical complications [7]. In addition, errors on the occlusal and proximal sides of the resulting implant crown may occur, possibly lengthening the operating time for repairing the prosthesis or causing discomfort to the patient, or even requiring remanufacturing [8].

The high accuracy of optical scanners allows digital impressions to be applied in various fields of dentistry, not only to produce inlays, onlays, crowns, and fixed partial dentures, but also to fabricate implant prostheses by capturing the three-dimensional (3D) position of the implant [9,10]. Digital impression-taking has the advantages of creating a virtual model using an optical method, easy standardization, and high interoperator repeatability [11]. In particular, in the case of direct digitalization using an intraoral scanner, information in the oral cavity is acquired without the process of taking impressions and producing the work model. This makes the processing time efficient and also comfortable for the patient, particularly for those with a heightened gagging reflex [12,13].

In the digital implant impression process, instead of using an impression coping, an implant scan body (ISB) is connected to the implant fixture before performing the scanning process, and information, such as the depth or direction of the implant fixture placed in the alveolar bone, is obtained. ISBs have various sizes and shapes, and the scan region has an asymmetrical shape and contains important information about the angle and orientation of the implant [14]. The position of the ISB in the dentition is recorded through optical scanning, and the library information for the ISB and the implant is used to reproduce the position of the implant fixture connected to each ISB and the abutment using CAD (Computer Aided Design) software. The reproduced data are then used in CAD software to design a prosthesis that is subsequently produced using CAM (Computer Aided Manufacturing) [15].

Factors affecting the accuracy of digital implant impressions using intraoral scanners and ISBs include the angle and depth of the implant, the implant-to-implant distance, implant location, geometry variance, scanning method, and ISB materials and designs [16–23]. Most previous studies have investigated either complete or partial but multiple edentulous cases, and there have been very few studies on the accuracy of implant digital impressions according to the ISB orientation or scanning method in cases of single implants. One previous study found that the deficiency of the scanned image of the ISB affects the position of the virtual implant in the single implant case, but that study only considered a single oral scanner, and it simulated deficient scan images experimentally after completing the scanning procedure [24].

According to the International Organization for Standardization, accuracy consists of trueness and precision [25]. Trueness is the deviation of the test results from its reference value, whereas precision is the deviation between the test results. The methods of measuring the accuracy of the intraoral scanners have been either two-dimensional or three-dimensional, and the three-dimensional measuring method using superimposition is advantageous because it also evaluates local errors three-dimensionally [26]. In order to evaluate the trueness in three dimensions, data obtained by industrial optical or desktop scanners are required as a reference. On the other hand, since precision measures the repeatability between test results, the reference is not required, and it is sufficient to measure the deviation between the test results.

The purpose of the present study was to compare the trueness of digital implant impressions in a single implant case according to two variables: the ISB orientation and the scanning method. This was achieved by evaluating prealignment data containing the ISB on the virtual model, and postalignment data containing a virtual abutment reconstructed using the implant library. The first null hypothesis was that the trueness of prealignment and postalignment data obtained by the intraoral scanner is not affected by the type of intraoral scanner, ISB orientation, or scanning method. The second null hypothesis was that the trueness of prealignment and postalignment data obtained by a laboratory scanner is not affected by the ISB orientation.

2. Materials and Methods

The overall experimental process is summarized in Figure 1. The number of samples in each group was set to eight, and a post hoc sample power calculation was performed using the G-Power sample power calculator (University of Kiel, Kiel, Germany). The power of the sample with an effect size of 0.4 was determined to be 0.941 with an alpha of 0.05 [27].

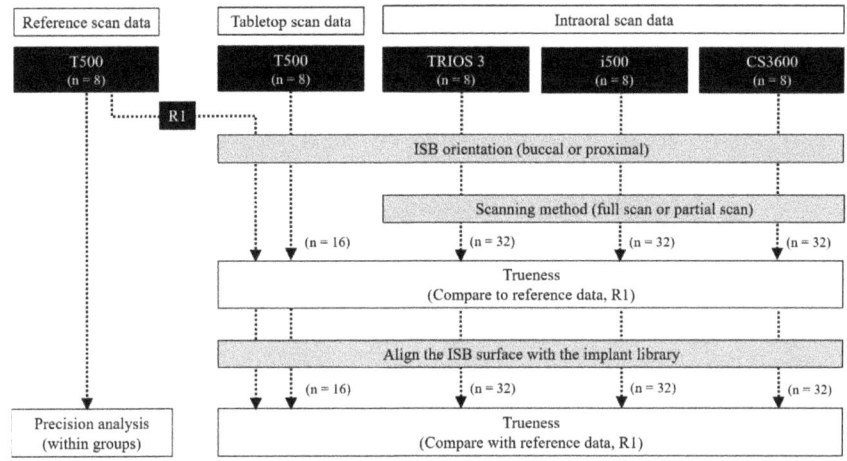

Figure 1. The overall workflow of the study. One dataset was selected randomly among the 8 reference scans.

2.1. Master Model Production

A maxillary full-arch dentate dental model (Dentiform, Nissin Dental Products, Kyoto, Japan) was scanned using a tabletop scanner (T500, Medit, Seoul, Korea), and then a dental CAD software (DentalCAD, exocad, Darmstadt, Germany) was used to modify and design the experimental model digitally. The unilateral half was removed from the full-arch model; the lateral incisor, first premolar, and first molar teeth were deleted; and the model was then modified into an edentulous ridge shape. The designed file was exported to a file in Standard Tessellation Language (STL) format, and the model was printed on a 3D printer (Form 2, Formlabs, Somerville, MA, USA) using a photocurable resin (standard gray resin, Formlabs). Three screw-type implants (length 10 mm, ø4.1 mm; Straumann, Basel, Switzerland) with a quadrangular internal structure were placed on the three edentulous areas at the bone level, with the implants' four antirotation (flat) surfaces facing in the buccal and proximal directions.

2.2. Implant Scan Body Connection and Scanning Procedure

2.2.1. Test Group Scanning with a Tabletop Scanner and Intraoral Scanners

This study used an ISB (SC-BLR, Geomedi, Gyeonggi-do, Korea) with a cylindrical shape and a flat surface, and one tabletop scanner (T500, Medit) and three oral scanners (CS3600, Carestream Dental, Atlanta, GA, USA; TRIOS 3, 3Shape, Copenhagen, Denmark; i500, Medit). Information about the scanners used in this study is provided in Table 1, and the experimental group design is summarized in Table 2.

All scanners were calibrated according to the manufacturer's instructions prior to starting the scans, and then the following experimental procedure was performed: The ISBs were connected to the fixtures at a torque of 15 Ncm and oriented so that their flat surfaces faced in the buccal direction (Figure 2A). The teeth were scanned first, and then the ISB portions were scanned. Scanning using the tabletop scanner was performed in the automatic scan mode provided by the equipment's own software ($n = 8$), while that using the intraoral scanners was performed over the entire area ($n = 8$) or only a partial area (n = 8). Scanning the entire areas of the ISBs involved scanning all sides of the ISBs without any gaps, whereas scanning under the partial-area condition was performed mainly on the buccal and lingual surfaces. The connection direction of the ISBs was then changed so that their flat surfaces faced the proximal direction (Figure 2B), and the same scanning procedure was repeated. Each set of prealignment data was then converted into postalignment data containing the virtual implants and the abutments.

Table 1. Scanners used in this study.

Scanner	Manufacturer	Scanning Technology	Scanning Tip Size
T500	Medit	Phase-shifting optical triangulation	-
TRIOS 3	3Shape	Confocal microscopy, continuous imaging	16 mm × 20 mm
CS3600	Carestream Dental	Structured light-active Speed 3D Video™	16 mm × 12 mm
i500	Medit	3D-in-motion video technology	19 mm × 15.2 mm

Table 2. Experimental group design.

Scanner	ISB Orientation	Scanning Method
T500	Buccal	Automatic scan
	Proximal	Automatic scan
TRIOS 3	Buccal	Full scan
CS3600	Proximal	Partial scan
i500	Buccal	Full scan
	Proximal	Partial scan

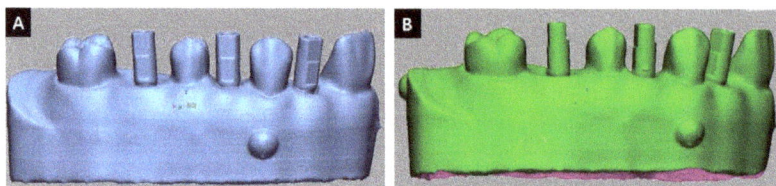

Figure 2. In order to compare the trueness according to the ISB orientation, the flat surfaces of the ISBs faced either the buccal (**A**) or proximal (**B**) direction.

2.2.2. Reference Scanning with Tabletop Scanner

After performing the test scans, the marginal gingival part of the model was ground to expose the ISBs completely, the ISBs were connected to the buccal or proximal surface, and eight scans were performed using the tabletop scanner in each orientation.

2.3. Data Processing and Assessment

In order to evaluate the trueness of each test group, the trueness of the prealignment and postalignment data were evaluated. The reference file and each test file were aligned with a best-fit algorithm in 3D analysis software (Geomagic Control X, 3D Systems, Morrisville, SC, USA) to perform superimposition. After alignment, ISB areas in the prealignment data and abutment areas in the postalignment data were extracted to obtain the root-mean-square error (RMSE) value calculated according to the following formula:

$$\text{RMSE} = \frac{1}{\sqrt{n}} * \sqrt{\sum_{i=1}^{n} (\chi_{1,i} - \chi_{2,i})^2}$$

where $\chi_{1,i}$ is the reference scan value at measurement point i, $\chi_{2,i}$ is the evaluated scan value at measurement point i, and n is the total number of measurement points in the analysis.

2.4. Statistical Analysis

Statistical analysis was performed using SPSS software (version 25.0, IBM SPSS Statistics, Chicago, IL, USA). All acquired data were subjected to Levene's test to evaluate its homoscedasticity and to the Shapiro–Wilk test to test for normality ($\alpha = 0.05$). Three-way ANOVA was used to evaluate the prealignment and postalignment data, and the effects of the type of oral scanner, the ISB orientation, and the scanning method and their interactions on the RMSE values were analyzed ($\alpha = 0.05$). One-way ANOVA and post hoc Bonferroni testing were performed to analyze the effects of combinations of ISB orientation and the scanning method for each scanner on the RMSE ($\alpha = 0.05$). The comparative analysis of the RMSE according to the ISB orientation of the T500 scan data was performed using a Student's t-test ($\alpha = 0.05$).

3. Results

The precision of the reference scan was 7.23 ± 0.34 μm (mean $\pm$ SD) when the flat surface of the ISB faced the buccal direction, and 6.84 ± 0.34 μm when it faced the proximal direction. One of these data was randomly selected as the reference data for the trueness evaluation of the test data.

Prealignment data on trueness according to the ISB orientation, scanning method, and type of intraoral scanner are shown in Figure 3. The three-way ANOVA of prealignment data revealed that all main effects of ISB orientation ($F = 65.493$, $p < 0.001$), scanning method ($F = 137.794$, $p < 0.001$), and scanner type were statistically significant ($F = 47.865$, $p < 0.001$). Analysis of two-way interactions revealed significant interaction effects of the scanning method and the scanner type ($F = 8.177$, $p = 0.001$), while the other interaction effects were not statistically significant (ISB orientation and scanning method: $F = 3.343$, $p = 0.071$; ISB orientation and scanner type: $F = 0.015$, $p = 0.985$). The three-way interaction effect of the ISB orientation, scanning method, and scanner type was not statistically significant ($F = 2.445$, $p = 0.093$). The overall RMSE according to the ISB orientation and scanning methods was lower in the buccal groups (67.50 ± 18.56 μm) than in the proximal groups (82.80 ± 16.73 μm), and lower in the full-scan groups (64.05 ± 14.74 μm) than in the partial-scan groups (86.24 ± 16.59 μm). RMSE values for the overall prealignment data according to the type of intraoral scanner were significantly lower for the TRIOS 3 device (62.46 ± 11.51 μm) than for the CS3600 (78.73 ± 20.76 μm, $p < 0.001$) and i500 (84.25 ± 17.30 μm, $p < 0.001$) devices.

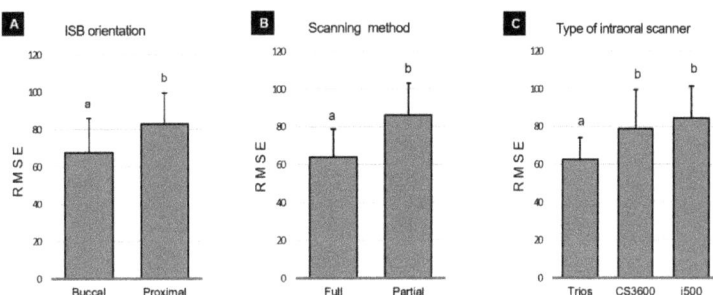

Figure 3. Overall trueness in the prealignment data according to (**A**) ISB orientation, (**B**) scanning method, and (**C**) type of intraoral scanner. Data are mean and SD values. Different letters indicate significant differences.

Postalignment data on trueness according to the ISB orientation, scanning method, or type of intraoral scanner are shown in Figure 4. The three-way ANOVA of postalignment data revealed that there were significant main effects of the ISB orientation ($F = 4.811$, $p = 0.031$) and scanning method ($F = 6.022, p = 0.016$), but not of the scanner type ($F = 3.104$, $p = 0.050$). Analysis of two-way interactions revealed that there were no significant interaction effects of the ISB orientation and scanning method ($F = 2.446 \ p = 0.122$), ISB orientation and scanner type ($F = 1.061, p = 0.351$), or scanning method and scanner type ($F = 1.241, p = 0.294$). The three-way interaction effect of the ISB orientation, scanning method, and scanner type was not statistically significant ($F = 0.454, p = 0.636$). The overall RMSE according to the ISB orientation and scanning methods was significantly lower in the buccal groups (28.15 ± 8.87 μm) than in the proximal groups (31.94 ± 8.95 μm), and significantly lower in the full-scan groups (27.92 ± 10.80 μm) than in the partial-scan groups (32.16 ± 6.35 μm). RMSE values for the overall postalignment data according to the type of intraoral scanner were significantly lower for the TRIOS 3 device (27.61 ± 8.33 μm) than for the i500 device (32.84 ± 8.13 μm, $p = 0.040$).

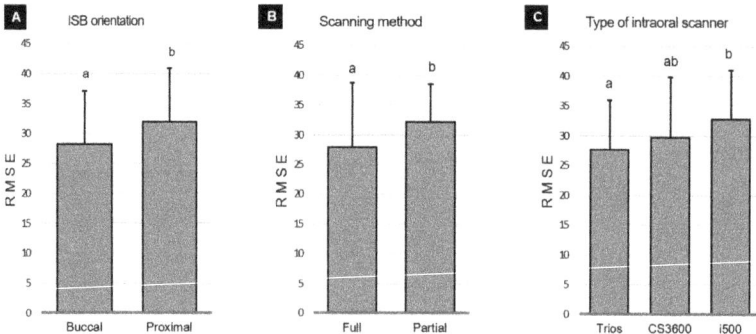

Figure 4. Overall trueness in the postalignment data according to (**A**) ISB orientation, (**B**) scanning method, and (**C**) type of intraoral scanner. Data are mean and SD values. Different letters indicate significant differences.

Prealignment data on trueness according to combinations of the ISB orientation and scanning method for each scanner are shown in Figure 5. For the T500 scanner, the RMSE was significantly lower in the buccal groups (33.45 ± 1.50 μm) than in the proximal groups (56.91 ± 3.60 μm, $F = 4.088, p < 0.001$). The TRIOS 3 scanner showed significant differences in one-way analysis according to ISB orientation ($F = 32.923, p < 0.001$). The RMSE was lowest for the ISB with its flat surface facing the buccal direction and full scanning (buccal–full:47.02 ± 5.91 μm), and highest for the ISB with its flat surface facing the proximal direction and partial scanning (proximal–partial: 74.91 ± 3.99 μm). The CS3600 scanner also showed significant differences in one-way analysis ($F = 25.929, p < 0.001$), with the RMSE being lowest for buccal–full (56.09 ± 7.74 μm) and proximal–full (69.79 ± 11.18 μm), and highest for proximal–partial (102.79 ± 9.22 μm). The i500 scanner also showed a significant difference in one-way analysis ($F = 22.046, p < 0.001$), with the RMSE being lowest for buccal–full (60.91 ± 10.74 μm). The common result for all scanners was that in the case of prealignment data, the RMSE was the lowest for buccal–full and the highest for proximal–partial.

Postalignment data on trueness according to combinations of the ISB orientation and scanning method for each scanner are shown in Figure 6. For the T500 scanner, the RMSE was lower in the buccal groups (14.34 ± 0.89 μm) than in the proximal groups (29.35 ± 1.15 μm, $p < 0.001$). The TRIOS 3 scanner showed significant differences in one-way analysis according to the ISB orientation and scanning method ($F = 5.342, p < 0.005$), with the RMSE being lower for buccal–full (19.45 ± 8.42 μm) than for buccal–partial (31.89 ± 6.07 μm) and proximal–partial (31.20 ± 6.70 μm). For the CS3600 scanner, the RMSE values did not differ between the groups ($F = 0.059, p = 0.981$). The i500 scanner showed significant differences in one-way analysis ($F = 3.369, p = 0.032$), with the RMSE being lower for buccal–full (26.18 ± 10.11 µm) and buccal–partial (32.69 ± 7.31 µm) than for proximal–partial (36.54 ± 3.08 µm).

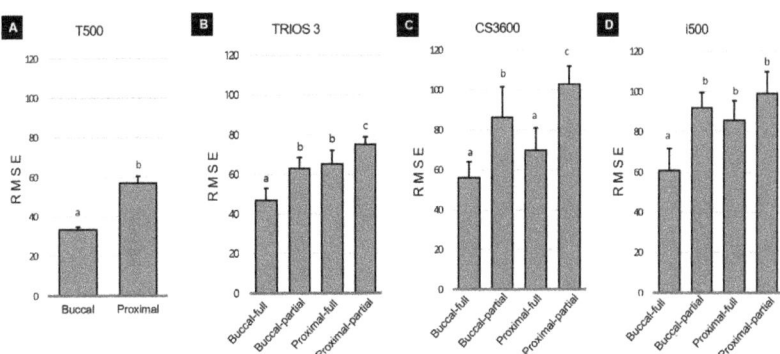

Figure 5. Trueness in the prealignment data for each scanner according to combinations of the ISB orientation and scanning method: (**A**) T500, (**B**) TRIOS 3, (**C**) CS3600, and (**D**) i500. Data are mean and SD values. Different letters indicate significant differences.

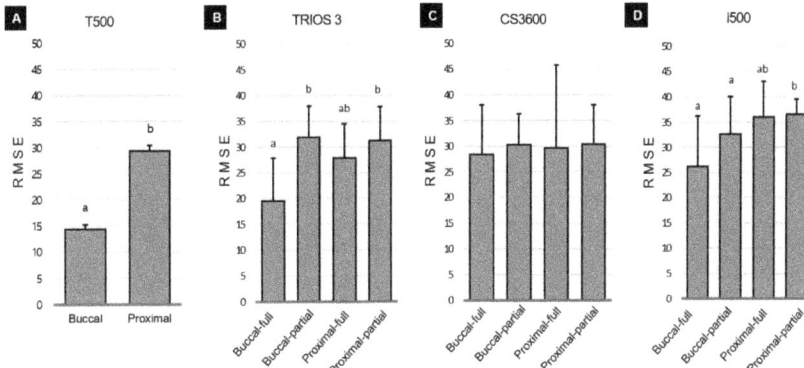

Figure 6. Trueness in the postalignment data for each scanner according to combinations of the ISB orientation and scanning method: (**A**) T500, (**B**) TRIOS 3, (**C**) CS3600, and (**D**) i500. Data are mean and SD values. Different letters indicate significant differences.

Figures 7 and 8 show representative images from the trueness evaluation of test data for the i500 scanner. Figure 7 shows prealignment data for the deviation of the ISB areas, which was higher in the proximal groups (Figure 7C,D) than in the buccal groups (Figure 7A,B), and higher in the partial-scan groups (Figure 7B,D) than in the full-scan groups (Figure 7A,C). Figure 8 shows postalignment data for the deviation of the abutment areas, which was higher in the proximal groups (Figure 8C,D) than in the buccal groups (Figure 8A,B), and higher in the partial-scan groups (Figure 8B,D) than in the full-scan groups (Figure 8A,C). Comparing the prealignment and postalignment images reveals that the degree of deviation tended to be lower in the postalignment data.

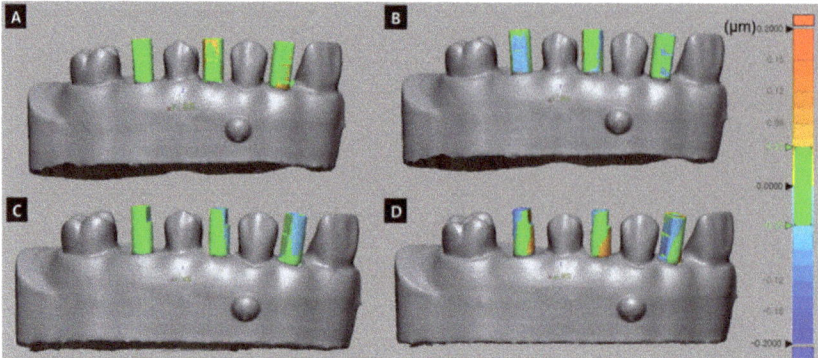

Figure 7. After connecting the ISB, scanning procedures were performed to obtain prealignment data, and the trueness was evaluated by superimposing the reference scan data and extracting the ISB areas. The deviation tended to be lower in the buccal groups than in the proximal groups, and lower in the full-scan groups than in the partial-scan groups: (**A**) buccal–full group, (**B**) buccal–partial group, (**C**) proximal–full group, and (**D**) proximal–partial group.

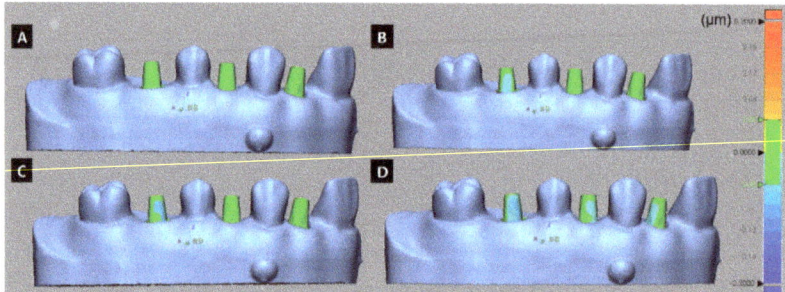

Figure 8. The postalignment data in which the virtual abutments were created by aligning using the implant library, and the trueness was evaluated by superimposing the reference scan data and extracting the abutment areas. The deviation tended to be lower in the buccal groups than in the proximal groups, and lower in the full-scan groups than in the partial-scan groups. The deviation tended to decrease relative to the prealignment data: (**A**) buccal–full group, (**B**) buccal–partial group, (**C**) proximal–full group, and (**D**) proximal–partial group.

4. Discussion

This study compared the trueness of digital implant impressions according to the ISB orientation and scanning method in the cases of a single implant in the presence of adjacent teeth. For two of the three intraoral scanners, there were significant differences according to the ISB orientation and the scanning method. For the tabletop scanner, it was found to show higher trueness to connect the ISB with its flat surface facing the buccal direction; that is, the null hypothesis of this study was partially rejected for three types of intraoral scanner, and rejected for one laboratory scanner.

For the prealignment data, the overall RMSE was significantly lower in the buccal group than in the proximal group for the three intraoral scanners. Deep, undercut, angled, inclined, or crowded surfaces of surrounding structures are difficult to scan and hence cause inaccurate point clouds, which may decrease the scan accuracy in proximal areas [28,29]. This difference in ease of scanning between the buccal and proximal surfaces would have influenced the trueness according to the ISB orientation.

For the postalignment data, the RMSE was lower when the flat surface of the ISB faced the buccal direction and a full scan was performed. The effects of the ISB orientation and scanning method do not seem to be completely compensated for even in the process of aligning with a virtual implant, which seems to have a subtle effect on the completion of the process of aligning library data. In the case of fabricating restorations from natural teeth, it is important to capture the details of the teeth well, including in the margin area. However, in the case of implants, only the location of the ISB is important, resulting in differences in the reported importance of the scanning method [30]. However, the present study confirmed that a meticulous full scan of the entire areas of the ISBs is important even when scanning an implant case using ISBs. This is consistent with the finding of Park et al. that the imaging deficiency of the ISB influenced the position of the virtual implant; these authors suggested that a surface area deficiency of more than 10% in an ISB should be avoided [24].

The present study found that both prealignment and postalignment data showed differences in RMSE values according to the ISB orientation and scanning method for different scanners. For the implant, after data are acquired by scanning, mesh reconstruction is performed using an implant library, and a virtual implant is created by surface matching with the digital implant library [9]. Therefore, not only the scan quality but also the shape-matching algorithm affect the accuracy. The differences in trueness according to scanner types in the present study may have resulted from not only the scanning process itself but also during data processing. Previous studies have found that the accuracy when using different intraoral scanner systems varies with factors such as the familiarity of the operator, learning curve, ergonomic design of the handheld camera, design of hardware and software, and the research method and design [31]. Therefore, future comparisons of the accuracy of scanners for digital implant impressions will require the establishment of a standardized research model [31].

The T500 device is a laboratory scanner, and unlike intraoral scanners that acquire small images using a small scanner head and stitch these images together to obtain the entire image, the overall accuracy is higher for a laboratory scanner because it obtains a whole image of the entire area and scans by rotating the model table [32]. The present study found that the accuracy of the T500 scanner was higher when the flat surface of the ISB facing the buccal direction in both the prealignment and postalignment data. The model table was scanned within the limit that allowed rotation, so the flat surface of the ISB faced the buccal direction, and the scan accessibility of the flat surface was higher, which would have contributed to increased trueness.

This was an in vitro study, and real clinical scanning procedures are further influenced by patient movements (e.g., breathing), humidity, and the restricted intraoral space [33]. Therefore, future studies need to reproduce the in vivo environment of the oral cavity. Additionally, the present study analyzed the trueness by matching a reference file and the test file using a best-fit algorithm to obtain RMSE values. This method presents negative and positive deviations for each region as a color map in the scan file in three dimensions, and provides an average deviation value for the entire area as an RMSE value; however, a limitation is that it does not indicate the accuracy of the actual implant position. Future studies should, therefore, evaluate linear and angular discrepancies in the positions of implant fixtures, and also the final restorations in order to assess clinically significant differences. Moreover, the ISBs used in this study had a cylindrical shape with a flat surface and were made of polyether ether ketone. Since clinicians use various types of ISBs in clinical practice, it is necessary to conduct additional research into the effects of different materials and types of ISBs [22]. Finally, since scanning results are also affected by the individual's experience, it is also necessary to investigate outcomes for several researchers to determine the intra- and interoperator reliabilities [34].

Previous studies on the accuracy of digital implant impressions have mainly involved edentulous cases or multiple cases [16–23]. In contrast, this study focused on partial-arch models with single implants in the presence of adjacent teeth. In particular, the effect of ISB orientation and the scanning method was examined. Clinically, the operator must invest additional time and effort to completely scan all areas, including the proximal surface of the ISB. The results of this study indicate that when performing oral scanning, the operator should connect the ISB so that its flat surface faces the buccal direction, and should try to scan the full area. It was also found that it is advantageous to connect the ISBs buccally when using a tabletop scanner.

5. Conclusions

Within the limitations of this in vitro study, when taking a digital implant impression using an intraoral scanner in a single implant case in the presence of adjacent teeth, connecting the ISBs so that their flat surfaces faced the buccal direction and scanning the full area produced more accurate results. When using the laboratory scanner, the trueness was higher when connecting the ISB buccally rather than proximally.

Author Contributions: Conceptualization, J.-E.K.; data curation, B.L. and N.-E.N.; formal analysis, B.L., N.-E.N., S.-H.S., J.-H.L. and J.-E.K.; methodology, B.L., N.-E.N. and J.-E.K.; resources, J.-E.K. and J.-S.S.; software, N.-E.N. and S.-H.S.; supervision, J.-E.K.; validation, J.-E.K. and J.-S.S.; visualization, B.L., N.-E.N. and J.-E.K.; writing—original draft preparation, B.L. and J.-E.K.; writing—review and editing, B.L., N.-E.N., S.-H.S., J.-H.L., J.-E.K. and J.-S.S. All authors have read and agreed to the published version of the manuscript.

Funding: This research was supported by a grant from the Korea Health Technology R&D Project through the Korea Health Industry Development Institute (KHIDI), funded by the Ministry of Health & Welfare, Republic of Korea (grant number: HI20C0127).

Institutional Review Board Statement: Not applicable.

Informed Consent Statement: Not applicable.

Data Availability Statement: The data presented in this study are available on request from the corresponding author.

Conflicts of Interest: The authors declare no conflict of interest.

References

1. Gonçalves, F.S.; Popoff, D.A.V.; Castro, C.D.L.; Silva, G.C.; Magalhães, C.S.; Moreira, A.N. Dimensional stability of elastomeric impression materials: A critical review of the literature. *Eur. J. Prosthodont. Restor. Dent.* **2011**, *19*, 163–166.
2. Corso, M.; Abanomy, A.; Di Canzio, J.; Zurakowski, D.; Morgano, S.M. The effect of temperature changes on the dimensional stability of polyvinyl siloxane and polyether impression materials. *J. Prosthet. Dent.* **1998**, *79*, 626–631. [CrossRef]
3. Lacy, A.; Fukui, H.; Bellman, T.; Jendresen, M.D. Time-dependent accuracy of elastomer impression materials. Part II: Polyether, polysulfides, and polyvinylsiloxane. *J. Prosthet. Dent.* **1981**, *45*, 329–333. [CrossRef]
4. Pratten, D.; Craig, R. Wettability of a hydrophilic addition silicone impression material. *J. Prosthet. Dent.* **1989**, *61*, 197–202. [CrossRef]
5. Reddy, N.S.; Reddy, G.V.; Ittigi, J. A Comparative Study to Determine the Wettability and Castability of Different Elastomeric Impression Materials. *J. Contemp. Dent. Pract.* **2012**, *13*, 356–363. [CrossRef]
6. Martin, N.; Martin, M.; Jedynakiewicz, N. The dimensional stability of dental impression materials following immersion in disinfecting solutions. *Dent. Mater.* **2007**, *23*, 760–768. [CrossRef] [PubMed]
7. Katsoulis, J.; Takeichi, T.; Gaviria, A.S.; Peter, L.; Katsoulis, K. Misfit of implant prostheses and its impact on clinical outcomes. Definition, assessment and a systematic review of the literature. *Eur. J. Oral Implant.* **2017**, *10* (Suppl. 1), 121–138.
8. Mühlemann, S.; Greter, E.A.; Park, J.-M.; Hämmerle, C.H.F.; Thoma, D.S. Precision of digital implant models compared to conventional implant models for posterior single implant crowns: A within-subject comparison. *Clin. Oral Implant. Res.* **2018**, *29*, 931–936. [CrossRef]
9. Mangano, F.; Gandolfi, A.; Luongo, G.; Logozzo, S. Intraoral scanners in dentistry: A review of the current literature. *BMC Oral Heal.* **2017**, *17*, 149. [CrossRef] [PubMed]
10. Van Der Meer, W.J.; Andriessen, F.S.; Wismeijer, D.; Ren, Y. Application of Intra-Oral Dental Scanners in the Digital Workflow of Implantology. *PLoS ONE* **2012**, *7*, e43312. [CrossRef]
11. Kamimura, E.; Tanaka, S.; Takaba, M.; Tachi, K.; Baba, K. In vivo evaluation of inter-operator reproducibility of digital dental and conventional impression techniques. *PLoS ONE* **2017**, *12*, e0179188. [CrossRef]
12. Joda, T.; Lenherr, P.; Dedem, P.; Kovaltschuk, I.; Bragger, U.; Zitzmann, N.U. Time efficiency, difficulty, and operator's preference comparing digital and conventional implant impressions: A randomized controlled trial. *Clin. Oral Implant. Res.* **2017**, *28*, 1318–1323. [CrossRef]
13. Yuzbasioglu, E.; Kurt, H.; Turunc, R.; Bilir, H. Comparison of digital and conventional impression techniques: Evaluation of patients' perception, treatment comfort, effectiveness and clinical outcomes. *BMC Oral Health* **2014**, *14*, 10. [CrossRef]

14. Mizumoto, R.M.; Yilmaz, B. Intraoral scan bodies in implant dentistry: A systematic review. *J. Prosthet. Dent.* **2018**, *120*, 343–352. [CrossRef]
15. Duello, G.V. Intraoral Scanning for Single-Tooth Implant Prosthetics: Rationale for a Digital Protocol. *Compend. Contin. Educ. Dent.* **2018**, *39*, 28–34.
16. Chia, V.A.; Esguerra, R.J.; Teoh, K.H.; Teo, J.W.; Wong, K.M.; Tan, K.B. In Vitro Three-Dimensional Accuracy of Digital Implant Impressions: The Effect of Implant Angulation. *Int. J. Oral Maxillofac. Implant.* **2017**, *32*, 313–321. [CrossRef]
17. Giménez, B.; Özcan, M.; Martínez-Rus, F.; Pradíes, G. Accuracy of a Digital Impression System Based on Parallel Confocal Laser Technology for Implants with Consideration of Operator Experience and Implant Angulation and Depth. *Int. J. Oral Maxillofac. Implant.* **2014**, *29*, 853–862. [CrossRef]
18. Gimenez-Gonzalez, B.; Hassan, B.; Özcan, M.; Pradíes, G. An In Vitro Study of Factors Influencing the Performance of Digital Intraoral Impressions Operating on Active Wavefront Sampling Technology with Multiple Implants in the Edentulous Maxilla. *J. Prosthodont.* **2017**, *26*, 650–655. [CrossRef]
19. Mizumoto, R.M.; Alp, G.; Özcan, M.; Yilmaz, B. The effect of scanning the palate and scan body position on the accuracy of complete-arch implant scans. *Clin. Implant. Dent. Relat. Res.* **2019**, *21*, 987–994. [CrossRef]
20. Iturrate, M.; Eguiraun, H.; Solaberrieta, E. Accuracy of digital impressions for implant-supported complete-arch prosthesis, using an auxiliary geometry part—An in vitro study. *Clin. Oral Implant. Res.* **2019**, *30*, 1250–1258. [CrossRef]
21. Motel, C.; Kirchner, E.; Adler, W.; Wichmann, M.; Matta, R.E. Impact of Different Scan Bodies and Scan Strategies on the Accuracy of Digital Implant Impressions Assessed with an Intraoral Scanner: An In Vitro Study. *J. Prosthodont.* **2020**, *29*, 309–314. [CrossRef]
22. Arcuri, L.; Pozzi, A.; Lio, F.; Rompen, E.; Zechner, W.; Nardi, A. Influence of implant scanbody material, position and operator on the accuracy of digital impression for complete-arch: A randomized in vitro trial. *J. Prosthodont. Res.* **2020**, *64*, 128–136. [CrossRef] [PubMed]
23. Revilla-León, M.; Fogarty, R.; Barrington, J.J.; Zandinejad, A.; Özcan, M. Influence of scan body design and digital implant analogs on implant replica position in additively manufactured casts. *J. Prosthet. Dent.* **2020**, *124*, 202–210. [CrossRef]
24. Park, S.-W.; Choi, Y.-D.; Lee, D.-H. The effect of the improperly scanned scan body images on the accuracy of virtual implant positioning in computer-aided design software. *J. Adv. Prosthodont.* **2020**, *12*, 107–113. [CrossRef] [PubMed]
25. *ISO I: 5725-1: 1994 Accuracy (Trueness and Precision) of Measurement Methods and Results-Part 1: General Principles and Definitions*; International Organization for Standardization: Geneva, Switzerland, 1994.
26. Ender, A.; Mehl, A. Influence of scanning strategies on the accuracy of digital intraoral scanning systems. *Int. J. Comput. Dent.* **2013**, *16*, 11–21. [PubMed]
27. Cohen, J. *Statistical Power Analysis for the Behavioral Science*, 2nd ed.; Lawrence Erlbaum Associates: Mahwah, NJ, USA, 1988; pp. 274–288.
28. Chan, D.C.N.; Chung, A.-H.; Haines, J.; Yau, E.-T.; Kuo, C.-C. The Accuracy of Optical Scanning: Influence of Convergence and Die Preparation. *Oper. Dent.* **2011**, *36*, 486–491. [CrossRef]
29. Lin, W.-S.; Harris, B.T.; Elathamna, E.N.; Abdel-Azim, T.; Morton, D. Effect of implant divergence on the accuracy of definitive casts created from traditional and digital implant-level impressions: An in vitro comparative study. *Int. J. Oral Maxillofac. Implant.* **2015**, *30*, 102–109. [CrossRef]
30. Keeling, A.; Wu, J.; Ferrari, M. Confounding factors affecting the marginal quality of an intra-oral scan. *J. Dent.* **2017**, *59*, 33–40. [CrossRef]
31. Abduo, J.; Elseyoufi, M. Accuracy of Intraoral Scanners: A Systematic Review of Influencing Factors. *Eur. J. Prosthodont. Restor. Dent.* **2018**, *26*, 101–121.
32. Son, K.; Lee, K.-B. Effect of Tooth Types on the Accuracy of Dental 3D Scanners: An In Vitro Study. *Materials* **2020**, *13*, 1744. [CrossRef]
33. Sun, L.; Lee, J.-S.; Choo, H.-H.; Hwang, H.-S.; Lee, K.-M. Reproducibility of an intraoral scanner: A comparison between in-vivo and ex-vivo scans. *Am. J. Orthod. Dentofac. Orthop.* **2018**, *154*, 305–310. [CrossRef]
34. Kim, J.; Park, J.-M.; Kim, M.; Heo, S.-J.; Shin, I.H.; Kim, M. Comparison of experience curves between two 3-dimensional intraoral scanners. *J. Prosthet. Dent.* **2016**, *116*, 221–230. [CrossRef]

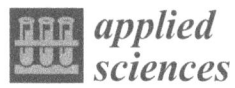

Article

Accuracy of Implant Level Intraoral Scanning and Photogrammetry Impression Techniques in a Complete Arch with Angled and Parallel Implants: An In Vitro Study

Hani Tohme [1,*], Ghida Lawand [2], Rita Eid [3], Khaled E. Ahmed [4], Ziad Salameh [5] and Joseph Makzoume [1]

[1] Department of Removable Prosthodontics, Faculty of Dental Medicine, Saint Joseph University, Beirut 1107, Lebanon; joseph.makzoume@usj.edu.lb
[2] Department of Prosthodontics and Esthetic Dentistry, Faculty of Dental Medicine, Saint Joseph University, Beirut 1107, Lebanon; ghida.lawand@net.usj.edu.lb
[3] Department of Prosthodontics, Faculty of Dental Medicine, Lebanese University, Beirut 1107, Lebanon; ritaeid@ul.edu.lb
[4] School of Medicine and Dentistry, Griffith University, Gold Coast 4000, Australia; khaled.ahmed@griffith.edu.au
[5] Faculty of Dental Medicine, Lebanese University, Beirut 1107, Lebanon; ziad.salameh@ul.edu.lb
* Correspondence: hani@tohmeclinic.com; Tel.: +961-330-7910

Citation: Tohme, H.; Lawand, G.; Eid, R.; Ahmed, K.E.; Salameh, Z.; Makzoume, J. Accuracy of Implant Level Intraoral Scanning and Photogrammetry Impression Techniques in a Complete Arch with Angled and Parallel Implants: An In Vitro Study. *Appl. Sci.* **2021**, *11*, 9859. https://doi.org/10.3390/app11219859

Academic Editor: Ricardo Castro Alves

Received: 9 October 2021
Accepted: 20 October 2021
Published: 22 October 2021

Publisher's Note: MDPI stays neutral with regard to jurisdictional claims in published maps and institutional affiliations.

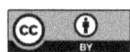

Copyright: © 2021 by the authors. Licensee MDPI, Basel, Switzerland. This article is an open access article distributed under the terms and conditions of the Creative Commons Attribution (CC BY) license (https://creativecommons.org/licenses/by/4.0/).

Abstract: (1) Background: Stereophotogrammetry has recently been investigated showing high accuracy in complete implant supported cases but has scarcely been investigated in cases of tilted implants. The aim of this in vitro study was to compare the accuracy of digital impression techniques (intraoral scanning and photogrammetry) at the level of intraoral scan bodies in terms of angular deviations and 3D discrepancies. (2) Methods: A stone master cast representing an edentulous maxilla using four implant analogs was fabricated. The two anterior implants were parallel to each other, and the two posterior implants were at an angulation of 17 degrees. Digital intraoral scanning (DIOS) impressions were taken after connecting implant level scan bodies to the master cast and STL files were exported ($n = 15$). Digital photogrammetry (DPG) impressions were captured using a PiC Camera after tightening implant level PiC optical markers and STL files were exported ($n = 15$). Superimposition was carried out by a software for determining the accuracy of both. (3) Results: Significant angular discrepancies (ΔA) and 3D deviations of scan bodies were found among the groups in trueness with lower deviations for the DPG (p value < 0.001). However, trueness within ISBs varied between angular and 3D deviations and outcomes were not specific to determine the effect of implant angulation. In precision, no significant differences were detected within ISBs and among both groups in terms of angular deviation. However, DPG had less deviations than DIOS group in terms of 3D deviations (p value < 0.001). (4) Conclusion: Digital photogrammetry technique conveyed the utmost accuracy in both trueness and precision for the intraoral scan bodies among both impression methods assessed. In addition, implant angulation did not influence the precision of the impression techniques but affected their trueness without explicit conclusions.

Keywords: angulated implants; implant supported prosthesis; intraoral scanning; photogrammetry

1. Introduction

Digital technology in the dental field has been a game-changer ever since its introduction into surgical and prosthetic procedures [1,2]. Transforming workflows to cope up with this advancement necessitates the need of intraoral scanners (IOS)s, intraoral scan bodies (ISB)s, computer software, milling machines, and digital ceramic materials [3–5]. This new era has been met with great success facilitating the fabrication of crowns and bridges, restoration of missing teeth, planning, and prosthetically guiding implant placement [6–8]. It has also revealed higher predictability and consistency of results in contrast with conventional techniques that were considered as hosts to a wide assortment of human and technical errors [9,10]. From that time on, technology has revolutionized treatment modalities, especially in implant-supported cases.

However, there are still many lingering problems with scanning full arch implant prosthesis where a passive fit is still questionable. This is due to several factors affecting the accuracy when taking a digital impression such as implant position [11–14], scanning strategy [15], light intensity [16,17], and arch length [18]. Additionally, when performing scans of multiple implants, it may be hard for the IOS to distinguish identical ISBs and to recognize their locations [19]. The IOS in this case will analyze dissimilar scan bodies as only one and may fix images on top of each other [20]. In addition, obtaining consistent digital scans with edentulous patients is demanding since the scanned surface may lack reference points between point clouds that may accompany improper stitching of the images. Accordingly, the images may be stitched with compounding errors including imprecise and noisy mesh [21]. Also, the main parts of the scan may be recognized as redundant and eventually will be cut out by the software's post-processing algorithm [21–23].

The technological evolution did not stop with digital intraoral scanners (DIOS) but grew to bring forth a new digital technique called photogrammetry (DPG). This development is based on obtaining reliable information about physical objects through processes of recording, measuring, and interpreting photographic images and patterns and is devoid of any direct physical contact with the measured object [24]. In 1999, DPG was proposed by Jemt and Back as a technique for complete implant-supported impressions showing similar fidelity results with conventional procedures [25]. The supremacy of this technique lies in that the presence of blood, saliva, or any other residue does not affect the measurement precision [26]. Its camera is based on measuring angles and distances between prosthetic attachments allowing the patient total freedom of movement. In a randomized clinical trial, Peñarrocha-Diago et al. reported that stereophotogrammetric and traditional impressions showed no differences in implant success rate, marginal bone loss, or prosthesis survival after one year of follow-up [27]. In addition, numerous clinical reports also stated that this technique ensures optimum fit of the framework representing a predictable solution for complete implant-supported cases [28–33]. Although new technologies are based on the premise of achieving higher quality prosthesis, their direct comparison with digital intraoral scanning is still lacking robust evidence in the literature (specifically with tilted implants) [34–36].

Accuracy is a blend of precision and trueness according to the ISO standards [37]. Precision is the closeness of measurements to each other in a specific group which makes the results more expectable. However, trueness refers to how much these measurements are in accordance with fact [38,39]. To date, no article has investigated the fidelity of implant level impressions using DPG in comparison with DIOS in all on four cases with posteriorly tilted implants. Hence, the aim of this in vitro study was to assess and compare the accuracy in terms of trueness and precision of these methods and the effect of implant angulation through measuring the intraoral scan body 3D deviation and angular distortion. The first null hypothesis was that there was no significant difference in the accuracy (trueness and precision) between the DIOS and DPG groups. The second null hypothesis was that implant inclination would not affect the fidelity.

2. Materials and Methods

A scannable gypsum cast covered with pink gingiva used as the reference model (RM) was a representative of a fully edentulous maxilla with four implant analogs (RC Bone Level Implant Analog; Institut Straumann AG) located in right first premolar (RP), right lateral incisor (RLI), left first premolar (LFP), and left lateral incisor (LLI) regions demonstrating a typical clinical scenario. The two anterior analogs were parallel whereas those posteriorly situated were of 17 degrees angulation. This cast was obtained from an all-on-four acrylic model by taking a polyether (Impregum Polyether Impression Material; 3M ESPE, Seefeld, Germany) impression with splinted implant level impression copings (Implant level open tray impression post, D4.6 mm, Straumann, Basel, Switzerland). Autopolymerizing pattern resin (Pattern Resin LS; GC) was used to join the copings where it was sectioned and rejoined after 24 h of setting to minimize the resin polymerization shrinkage [40]. Light pink impression silicone (Gingifast Rigid; Zhermack, Badia Polisine, Italy) was first placed surrounding the impression copings to create the gingival mask. Then scannable plaster (CAM-Stone N; SILADENT, Goslar, Germany) was mixed according to the manufacturer's instructions and poured over the impression. To create control Standard Tessellation Language (STL) files for trueness comparison, new identical four implant level ISBs (Cares Mono Scanbody D4.6mm PEEK/TAN, Institut Straumann A/S, Basel, Switzerland) of the same diameter and height were chosen and prior to tightening, the pink silicone was covered with scanning powder. After that they were tightened at 15 N over the gypsum model and digitized with a desktop scanner (E3; 3Shape A/S, Copenhagen, Denmark) of 7 μm accuracy. This file was considered as a baseline scan acting as a standard to which all other scans would be compared.

On the part of the DIOS group, fifteen scans were obtained using a previously calibrated IOS (TRIOS3 Cart; 3Shape A/S) after tightening implant level scan bodies (Cares Mono Scanbody D4.6mm PEEK/TAN, Institut Straumann A/S) on the RM (Figure 1). To escape the impending adverse effects of practitioner fatigue, a 5-min break was scheduled between scans. The progress of the scanning strategy used was slow and constant where the practitioner started from the occlusal surface, continued to capture the buccal region, and then ended by registering the palatal area starting from the scan body of implant LFP and ending at that of implant RFP. The operator tried to capture all the details of each ISB, without asserting too much on them from the same angle, to prevent unnecessary reflection. All scans were captured in the same environmental conditions with ambient light of 1003 lux, without interference from any external light sources [16,17].

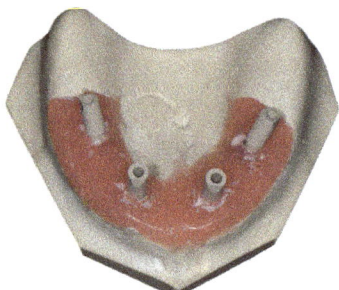

Figure 1. Implant level intraoral scan bodies tightened on the reference model.

For the DPG group, implant level Pic transfers (PiCabutment; PiC dental, Miami, FL, USA) were screwed on top of the analogs (Figures 2 and 3). A stereo-camera positioned 15–30 cm away from the reference cast with a supreme angle of 45 degrees with respect to the transfers was used to register implant positions (PiC camera; PiC dental). After defining the code of each Pic transfer, the information was captured and processed by a customized Pic program (Pic Cam Soft v1.1; PiC dental) that created vectors representing the implants' positions. From the Pic library file, ISBs having the same shape as the ones used for the RM were chosen to replace the vectors, and STL files were exported. Fifteen STL files were attained for this group.

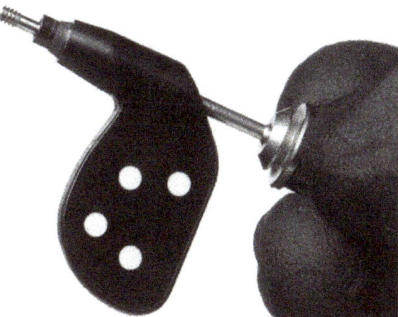

Figure 2. Implant level PiC transfer with an engaging configuration.

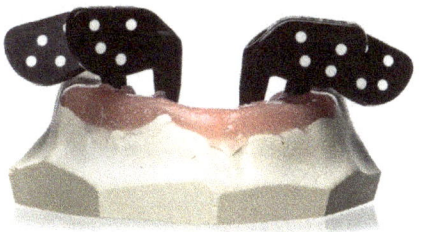

Figure 3. PiC transfers screwed on the reference model.

After all scans were captured, the reference file and the scans obtained from the DIOS group were trimmed using reverse engineering software (Geomagic Control X; 3D System, Boston, MA, USA) leaving the scan bodies only and disregarding the surrounding structures. This was carried out to have all files in resemblance with DPG captures that are devoid of surface scans ensuring a close number of point clouds between all registrations. After this, the scans were assessed and compared by the same software. For trueness, each scan of each group was compared with the reference. However, for precision, the scans of each group were superimposed randomly over each other [41]. Each alignment entailed two steps where the initial alignment option was carried out first to proceed to the final rough alignment through the best fit option ensuring a top-notch merging (Figure 4) [42–48]. Fifteen superimpositions were conducted for each group, for a total of thirty alignments for each of precision and trueness.

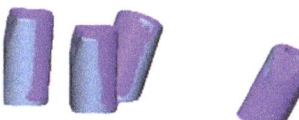

Figure 4. STL file to be measured superimposed over the reference STL file using best fit algorithm.

Congruence between the two superimposed scans was expressed quantitatively by measuring the 3D deviations (Figure 5) and angular deviations of each ISB. 3D comparison option was used to determine 3D distortions in mm. Then, means ± standard deviations (SD) of these distortions were calculated after obtaining the Root Mean Square (RMS) of each ISB that was unitless [49]. For the angular discrepancies, the geometrical deviation option in the software was implied after defining the geometrical shape to be cylindrical in this case due to the topography of the ISBs. The distortion level between the control and measured scans was calculated in degrees. Finally, for a better empirical evaluation of the 3D deviations between the files and interpretation of the directivity of the deviation, the software allowed engendering a colorimetric map (Figure 5). This map was generated for the ISB where the blue color was for inward defects, red for outward excesses, and green for minimal deformities. The surface tolerance was set with the scale ranging from a maximum deviation of +50 to −50 µm. This value was determined according to the maximum clinically acceptable framework misfit tolerance [50]. All of the data collected were included in datasheets used for statistical analysis. The sample size was determined adequate for the analysis by a professional statistician. The appropriate significance was set at 0.05 and the power level was set at 0.80. A sample size of 15 in each group would detect a significant difference with a standardized effect size of 1.080.

Figure 5. Colorimetric map showing the 3D deviation of intraoral scan bodies of an STL file obtained from digital intraoral scanning group.

The statistical analysis was performed with IBM SPSS Statistics (version 26.0, New York, NY, USA). The level of significance was set at p value ≤ 0.05. Kolmogorov-Smirnov and Shapiro-Wilk tests were used to assess the normal distribution of quantitative variables. Repeated-measure analyses of variance followed by univariates analysis and Bonferroni multiple comparisons tests were performed to compare the 3D deviation and angular deviations of precision and trueness between impression techniques and within ISBs. The Bonferroni test was performed to prevent data from incorrectly appearing to be statistically significant during multiple comparison testing since each comparison can impact other results creating multiple false positives.

3. Results

The results of the repeated-measure analyses of variance followed by univariates analyses and Bonferroni multiple comparisons tests for trueness are shown in Table 1 and Figure 6 and for precision in Table 2 and Figure 7.

Table 1. Means and standards deviations of angular distortions among implant level impression techniques in terms of trueness.

	Angular Deviation for Trueness (Mean ± SD) in Degrees (°)		
ISBs	DIOS (n = 15)	DPG (n = 15)	p Value
LFP	1.682 ± 0.205 [b]	0.586 ± 0.088 [a]	<0.001
LLI	1.907 ± 0.234 [c]	0.346 ± 0.038 [a]	<0.001
RLI	1.496 ± 0.142	1.293 ± 0.068	0.398
RFP	1.890 ± 0.293 [b]	0.672 ± 0.081 [a]	<0.001
Global	1.744 ± 0.175 [b]	0.724 ± 0.064 [a]	<0.001
p value	<0.001	<0.001	
	RLI < LFP < LLI = RFP	LLI < LFP < RFP < RLI	

[a–c] different letters indicate the presence of significant difference between impression techniques using post hoc tests. ISBs, intraoral scan-bodies; LFP, left first premolar; LLI, left lateral incisor; RLI, right lateral incisor; RFP, right first premolar; DIOS, digital intraoral scanning; DPG, digital photogrammetry.

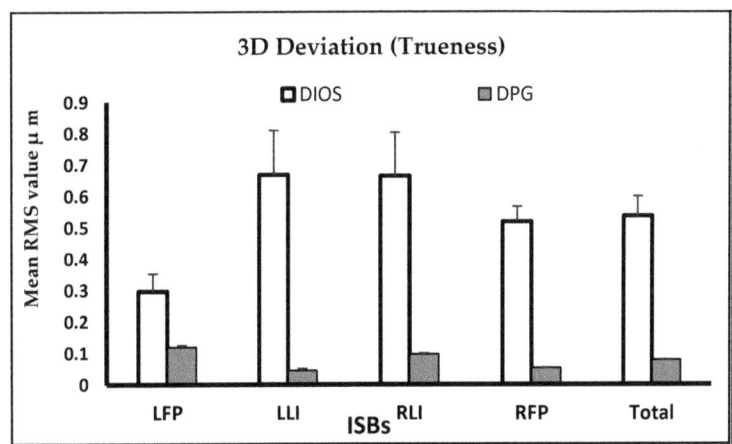

Figure 6. Trueness of intraoral scan bodies in terms of 3D deviation. RMS, root mean square; ISBs, intraoral scan-bodies; LFP, left first premolar; LLI, left lateral incisor; RLI, right lateral incisor; RFP, right first premolar; DIOS, digital intraoral scanning; DPG, digital photogrammetry.

Table 2. Means and standards deviations of RMS 3D distortions among implant level impression techniques in terms of precision.

	RMS 3D ISBs Deviation for Precision (Mean ± SD)		
ISBs	DIOS (n = 15)	DPG (n = 15)	p Value
LFP	0.042 ± 0.020 [a]	0.019 ± 0.015 [a]	<0.001
LLI	0.042 ± 0.016 [a]	0.020 ± 0.021 [a]	<0.001
RLI	0.032 ± 0.007 [a]	0.009 ± 0.007 [a]	<0.001
RFP	0.043 ± 0.012 [b]	0.010 ± 0.014 [a]	<0.001
Global	0.039 ± 0.009 [b]	0.014 ± 0.013 [a]	<0.001
p value	0.615	0.666	

[a,b] different letters indicate the presence of significant difference between impression techniques using post hoc tests. RMS, root mean square; ISBs, intraoral scan-bodies; LFP, left first premolar; LLI, left lateral incisor; RLI, right lateral incisor; RFP, right first premolar; DIOS, digital intraoral scanning; DPG, digital photogrammetry.

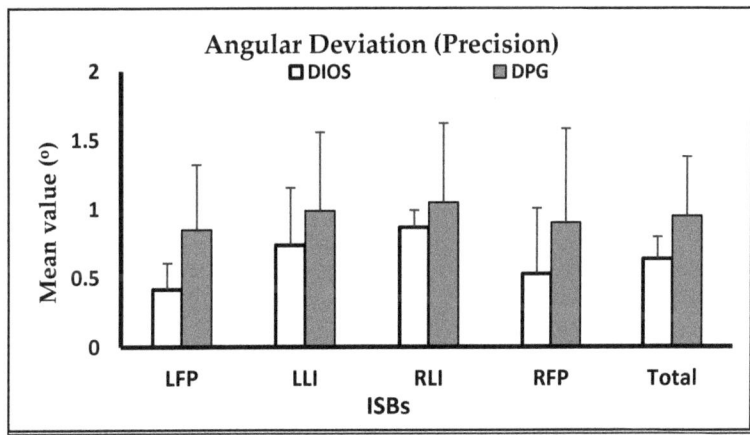

Figure 7. Mean values of angular deviations among impression techniques when evaluating precision. ISBs, intraoral scan-bodies; LFP, left first premolar; LLI, left lateral incisor; RLI, right lateral incisor; RFP, right first premolar; DIOS, digital intraoral scanning; DPG, digital photogrammetry.

For trueness, means and standard deviations for angular discrepancy were significantly different between impression techniques ($p < 0.001$); it was the lowest with DPG (0.724 ± 0.064°) and elevated for DIOS (1.744 ± 0.175°). With DIOS and DPG, the angular deviations within the ISBs were also significantly different. For DIOS, deviation was the highest on LLI and RFP, intermediary on LFP, and the smallest on RLI ($p < 0.001$) but no significant differences were found between LLI and RFP ($p = 1.000$). With DPG, it was smaller on LLI, intermediate on LFP followed by RFP and elevated on RLI ($p < 0.001$). The mean RMS 3D deviation was significantly different between impression techniques ($p < 0.001$); it was smaller with DPG (0.078 ± 0.001) and raised with DIOS (0.536 ± 0.063). The mean RMS 3D deviation within the ISBs was also significantly different ($p < 0.001$). With DIOS, it was elevated on LLI and RLI, intermediate on RFP, and smaller on LFP ($p < 0.001$). The difference was not significant between RLI and LLI ($p = 1.000$). With DPG, the 3D deviation was smaller on LLI, followed by RFP, RLI and finally elevated on LFP ($p < 0.001$).

For precision, the mean angular deviation was not significantly different between impression techniques ($p = 0.067$) and within ISBs for DIOS ($p = 0.090$), and DPG ($p = 0.725$). The mean RMS was significantly different between impression techniques ($p < 0.001$); it was smaller with DPG (0.014 ± 0.013) and elevated with DIOS (0.039 ± 0.009) The mean RMS for 3D deviation within ISBs was not significantly different for DIOS ($p = 0.615$) and DPG ($p = 0.666$).

4. Discussion

This study aimed to measure the trueness and precision of different implant level impression techniques in an all-on-four fully edentulous cast with anterior parallel implants and posteriorly tilted implants. The first null hypothesis was partially rejected. In terms of trueness, statistically significant differences were found between the DIOS and DPG groups in comparison with the true value. However, in terms of precision, scans were consistently reproducible within each group when analyzing angular deviations, yet DPG had fewer discrepancies when comparing 3D distortion datasets. The second null hypothesis was also partially rejected.

Trueness within ISBs revealed significant differences but did not have a clear direction since the results varied between parallel and angulated ISBs. However, parallel and distal implants were equally precise in terms of angular deviation and 3D deviation for both groups. This is important since the correlation between trueness and precision is a substantial aspect in choosing a proper impression technique for the intended application.

Several factors can influence impression accuracy which may project in the passivity of the prosthesis including implant angulation, implant depth, implant connection type, and inter-implant distance [11–13]. These factors were highlighted with conventional impressions in previous studies. However, different paths of results can be found when studying scans of digital impressions. With regards to implant angulation, the fidelity of digital impressions must not be affected by the angulation of implants as the worry of impression material distortion during removal, or movement of impression transfer is not a problem in this technique [11,12]. However, the results of this study showed no clear results for trueness when comparing parallel and distal implants where alternating values were recorded, having parallel implants more accurate in some cases and distal ones more legitimate in others. In the DIOS group, higher angular deviations were observed at scan body of the LLI and RFP followed by RLI and LFP. A possible analysis of this can be directional inaccuracy when bending the IOS as it approaches a different plane disfavoring the capture of scan bodies located at the curve. In other words, errors may depend not on implant angulation but rather on the arch shape and how the scanner is oriented to capture the needed image unlike photogrammetry system being fixed in a certain position and at a predetermined standardized distance is not influenced by motion or camera's inclination. However, this was not the case with 3D deviations of DIOS where RFP and LFP were truer than RLI and LLI. This means that implant angulation favors accuracy of

IOSs where results were consistent with Sallorenzo and Gómez-Polo [35]. In contrast, a systematic review by Carneiro Pereira et al. stated that angulations larger than 15 degrees can influence intraoral scanning accuracy [13].

It is important to note that differences in the results between 3D distortions and angular deviations are due to the lack of measurement uniformity between both variables despite the similarity of the purpose traced. 3D distortions are calculated from the surface of the ISB while the latter are calculated from the center axis projected by the software. In addition, RMS used to calculate the surface fit is more sensitive to outliers [48] than the mean absolute deviation used to calculate angular deviations. However, RMS was used instead of mean values since the best fit algorithm matching produces positive and negative deviations between reference and test objects which could lead to results canceling each other and not representing the real divergence [47].

The findings in this study did not relate directly to the previous work. Congruence is made difficult by the lack of standardization of measurement methodology, comparison programs, number of implants, origin of the reference dataset, and IOS and DPG technologies used. Although perfect superimposition is still difficult to obtain with digital comparison software, the technique using best-fit alignment significantly amended the merging accuracy and dwindled the quantification fallacy [42]. Also, many researchers quoted outcomes for measuring change using the best fit alignment [14,43–47] although other authors relied on the zero-method technique for calculating deviations [11,12,18,21,35]. The zero method relies on the implant center to calculate angulations and distance deviations. In addition, some preceding studies used a coordinate measuring machine (CMM) instead of desktop scanner [11,12,18,21,35]. Even though the CMM is a repeatable measuring method, it shows abbreviated exactitude in assessing small areas due to its probe size and shape [37]. In our previous work and in a similar study by Sallorenzo and Gómez-Polo similar conclusions were found showing favorable results for photogrammetry even when the latter used the zero-method technique [35,36]. In contrast, Revilla-León and her colleagues contradicted the results of this investigation and stood out among other previous clinical reports stating that photogrammetry provided the least accurate values, with the highest discrepancy [34]. It is critical to mention that a different DPG system called Icam Imetric was used, which may have a different capture complexity than Pic.

Despite the significant findings of this study, limitations do exist. Correlating findings of this in vitro study to clinical situation should be carried out with attentiveness as there are contributing factors that although standardized are different in the oral environment [9]. This includes different light reflectivity, presence of saliva, and limited access during scanning. In addition, upon importing the STL files into Geomagic software, inconsistencies in the mesh quality were noticed between the groups. Since DPG STL files were imported from Pic library, they had the least irregularities in comparison with DIOS. This may be the reason behind the underestimation of the intraoral scanning technology which may have influenced the RMS 3D deviation. However, angular deviations were sufficient to reflect the validity of the results. Further analysis should investigate the effect of mesh topography when weighing up STL files and determining accuracy. Also, the current study only attempted to assess the data acquisition step of the workflow and did not investigate what effect this may have on the manufacturing procedures, such as the processing and production of the definitive full arch framework. Challenges remain in identifying the appropriate methodology for comparing these techniques since alignment of datasets is still highly prone to errors and these techniques vary in their workflow and strategy. Future studies should be directed towards evaluating the influence of various comparison methodologies, implant angulation, photogrammetry systems, and ISBs on the legitimacy of the impression techniques.

5. Conclusions

Within the limitations of this in vitro study, the following conclusions can be drawn. Digital photogrammetry impressions were truer than the digital intraoral scanning ones but were of similar precision in terms of angular deviation.

Implant angulation had little effect on precision in both techniques. In terms of trueness, angulated implants had less 3D distortions in the digital intraoral scanning group than parallel implants. However, no clear results were observed for both techniques when angular deviations were evaluated.

Author Contributions: Conceptualization, H.T.; methodology, H.T. and G.L.; software, G.L.; validation, H.T. and G.L.; formal analysis, H.T. and G.L.; investigation, H.T. and G.L.; resources, G.L.; data curation, R.E.; writing—original draft preparation, H.T. and G.L.; writing—review and editing, H.T. and G.L.; visualization, H.T.; supervision, J.M., K.E.A. and Z.S.; project administration, J.M., K.E.A. and Z.S. All authors have read and agreed to the published version of the manuscript.

Funding: This research received no external funding.

Institutional Review Board Statement: Not applicable.

Informed Consent Statement: Not applicable.

Data Availability Statement: Not applicable.

Acknowledgments: The authors would like to thank Straumann Group and Prodent SARL for providing the needed materials, Nadine Saade for her assistance in extraorally scanning the models, and Kris Chmielewski for his support in terms of providing the Pic stereo-photogrammetry system.

Conflicts of Interest: The authors declare no conflict of interest.

References

1. Moreira, A.H.; Rodrigues, N.F.; Pinho, A.C.; Fonseca, J.C.; Vilaça, J.L. Accuracy comparison of implant impression techniques: A systematic review. *Clin. Implant Dent. Relat. Res.* **2015**, *17*, e751–e764. [CrossRef] [PubMed]
2. Joda, T.; Ferrari, M.; Gallucci, G.O.; Wittneben, J.G.; Brägger, U. Digital technology in fixed implant prosthodontics. *Periodontology 2000* **2016**, *73*, 178–192. [CrossRef] [PubMed]
3. Mangano, F.; Gandolfi, A.; Luongo, G.; Logozzo, S. Intraoral scanners in dentistry: A review of the current literature. *BMC Oral Health* **2017**, *17*, 1–11. [CrossRef] [PubMed]
4. Mizumoto, R.M.; Yilmaz, B. Intraoral scan bodies in implant dentistry. A systematic review. *J. Prosthet. Dent.* **2018**, *120*, 343–352. [CrossRef] [PubMed]
5. Pyo, S.W.; Kim, D.J.; Han, J.S.; Yeo, I.L. Ceramic materials and technologies applied to digital works in implant-supported restorative dentistry. *Materials* **2020**, *13*, 1964. [CrossRef] [PubMed]
6. Papadiochou, S.; Pissiotis, A.L. Marginal adaptation and CAD-CAM technology: A systematic review of restorative material and fabrication techniques. *J. Prosthet. Dent.* **2018**, *119*, 545–551. [CrossRef] [PubMed]
7. Hultin, M.; Svensson, K.G.; Trulsson, M. Clinical advantages of computer-guided implant placement: A systematic review. *Clin. Oral Implant. Res.* **2012**, *6*, 124–135. [CrossRef] [PubMed]
8. Bover-Ramos, F.; Viña-Almunia, J.; Cervera-Ballester, J.; Peñarrocha-Diago, M.; García-Mira, B. Accuracy of implant placement with computer-guided surgery: A systematic review and meta-analysis comparing cadaver, clinical, and in vitro studies. *Int. J. Oral Maxillofac. Implant.* **2018**, *33*, 101–115. [CrossRef] [PubMed]
9. Keul, C.; Güth, J.F. Accuracy of full-arch digital impressions: An in vitro and in vivo comparison. *Clin. Oral Investig.* **2020**, *24*, 735–745. [CrossRef] [PubMed]
10. Aragón, M.L.; Pontes, L.F.; Bichara, L.M.; Flores-Mir, C.; Normando, D. Validity and reliability of intraoral scanners compared to conventional gypsum models measurements: A systematic review. *Eur. J. Orthod.* **2016**, *38*, 429–434. [CrossRef] [PubMed]
11. Giménez, B.; Özcan, M.; Martínez-Rus, F.; Pradíes, G. Accuracy of a digital impression system based on parallel confocal laser technology for implants with consideration of operator experience and implant angulation and depth. *Int. J. Oral Maxillofac. Implant.* **2014**, *29*, 853–862. [CrossRef] [PubMed]
12. Alikhasi, M.; Siadat, H.; Nasirpour, A.; Hasanzade, M. Three-dimensional accuracy of digital impression versus conventional method: Effect of implant angulation and connection type. *Int. J. Dent.* **2018**, *2018*, 3761750. [CrossRef] [PubMed]
13. Carneiro Pereira, A.L.; Medeiros, V.R.; da Fonte Porto Carreiro, A. Influence of implant position on the accuracy of intraoral scanning in fully edentulous arches: A systematic review. *J. Prosthet. Dent.* **2020**. [CrossRef] [PubMed]
14. Arcuri, L.; Pozzi, A.; Lio, F.; Rompen, E.; Zechner, W.; Nardi, A. Influence of implant scanbody material, position and operator on the accuracy of digital impression for complete-arch: A randomized in vitro trial. *J. Prosthodont. Res.* **2020**, *64*, 128–136. [CrossRef] [PubMed]

15. Müller, P.; Ender, A.; Joda, T.; Katsoulis, J. Impact of digital intraoral scan strategies on the impression accuracy using the TRIOS Pod scanner. *Quintessence Int.* **2016**, *47*, 343–349. [PubMed]
16. Revilla-León, M.; Jiang, P.; Sadeghpour, M.; Piedra-Cascón, W.; Zandinejad, A.; Özcan, M.; Krishnamurthy, V.R. Intraoral digital scans-Part 1: Influence of ambient scanning light conditions on the accuracy (trueness and precision) of different intraoral scanners. *J. Prosthet. Dent.* **2020**, *124*, 372–378. [CrossRef] [PubMed]
17. Revilla-León, M.; Jiang, P.; Sadeghpour, M.; Piedra-Cascón, W.; Zandinejad, A.; Özcan, M.; Krishnamurthy, V.R. Intraoral digital scans: Part 2-influence of ambient scanning light conditions on the mesh quality of different intraoral scanners. *J. Prosthet. Dent.* **2020**, *124*, 575–580. [CrossRef] [PubMed]
18. Tan, M.Y.; Yee, S.H.X.; Wong, K.M.; Tan, Y.H.; Tan, K.B.C. Comparison of three-dimensional accuracy of digital and conventional implant impressions: Effect of interimplant distance in an edentulous arch. *Int. J. Oral Maxillofac. Implant.* **2019**, *34*, 366–380. [CrossRef] [PubMed]
19. Fluegge, T.; Att, W.; Metzger, M.; Nelson, K. A novel method to evaluate precision of optical implant impressions with commercial scan bodies-an experimental approach. *J. Prosthodont.* **2017**, *26*, 34–41. [CrossRef] [PubMed]
20. Andriessen, F.S.; Rijkens, D.R.; van der Meer, W.J.; Wismeijer, D.W. Applicability and accuracy of an intraoral scanner for scanning multiple implants in edentulous mandibles: A pilot study. *J. Prosthet. Dent.* **2014**, *111*, 186–194. [CrossRef] [PubMed]
21. Giménez, B.; Pradíes, G.; Martínez-Rus, F.; Özcan, M. Accuracy of two digital implant impression systems based on confocal microscopy with variations in customized software and clinical parameters. *Int. J. Oral Maxillofac. Implant.* **2015**, *30*, 56–64. [CrossRef] [PubMed]
22. Goodacre, B.J.; Goodacre, C.J.; Baba, N.Z. Using intraoral scanning to capture complete denture impressions, tooth positions, and centric relation records. *Int. J. Prosthodont.* **2018**, *31*, 377–381. [CrossRef] [PubMed]
23. Rhee, Y.K.; Huh, Y.H.; Cho, L.R.; Park, C.J. Comparison of intraoral scanning and conventional impression techniques using 3-dimensional superimposition. *J. Adv. Prosthodont.* **2015**, *7*, 460–467. [CrossRef] [PubMed]
24. Petriceks, A.H.; Peterson, A.S.; Angeles, M.; Brown, W.P.; Srivastava, S. Photogrammetry of human specimens: An innovation in anatomy education. *J. Med. Educ. Curric. Dev.* **2018**, *5*. [CrossRef] [PubMed]
25. Jemt, T.; Bäck, T.; Petersson, A. Photogrammetry-an alternative to conventional impressions in implant dentistry? A clinical pilot study. *Int. J. Prosthodont.* **1999**, *12*, 363–368. [PubMed]
26. Peñarrocha-Oltra, D.; Agustín-Panadero, R.; Bagán, L.; Giménez, B.; Peñarrocha, M. Impression of multiple implants using photogrammetry: Description of technique and case presentation. *Med. Oral Patol. Oral Cir. Bucal* **2014**, *19*, e366. [CrossRef] [PubMed]
27. Peñarrocha-Diago, M.; Balaguer-Martí, J.C.; Peñarrocha-Oltra, D.; Balaguer-Martínez, J.F.; Peñarrocha-Diago, M.; Agustín-Panadero, R. A combined digital and stereophotogrammetric technique for rehabilitation with immediate loading of complete-arch, implant-supported prostheses: A randomized controlled pilot clinical trial. *J. Prosthet. Dent.* **2017**, *118*, 596–603. [CrossRef] [PubMed]
28. Pradíes, G.; Ferreiroa, A.; Özcan, M.; Giménez, B.; Martínez-Rus, F. Using stereophotogrammetric technology for obtaining intraoral digital impressions of implants. *J. Am. Dent. Assoc.* **2014**, *145*, 338–344. [CrossRef] [PubMed]
29. Peñarrocha-Oltra, D.; Agustín-Panadero, R.; Pradíes, G.; Gomar-Vercher, S.; Peñarrocha-Diago, M. Maxillary Full-Arch Immediately Loaded Implant-Supported Fixed Prosthesis Designed and Produced by Photogrammetry and Digital Printing: A Clinical Report. *J. Prosthodont.* **2017**, *26*, 75–81. [CrossRef] [PubMed]
30. Agustín-Panadero, R.; Peñarrocha-Oltra, D.; Gomar-Vercher, S.; Peñarrocha-Diago, M. Stereophotogrammetry for Recording the Position of Multiple Implants: Technical Description. *Int. J. Prosthodont.* **2015**, *28*, 631–636. [CrossRef] [PubMed]
31. Sánchez-Monescillo, A.; Sánchez-Turrión, A.; Vellon-Domarco, E.; Salinas-Goodier, C.; Prados-Frutos, J.C. Photogrammetry Impression Technique: A Case History Report. *Int. J. Prosthodont.* **2016**, *29*, 71–73. [CrossRef] [PubMed]
32. Sánchez-Monescillo, A.; Hernanz-Martín, J.; González-Serrano, C.; González-Serrano, J.; Duarte, S., Jr. All-on-four rehabilitation using photogrammetric impression technique. *Quintessence Int.* **2019**, *50*, 288–293. [CrossRef] [PubMed]
33. Molinero-Mourelle, P.; Lam, W.; Cascos-Sánchez, R.; Azevedo, L.; Gómez-Polo, M. Photogrammetric and intraoral digital impression technique for the rehabilitation of multiple unfavorably positioned dental implants: A clinical report. *J. Oral Implantol.* **2019**, *45*, 398–402. [CrossRef] [PubMed]
34. Revilla-León, M.; Att, W.; Özcan, M.; Rubenstein, J. Comparison of conventional, photogrammetry, and intraoral scanning accuracy of complete-arch implant impression procedures evaluated with a coordinate measuring machine. *J. Prosthet. Dent.* **2021**, *125*, 470–478. [CrossRef] [PubMed]
35. Sallorenzo, A.; Gómez-Polo, M. Comparative study of the accuracy of an implant intraoral scanner and that of a conventional intraoral scanner for complete-arch fixed dental prostheses. *J. Prosthet. Dent.* **2021**. [CrossRef] [PubMed]
36. Tohme, H.; Lawand, G.; Chmielewska, M.; Makhzoume, J. Comparison between stereophotogrammetric, digital, and conventional impression techniques in implant-supported fixed complete arch prostheses: An in vitro study. *J. Prosthet. Dent.* **2021**. [CrossRef] [PubMed]
37. ISO 5725-1. *Accuracy (Trueness and Precision) of Measuring Methods and Results. Part-I: General Principles and Definitions*; Beuth Verlag GmbH: Berlin, Germany, 1994.
38. Ender, A.; Mehl, A. Accuracy of complete-arch dental impressions: A new method of measuring trueness and precision. *J. Prosthet. Dent.* **2013**, *109*, 121–128. [CrossRef]

39. Giachetti, L.; Sarti, C.; Cinelli, F.; Russo, D.S. Accuracy of digital impressions in fixed prosthodontics: A systematic review of clinical studies. *Int. J. Prosthodont.* **2020**, *33*, 192–201. [CrossRef] [PubMed]
40. Wenz, H.J.; Hertrampf, K. Accuracy of impressions and casts using different implant impression techniques in a multi-implant system with an internal hex connection. *Int. J. Oral Maxillofac. Implant.* **2008**, *23*, 39–47.
41. Mangano, F.G.; Hauschild, U.; Veronesi, G.; Imburgia, M.; Mangano, C.; Admakin, O. Trueness and precision of 5 intraoral scanners in the impressions of single and multiple implants: A comparative in vitro study. *BMC Oral Health* **2019**, *19*, 101. [CrossRef] [PubMed]
42. Tantbirojn, D.; Pintado, M.R.; Versluis, A.; Dunn, C.; Delong, R. Quantitative analysis of tooth surface loss associated with gastroesophageal reflux disease: A longitudinal clinical study. *J. Am. Dent. Assoc.* **2012**, *143*, 278–285. [CrossRef] [PubMed]
43. O'Toole, S.; Osnes, C.; Bartlett, D.; Keeling, A. Investigation into the accuracy and measurement methods of sequential 3D dental scan alignment. *Dent. Mater.* **2019**, *35*, 495–500. [CrossRef] [PubMed]
44. Kim, R.J.; Benic, G.I.; Park, J.M. Trueness of digital intraoral impression in reproducing multiple implant position. *PLoS ONE* **2019**, *14*, e0222070. [CrossRef] [PubMed]
45. Iturrate, M.; Eguiraun, H.; Solaberrieta, E. Accuracy of digital impressions for implant-supported complete-arch prosthesis, using an auxiliary geometry part-An in vitro study. *Clin. Oral Implant. Res.* **2019**, *30*, 1250–1258. [CrossRef] [PubMed]
46. Mizumoto, R.M.; Alp, G.; Özcan, M.; Yilmaz, B. The effect of scanning the palate and scan body position on the accuracy of complete-arch implant scans. *Clin. Implant Dent. Relat. Res.* **2019**, *21*, 987–994. [CrossRef] [PubMed]
47. Papaspyridakos, P.; Gallucci, G.O.; Chen, C.J.; Hanssen, S.; Naert, I.; Vandenberghe, B. Digital versus conventional implant impressions for edentulous patients: Accuracy outcomes. *Clin. Oral Implant. Res.* **2016**, *27*, 465–472. [CrossRef] [PubMed]
48. Amin, S.; Weber, H.P.; Finkelman, M.; El Rafie, K.; Kudara, Y.; Papaspyridakos, P. Digital vs. conventional full-arch implant impressions: A comparative study. *Clin. Oral Implant. Res.* **2017**, *28*, 1360–1367. [CrossRef] [PubMed]
49. Chai, T.; Draxler, R.R. Root mean square error (RMSE) or mean absolute error (MAE)? e Arguments against avoiding RMSE in the literature. *Geosci. Model Dev.* **2014**, *7*, 1247–1250. [CrossRef]
50. Pereira, L.M.S.; Sordi, M.B.; Magini, R.S.; Calazans Duarte, A.R.; Souza, J.C.M. Abutment misfit in implant-supported prostheses manufactured by casting technique: An integrative review. *Eur. J. Dent.* **2017**, *11*, 553–558. [CrossRef] [PubMed]

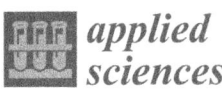

Technical Note

Alteration of the Occlusal Vertical Dimension for Prosthetic Restoration Using a Target Tracking System

Hwa-Jung Lee, June-Sung Shim, Hong-Seok Moon and Jong-Eun Kim *

Department of Prosthodontics, Yonsei University College of Dentistry, Yonsei-ro 50-1, Seodaemun-gu, Seoul 03722, Korea; hjlee0227@yuhs.ac (H.-J.L.); jfshim@yuhs.ac (J.-S.S.); hsm5@yuhs.ac (H.-S.M.)
* Correspondence: gomyou@yuhs.ac; Tel.: +82-2-2228-3160

Citation: Lee, H.-J.; Shim, J.-S.; Moon, H.-S.; Kim, J.-E. Alteration of the Occlusal Vertical Dimension for Prosthetic Restoration Using a Target Tracking System. *Appl. Sci.* 2021, *11*, 6196. https://doi.org/10.3390/app11136196

Academic Editors: José João Mendes, Ricardo Castro Alves, Ana Cristina Mano Azul and Alessandra Lucchese

Received: 27 April 2021
Accepted: 30 June 2021
Published: 4 July 2021

Publisher's Note: MDPI stays neutral with regard to jurisdictional claims in published maps and institutional affiliations.

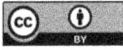

Copyright: © 2021 by the authors. Licensee MDPI, Basel, Switzerland. This article is an open access article distributed under the terms and conditions of the Creative Commons Attribution (CC BY) license (https://creativecommons.org/licenses/by/4.0/).

Abstract: Clinicians and researchers have used various methods to reproduce the maxillomandibular relationship and mandibular movement of individual patients using an articulator, with efforts being made to reduce errors associated with the conventional technique. When a change to a vertical dimension is required during the conventional prosthesis construction process, the maxillary and mandibular casts are mounted on the mechanical articulator using a facebow and bite registration and the elevation of the anterior guide pin of the articulator is used. However, this can inevitably cause errors due to differences between the articulator hinge movement and the actual trajectory of the patient. There has recently been increasing interest in tracking the trajectory of jaw motion of a patient, and this paper presents a new technique for altering the vertical dimension based on the measured trajectory. Target materials for performing tracking are attached to the maxillary and mandibular anterior teeth to record opening and closing movements of the patient's mouth in real time and align the patient's scanned intraoral data or cast data. The movements of the targets are replaced with the movement of the patient's oral scan data. Additionally, then the occlusal vertical dimension is set to a new position based on the obtained trajectory. After determining the optimal vertical dimension with consideration of the space required for restoration, maxillary and mandibular STL files are exported and the designed cast is created using a 3D printer. The printed cast is mounted on an articulator for subsequent procedures. This approach maintains the patient's actual maxillomandibular relationship at various vertical heights and can also reduce the chair time required when adjusting for errors.

Keywords: target tracking; digital dentistry; CAD-CAM; occlusal vertical dimension; maxillomandibular relationship

1. Introduction

The loss of posterior teeth loss results in the occlusal plane collapsing due to the extraction of the antagonist teeth and the lack of posterior support results in severe wearing of the remaining teeth. When there is insufficient space for a prosthesis due to excessive tooth wear, prosthetic restoration is necessary at the position where the original vertical dimension needs to be restored. The interventions in such cases require consideration of various of factors, including accurate assessment and diagnosis of the vertical dimension, the status of the remaining teeth, and the history of temporomandibular joint disease [1,2]. Determination of vertical dimension is important for fabrication of all restorations. Many techniques have been used for the measurement of the vertical dimension of occlusion such as facial landmarks, swallowing, phonetics, oscilloscope, freeway space, and cephalometric radiographs. There has been much debate in the dental literature concerning whether or not it is permissible to alter the occlusal vertical dimension (OVD). Physiologic OVD can better be described as a range instead of a fixed point or position for most subjects and the width of that comfort zone may vary among individuals according to their adaptive capacity [3]. From the clinical perspective, it is advantageous to consider altering the vertical dimension for restorative material, enhancing the esthetic tooth display and allowing for re-establishment of physiologic occlusion [4]. When the orthodontic force is applied to the teeth, periodontal ligament and alveolar bone change occurs abruptly due to the biochemical adaptive response [5,6]. Therefore, it is important to alter the vertical dimension as little as necessary after obtaining an accurate maxillomandibular relationship so that the residual teeth are not affected. Additionally, it is of paramount to mount the study casts in centric relation.

In the traditional method, an impression acquisition process is used to create a plaster cast that reproduces the patient's oral condition, which records the maxillary position based on the patient's cranial base. A facebow and the check-bite in centric relation position are used to transfer the cast to the articulator. A temporary dental prosthesis is then fabricated based on the newly set vertical dimension by raising the incisal guide pin of the articulator [4]. However, for convenience, facebows are not based on the patient's true hinge axis points. In addition, since the patient may have a centric relation–maximum intercuspation (CR–MI) discrepancy, the difference in the positions of the maxilla and mandible may occur when the gypsum model is mounted on the articulator. Therefore, the position and the maxilla-to-mandible vertical dimension of the cast may differ from the patient's actual dimensions [7], and errors may accumulate in the prosthesis being constructed based on this position.

Recent technological advances in digital dentistry have led to various methods for tracking jaw movement being proposed. A target-based method for tracking the movement of a specific reference point using an optical scanner is simpler than other tracking methods that involve mounting bulky and inconvenient equipment on the head, and has the additional advantage of recording the natural movements of patients [8–10].

This article proposes a process for transferring the gypsum cast or three-dimensional (3D) printed cast to the articulator that includes alteration of the vertical dimension. This alteration is determined using a target tracking method that can record the actual jaw motion in patients exhibiting a reduced vertical dimension due to the loss of posterior tooth support and overall wearing of the remaining teeth.

2. Materials and Methods

2.1. Attaching Target Materials to the Anterior Tooth and Tracking Jaw Movements

Before performing the target tracking process, a patient's remaining teeth, the presence of temporomandibular joint(TMJ) disease, the muscular system, and the current occlusal vertical dimension were evaluated. In the present example, a patient with extreme worn dentition due to the loss of posterior tooth support needed treatment for rehabilitation and did not have any TMJ disease selected. Four 3-mm-diameter non-reflective double circle targets (Target Sticker; Medit Corporation, Seoul, Korea) were attached to the maxillary and mandibular anterior teeth of the patient (Figure 1). Targets were attached after retracting the patient's cheeks using a mouth retractor and drying teeth surface sufficiently. The temporary filling material (Quicks Blue; Denkist, Gyeonggi, Korea) was additionally applied to enhance the adhesive force of the targets.

The anterior dentition is scanned using an intraoral scanner (i500; Medit Corporation, Seoul, Korea) to record the relationship between the targets and the teeth. Casts of the maxillary and mandibular arches using alginate impressions are each scanned and in the maximum intercuspal relationship using a 3D tabletop scanner (Identica Blue; Medit Corporation, Seoul, Korea). An optical scanner (Rexcan CS2; Medit Corporation, Seoul, Korea) is then positioned with its focal length at the patient's anterior dentition to detect the positions of the targets for tracking. The trajectories of the target movements are then tracked continuously with the optical scanner while the patient opens and closes their mouth repeated. After scanning the patient's mouth and cast of the full arch and completing the alignment using the scanned data of the target, the movements of the targets are replaced with the movement of the patient's oral scan data (Figure 2).

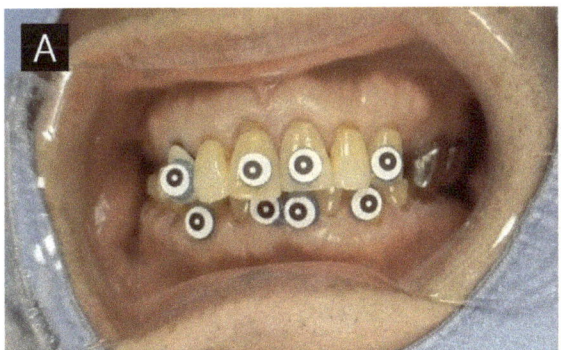 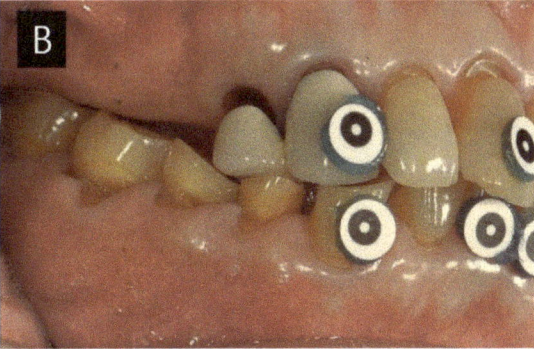

Figure 1. (**A**) Target tracking materials are attached to the labial surface of the upper and lower anterior teeth. (**B**) The restoration space is insufficient on the lateral side after losing the antagonist teeth.

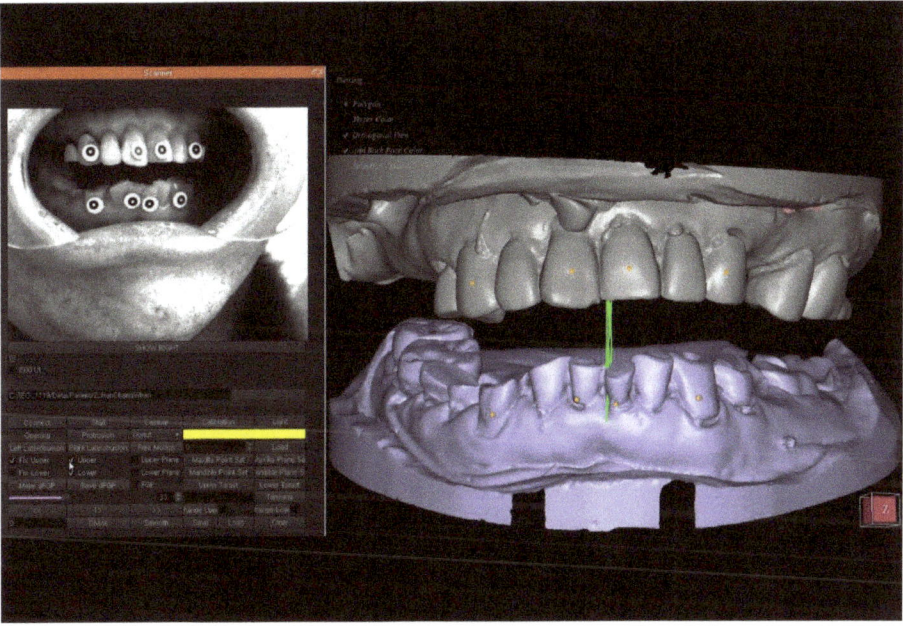

Figure 2. The mandibular movement is recorded in real time and replaced with data of the entire arch model.

The procedure of oral scanning after attaching the targets, target tracking of the anterior teeth using an optical scanner, and replacement of the entire arch data were performed in this case by aligning with referenced target stickers and the same position in the cast [11].

2.2. Confirmation of CR–MI Discrepancy

When the patient closes his mouth to the tooth contact position, it is possible to check whether a sliding motion occurs at the first contact position and the presence of CR–MI discrepancy can be checked (Figure 3A). If such a discrepancy is present, a horizontal trajectory (between two green dots) appears and its size can be measured by tracking software (Ezscan8; Medit Corporation, Seoul, Korea). Additionally, then it can be exported by specifying the positions of the maxilla and mandible in the centric relation position (Figure 3B). The centric relation recording followed the chin-point guidance method among the traditional methods and the target tracking method was used instead of the bite registration material in the step of recording the relationship between the maxilla and the mandible at the CR position.

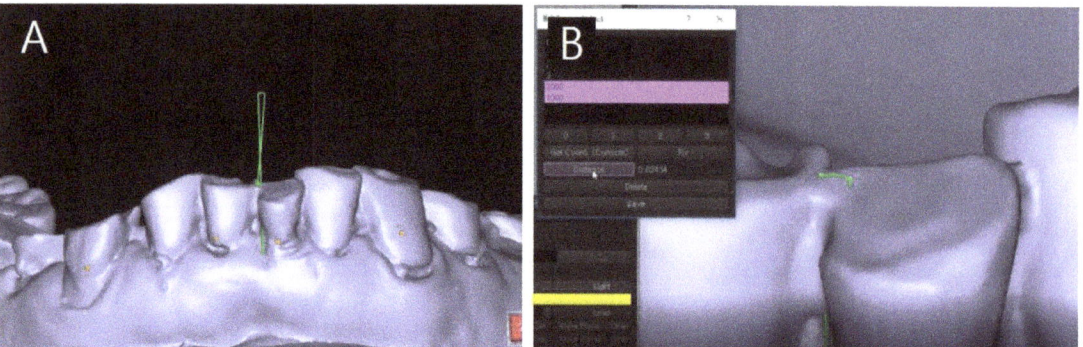

Figure 3. (**A**) Closing the mouth so that the teeth are in contact can reveal lateral sliding and the presence of a CR–MI discrepancy. (**B**) Prototype software confirmed that the difference was about 0.6 mm in this case.

2.3. Vertical Dimension Alteration

When adjustment of the occlusal vertical dimension is necessary during prosthetic restoration, the STL file produced based on the opening and closing movements of the patient's mouth can be exported after determining the optimal vertical dimension from consideration of the space required for restoration (Figure 4). Considering the patient's facial height and freeway space, alteration should be the minimum necessary to harmonize dento-facial esthetics and improve the occlusal relationship. Clinicians can select the optimal vertical dimension on a point of the trajectories of jaw motion. Maxillary and mandibular STL files were imported into 3D CAD software (Exocad dentalCAD; Exocad GmbH, Darmstadt, Germany) to reproduce the positional relationship in the digital model with the altered vertical dimension (Figure 5).

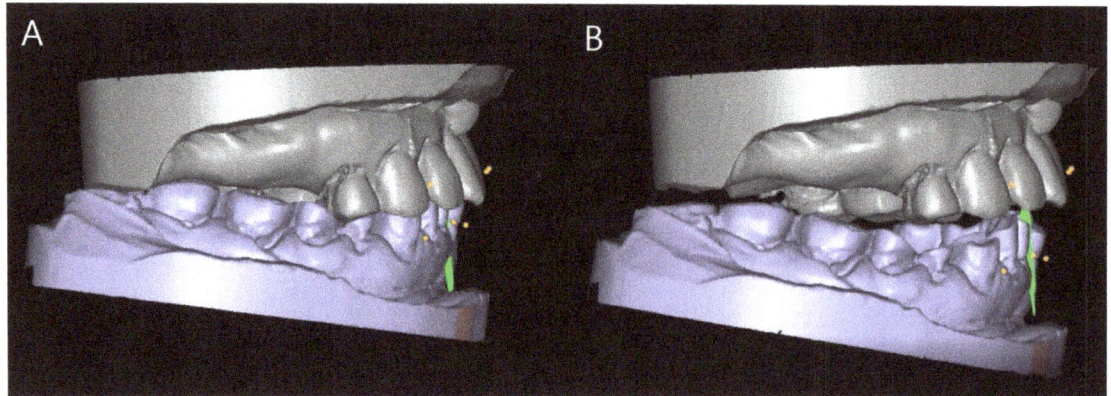

Figure 4. (**A**) Relationship between maxillary and mandibular arches in the state of maximum intercuspation. (**B**) An image showing the attempted alteration of the occlusal vertical dimension using digital software.

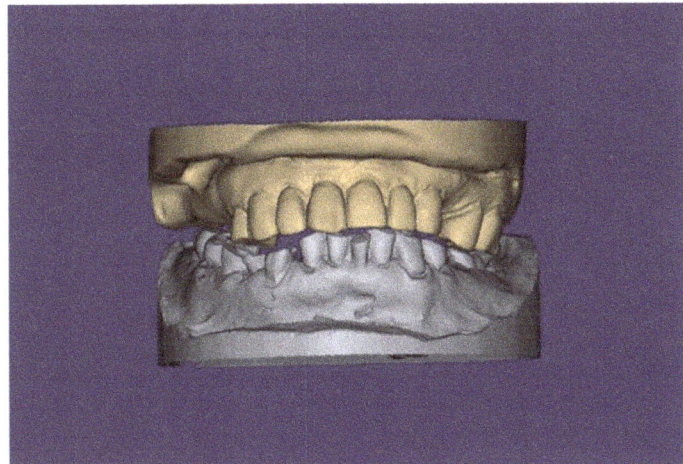

Figure 5. Images loaded from CAD software after exporting data and the relationship between the two arches with the desired occlusal vertical dimension.

2.4. Fabrication and Mounting of a 3D Printed Cast

A 3D printed cast was created using the obtained data. In order to physically relocate the position of the cast with the altered vertical dimension, a cast base and mounting pin should be designed using software (Model Creator; Exocad GmbH, Darmstadt, Germany) (Figure 6A). The designed cast was produced using a 3D printer (Form2; Formlabs, Somerville, MA, USA) and 3D printing resin (Grey Resin; Formlabs, Somerville, MA, USA) (Figure 6B).

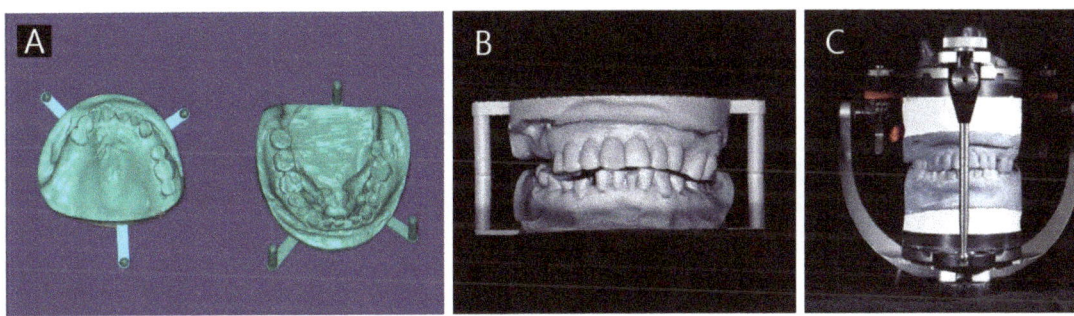

Figure 6. (**A**) A 3D printed model constructed using the exported data. Three mounting pins were designed to maintain the altered vertical dimension. (**B**) The 3D printed cast with altered vertical dimension. (**C**) The 3D printed cast is mounted on the mechanical articulator.

The printed cast with the optimal vertical dimension was mounted on a mechanical articulator while taking into account the positional relationships of the mounting pins (Figure 6C). Diagnostic wax modeling can be put on the cast or the case can be virtually waxed-up before printing the cast and the required prosthesis was then constructed.

2.5. Mounting Process of the Existing Plaster Cast

If the existing gypsum cast mounting is required for the laboratory process, a jig for mounting the gypsum cast can be fabricated using the data associated with the optimal vertical dimension (Figure 7A). After designing the jig using the bite splint module of the CAD software (Exocad dentalCAD; Exocad GmbH, Darmstadt, Germany), the jig was printed using the 3D printer (Form2; Formlabs, Somerville, MA, USA) and flexible 3D printing resin (Flexible Resin; Formlabs, Somerville, MA, USA) (Figure 7B).

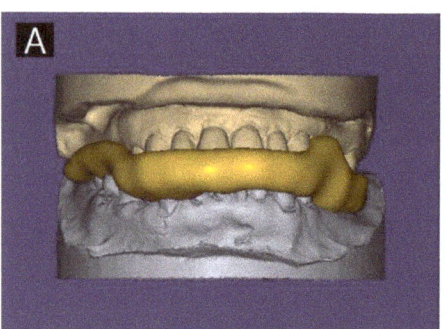 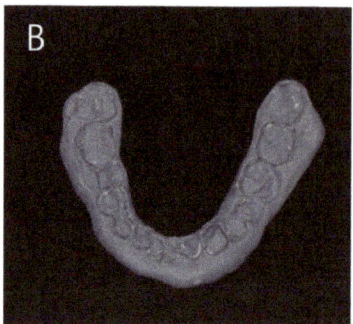 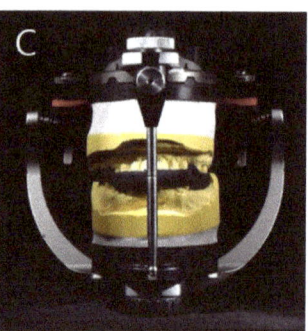

Figure 7. (**A**) Designing a flexible bite jig consistent with the altered vertical dimension for mounting the plaster cast. (**B**) The 3D printed bite jig for the gypsum cast mounting process constructed from flexible resin. (**C**) Mounting the plaster model on the mechanical articulator using the flexible bite jig.

The plaster cast was mounted on the articulator using the printed jig (Figure 7C). Wax was added to the cast for a diagnostic purpose and the required prosthesis was constructed.

2.6. Preliminary Study for Evaluating Tracking Accuracy

Preliminary study data for evaluating tracking accuracy according to the arrangement of targets were presented. The static model mounted on the articulator was recorded using the optical scanner while closed position and 4 mm (distance of tip of upper and lower central incisors) opened position. Targets were attached to the maxillary and mandibular central incisors and canines. The accuracy of target tracking was evaluated at maxillary and mandibular anteriors and the mesio-buccal cusp of the 2nd molars (Figure 8). Tracking data for 7 s at 50 frames per second was acquired and a total of 350 frames of data were recorded and compared with reference coordinates.

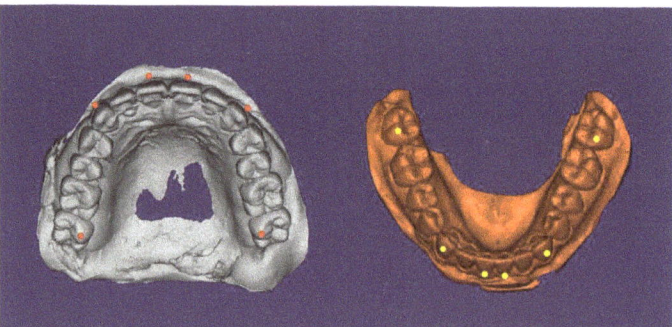

Figure 8. The accuracy of target tracking was evaluated at maxillary and mandibular anterior targets and the mesio-buccal cusp of the 2nd molars.

3. Results

The jaw movements of a patient were successfully tracked. Even a small CR–MI discrepancy within 1 mm could be detected and the optimal occlusal vertical dimension could be determined based on the opening and closing movements of the patient's mouth. A 3D printed model or an existing plaster model consistent with the newly set occlusal vertical dimension within jaw motion trajectories could be used to mount the model on the articulator and subsequent procedures.

The mean deviation at the closing state was smaller than that of the 4 mm opening state. The mean deviation of maxillary and mandibular anterior points were smaller than that of the maxillary and mandibular 2nd molar. The accuracy of the tracking data was within 10 μm in the anterior target region and within 30 μm in the cusp of the second molar, confirming that it showed very high accuracy in all environments (Figure 9).

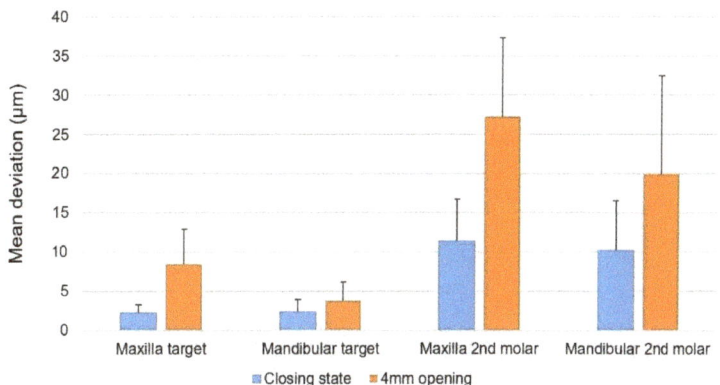

Figure 9. Mean deviation at the closing state was smaller than that of the 4 mm opening state (mean + standard deviation).

4. Discussion

The new technique presented here was able to reproduce the actual opening and closing movements of the patient's mouth, since the positions of the targets attached to the teeth were tracked using an optical scanner. A method was also proposed for confirming the CR–MI discrepancy and transferring the altered vertical dimension to the mechanical articulator. This can be used to fabricate the patient's prosthesis based on the observed trajectory, which allowed the actual maxillomandibular relationship to be maintained despite changes in the vertical dimension even when the patient had a CR–MI discrepancy. In the conventional technique, the facebow and semiadjustable articulator were manufactured based on the assumption that the patient's face and mandibular movements are symmetrical, and so errors can occur when the patient exhibits asymmetry. The occurrence of horizontal displacement during opening and closing trajectories is difficult to reproduce on the articulator. Our novel technique can overcome these limitations of the traditional method since it reproduces the detailed mandibular movements of the patient using digital software.

Another disadvantage of the conventional method is that converting between the digital cast and the physical cast is difficult on the digital articulator embedded in the CAD software. However, in the proposed technique, a 3D printed jig can be used to mount the patient's actual plaster cast in addition to the 3D printed cast. This approach can be very useful in cases that require an existing gypsum cast for the production of different kinds of prosthesis, such as a removable dental or implant prosthesis.

However, our technique also has some limitations. While it is only necessary to attach targets on the anterior teeth for target tracking, which is performed using an optical scanner, the retractor required to keep the targets exposed can interfere with the patient's natural jaw movement. It is important that the targets are in the same position without falling out even during jaw movement. If the position of the targets changes while tracking jaw motion, errors are generated and clinicians have to start over again. There are also limitations associated with the need to have access to optical scanner equipment. In order to fit exactly into the existing plaster casts without any damages, the bite jig needs to be flexible. However, there is a possibility that errors may occur due to the flexibility of the bite jig at the same time. It is necessary to confirm that the bite jig should be in the correct position when mounting the casts. Additionally, when flexible materials become too thick, occlusal errors may occur due to the elasticity of the material.

Future studies should assess the accuracy and reproducibility of our new method for altering the vertical dimension and the associated mounting procedure, and consider its compatibility with existing CAD software. The results obtained could lead to this technique having wide clinical applications.

5. Conclusions

The present dental technique records the actual mandibular movement of the patient in real time using targets attached to the maxillary and mandibular anterior teeth in patients with reduced vertical occlusion resulting from the loss of posterior teeth and wearing of the remaining teeth. The 3D printed maxillary and mandible casts can be mounted or a flexible bite jig can be constructed with increased vertical dimension to enable mounting of the existing gypsum cast.

Author Contributions: Conceptualization, H.-J.L. and J.-E.K.; methodology, J.-E.K.; software, H.-J.L. and J.-E.K.; validation, H.-J.L., H.-S.M. and J.-S.S.; formal analysis, J.-E.K.; investigation, H.-J.L.; resources, J.-S.S.; writing—original draft preparation, H.-J.L. and J.-E.K.; writing—review and editing, H.-J.L. and J.-E.K.; visualization, H.-J.L. and H.-S.M.; supervision, J.-E.K.; project administration, J.-E.K. All authors have read and agreed to the published version of the manuscript.

Funding: This research was supported by Basic Science Research Program through the National Research Foundation of Korea (NRF) funded by the Ministry of Education (NRF- 2019R1I1A1A01062792).

Institutional Review Board Statement: Not applicable.

Informed Consent Statement: Not applicable.

Data Availability Statement: The data presented in this study are available on request from the corresponding author.

Acknowledgments: The authors thank Soobok Lee and Sungbin Im from Medit Corporation for providing technical support.

Conflicts of Interest: The authors declare that they have no conflict of interest.

References

1. Verrett, R.G. Analyzing the etiology of an extremely worn dentition. *J. Prosthodont.* **2001**, *10*, 224–233. [CrossRef] [PubMed]
2. Turner, K.A.; Missirlian, D.M. Restoration of the extremely worn dentition. *J. Prosthet. Dent.* **1984**, *52*, 467–474. [CrossRef]
3. Rivera-Morales, W.C.; Mohl, N.D. Relationship of occlusal vertical dimension to the health of the masticatory system. *J. Prosthet. Dent.* **1991**, *65*, 547–553. [CrossRef]
4. Abduo, J. Safety of increasing vertical dimension of occlusion: A systematic review. *Quintessence Int.* **2012**, *43*, 369–380. [PubMed]
5. Matarese, G.; Isola, G.; Ramaglia, L.; Dalessandri, D.; Lucchese, A.; Alibrandi, A.; Fabiano, F.; Cordasco, G. Periodontal biotype: Characteristic, prevalence and dimensions related to dental malocclusion. *Minerva Stomatol.* **2016**, *65*, 231–238. [PubMed]
6. Rodriguez y Baena, R.; Pastorino, R.; Gherlone, E.F.; Perillo, L.; Lupi, S.M.; Lucchese, A. Histomorphometric Evaluation of two Different Bone Substitutes in Sinus Augmentation Procedures: A Randomized Controlled Trial in Humans. *Int. J. Oral. Maxillofac. Implants* **2017**, *32*, 188–194. [CrossRef] [PubMed]
7. Walker, P.M. Discrepancies between arbitrary and true hinge axes. *J. Prosthet. Dent.* **1980**, *43*, 279–285. [CrossRef]
8. Pinheiro, A.P.; Pereira, A.A.; Andrade, A.O.; Bellomo, D. Measurement of jaw motion: The proposal of a simple and accurate method. *J. Med. Eng. Technol.* **2011**, *35*, 125–133. [CrossRef] [PubMed]
9. Zafar, H.; Eriksson, P.O.; Nordh, E.; Häggman-Henrikson, B. Wireless optoelectronic recordings of mandibular and associated head–neck movements in man: A methodological study. *J. Oral. Rehabil.* **2000**, *27*, 227–238. [CrossRef] [PubMed]
10. Kim, J.E.; Park, J.H.; Moon, H.S.; Shim, J.S. Complete assessment of occlusal dynamics and establishment of a digital workflow by using target tracking with a three-dimensional facial scanner. *J. Prosthodont. Res.* **2019**, *63*, 120–124. [CrossRef] [PubMed]
11. Han, C.G.; Park, Y.B.; Shim, J.S.; Kim, J.E. Restorative Space Analysis by Jaw Motion Tracking Using a Template in Completely Edentulous Patients. *Appl. Sci.* **2021**, *11*, 3933. [CrossRef]

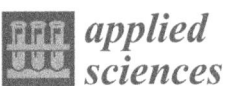

Technical Note

Digital Workflow to Fabricate Complete Dentures for Edentulous Patients Using a Reversing and Superimposing Technique

Hwa-Jung Lee [1], Jeongho Jeon [2], Hong Seok Moon [1] and Kyung Chul Oh [1,*]

[1] Department of Prosthodontics, Yonsei University College of Dentistry, Seoul 03722, Korea; hjlee0227@yuhs.ac (H.-J.L.); hsm5@yuhs.ac (H.S.M.)
[2] Central Dental Laboratory, Yonsei University Dental Hospital, Seoul 03722, Korea; denture@yuhs.ac
* Correspondence: kyungabc@yuhs.ac; Tel.: +82-2-22283168; Fax: +82-2-3123598

Featured Application: Digital complete denture.

Abstract: This technical procedure demonstrates a 4-step completely digital workflow for the fabrication of complete dentures in edentulous patients. The digital scan data of the edentulous arches were obtained using an intraoral scanner, followed by the fabrication of modeless trial denture bases using additive manufacturing. Using the trial denture base and a wax rim assembly, the interarch relationship was recorded. This record was digitized using an intraoral scanner and reversed for each maxillary and mandibular section individually. The digital scan data directly obtained using the intraoral scanner were superimposed over the reversed data, establishing a proper interarch relationship. The artificial teeth were arranged virtually and try-in dentures were additively manufactured. Subsequently, the gingival and tooth sections were additively manufactured individually and characterized. Thus, fabrication of digital complete dentures can be accomplished using digital data characteristics. The workflow includes data acquisition using an intraoral scanner, data processing using reverse engineering and computer-aided design software programs, and additive manufacturing.

Keywords: additive manufacturing; complete denture; computer-aided design; edentulism; interarch relationship registration; reversing and superimposing technique

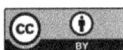

1. Introduction

Complete dentures have been manufactured using a conventional workflow, which requires multiple visits of the patients to a dental clinic and complex laboratory procedures [1,2]. With recent advances in computer-aided design and computer-aided manufacturing (CAD-CAM) technology, the digital design and fabrication of complete dentures have become an active area of research. The advantages of this workflow include the elimination of cumbersome denture tooth arrangement and subsequent resin injection or packing and reproducibility of the dentures, which can be attributed to the use of a digital workup; the designed data file can be stored in a backup device and reused later to manufacture the same denture [3].

Moreover, the performance of intraoral scanners has also dramatically increased; several studies and clinical reports have described the feasibility of intraoral scanners for obtaining digital scans in edentulous arches [4,5]. This direct digitization reduces chair time for impression making and enables real-time verification of the accuracy of the obtained impression through a monitor connected to the intraoral scanner. Nevertheless, a barrier for complete digitization is the inability to establish a three-dimensional (3D) interarch relationship using intraoral scanners. When using intraoral scanners, the interarch relationship is established by registering the bilateral buccal surfaces of the teeth; however, in cases of complete edentulism, this approach is not applicable since there are no teeth present to be registered [6].

The transformation of a negative imprint into a positive object is a fundamental concept of dentistry; for example, a definitive cast is fabricated by pouring dental stone into a negative dental impression. Commercial reverse engineering software programs have a similar function in a digital world; they enable free transformation of the 3D scan data between positive and negative shapes. This paper presents a digital workflow to register the interarch relationship by using a reversing and superimposing (RAS) technique.

2. Materials and Methods

The digital intraoral scan data of both the maxillary and mandibular arches were obtained using an intraoral scanner (TRIOS 3; 3Shape A/S, Copenhagen, Denmark) (Figure 1A,B). The scanned data were saved in the standard tessellation language (STL) file format. Modeless trial denture bases were designed using a CAD software program (Meshmixer; Autodesk, San Rafael, CA, USA) and additively manufactured using a 3D printing material (NextDent Try-In TI2; 3D Systems, NextDent B.V., Soesterberg, The Netherlands) and a 3D printer (NextDent 5100; 3D Systems, NextDent B.V., Soesterberg, The Netherlands). A wax rim was subsequently placed on each of the trial denture bases (Figure 1C). The trial denture base and wax rim assemblies were placed in the patient's mouth. They could be adjusted, if needed, to achieve better esthetic and functional outcomes. The interarch relationship was recorded using an occlusal registration material (O-Bite; DMG, Hamburg, Germany). The obtained, united assembly was scanned using the same intraoral scanner (TRIOS 3; 3Shape A/S, Copenhagen, Denmark) (Figure 1D).

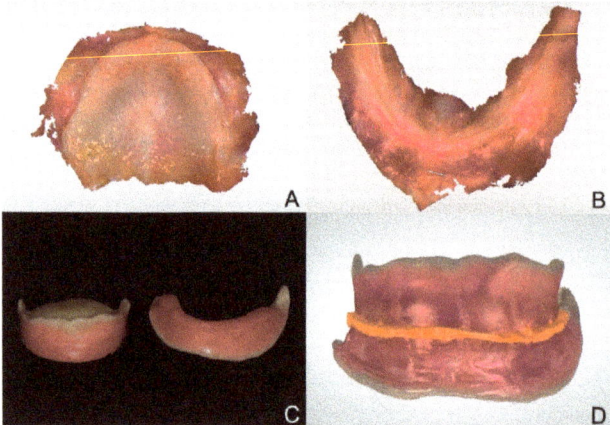

Figure 1. Impression making and bite registration for edentulous arches. (**A**) Digital intraoral scan data of a maxillary arch. (**B**) Digital intraoral scan data of a mandibular arch. (**C**) Trial denture base and wax rim assemblies. (**D**) Scan data of the united assembly with registered interarch relationship.

The STL file of the scan data of the united assembly with a registered interarch relationship was imported into a metrology/inspection software program (Geomagic Control X version 2018.0.1, 3D Systems, Rock Hill, SC, USA) to reverse the maxillary and mandibular portions individually. Subsequently, each portion was saved as an individual STL file (Figure 2A,B). The maxillary STL file obtained using the intraoral scanner was superimposed onto the reversed maxillary STL file. The same procedure was performed with the mandibular STL file, thus, establishing the interarch relationship for the original STL files (those obtained using the intraoral scanner) (Figure 2C).

The artificial teeth were arranged using the transformed maxillary and mandibular STL files as well as the STL file (or the color format file (.dcm)) of the united assembly. The occlusal plane of the assembly could be viewed by adjusting the translucency of the .dcm file (Figure 2D). Try-in dentures were additively manufactured with a 3D printing material

(NextDent Try-In TI0; 3D Systems, NextDent B.V., Soesterberg, The Netherlands) and the 3D printer (NextDent 5100; 3D Systems, NextDent B.V., Soesterberg, The Netherlands) to evaluate esthetics and function (Figure 2E). Thereafter, the gingival and tooth sections were additively manufactured individually and characterized (Figure 2F). The digitally fabricated complete dentures were placed in the patient's mouth and evaluated for esthetics and function.

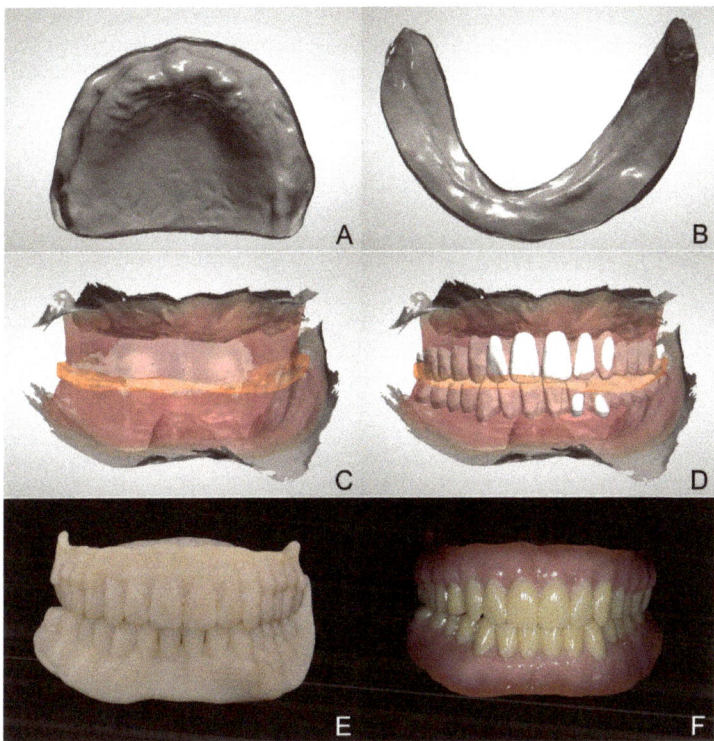

Figure 2. Computer-aided designing and additive manufacturing procedures to fabricate complete dentures. (**A**) Reversed maxillary data derived from the united assembly. (**B**) Reversed mandibular data derived from the united assembly. (**C**) Establishment of the interarch relationship for original standard tessellation language (STL) files. Translucency of the united assembly adjusted to visualize the interarch relationship. (**D**) Artificial tooth arrangement using STL files of the transformed edentulous maxillary and mandibular scan data and the united assembly data. Translucency of the united assembly was adjusted. (**E**) Additively manufactured try-in dentures. (**F**) Finalized digital complete dentures.

3. Discussion

Since the 1980s, fabrication of dental prostheses using CAD-CAM technology has become faster and more convenient than conventional methods, with the development of various scanning devices, software, and manufacturing machines [3]. Recently, an increasing number of studies have focused on reporting the methodologies and clinical cases for the fabrication of complete dentures using intraoral scanners and CAD-CAM systems. Presently, the edentulous area can be scanned using intraoral scanners without the aid of artificial indicators. Nevertheless, it was impossible to obtain the interarch relationship solely using intraoral scanners owing to the absence of distinct characteristics on the buccal side of the edentulous gingivae. By using this technique, a 4-step completely digital workflow for complete denture fabrication in edentulous patients was established: direct intraoral scanning, interarch relationship registration by the RAS technique, computer-aided designing, and additive manufacturing.

Russo et al. proposed a digital occlusal registration method, which overlaps the data obtained from facial scans with those obtained from occlusal rim scans using conventional methods [7]. However, errors may exist when using this method as the occlusal scan data are superimposed on the narrow, exposed surfaces when the patient smiles. The method proposed in the present study, i.e., the RAS technique, may be another effective option since it uses intaglio surfaces of each trial denture base for superimposition.

The present workflow is advantageous for the following reasons: First, a fully digital workflow is established, eliminating the need for making impressions that may cause discomfort to elderly edentulous patients, and the number of patient visits is reduced. Second, the technique can be expanded to the fabrication of new complete dentures using old complete dentures that exhibit decreased vertical dimension of occlusion (VDO). Old complete dentures can be relined to re-establish proper VDO, and the RAS technique can be applied by reversing the old complete dentures. This eliminates the step of remaking impressions of edentulous arches.

4. Conclusions

The present article describes a completely digital workflow for complete denture fabrication in edentulous patients. The workflow begins with data acquisition using an intraoral scanner, followed by data processing using reverse engineering and CAD software programs, and ends with additive manufacturing.

Author Contributions: Conceptualization, K.C.O.; methodology, H.S.M. and K.C.O.; software, J.J.; validation, K.C.O.; formal analysis, K.C.O.; investigation, H.-J.L. and J.J.; resources, K.C.O.; data curation, K.C.O.; writing—original draft preparation, H.-J.L. and J.J.; writing—review and editing, H.S.M. and K.C.O.; visualization, H.-J.L. and J.J.; supervision, H.S.M. and K.C.O.; project administration, K.C.O.; funding acquisition, K.C.O. All authors have read and agreed to the published version of the manuscript.

Funding: This research was funded by the National Research Foundation of Korea (NRF) grant funded by the Korea government (MSIT) (No. 2018R1C1B6005989).

Institutional Review Board Statement: Not applicable.

Informed Consent Statement: Not applicable.

Data Availability Statement: Not applicable.

Conflicts of Interest: The authors declare no conflict of interest.

References

1. Jacob, R.F. The traditional therapeutic paradigm: Complete denture therapy. *J. Prosthet. Dent.* **1998**, *79*, 6–13. [CrossRef]
2. Walmsley, A.; Pinsent, R.; Laird, W. Complete dentures: 1. Treatment planning and preliminary care. *Dent. Update* **1991**, *18*, 255, 257–260. [PubMed]
3. Beuer, F.; Schweiger, J.; Edelhoff, D. Digital dentistry: An overview of recent developments for CAD/CAM generated restorations. *Br. Dent. J.* **2008**, *204*, 505–511. [CrossRef] [PubMed]
4. Goodacre, B.J.; Goodacre, C.J. Using Intraoral Scanning to Fabricate Complete Dentures: First Experiences. *Int. J. Prosthodont.* **2018**, *31*, 166–170. [CrossRef] [PubMed]
5. Russo, L.L.; Salamini, A. Single-arch digital removable complete denture: A workflow that starts from the intraoral scan. *J. Prosthet. Dent.* **2018**, *120*, 20–24. [CrossRef] [PubMed]
6. Fang, Y.; Fang, J.H.; Jeong, S.M.; Choi, B.H. A technique for digital impression and bite registration for a single edentulous arch. *J. Prosthodont.* **2019**, *28*, e519–e523. [CrossRef] [PubMed]
7. Russo, L.L.; Salamini, A.; Troiano, G.; Guida, L. Digital dentures: A protocol based on intraoral scans. *J. Prosthet. Dent.* **2021**, *125*, 597–602. [CrossRef] [PubMed]

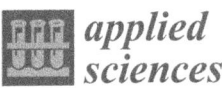

Case Report

Minimally Invasive Dentistry for Pre-Eruptive Enamel Lesions—A Case Series

Mariana Manaia [1], Larissa Rocha [1], José Saraiva [1], Ana Coelho [1,2,3], Inês Amaro [1], Carlos Miguel Marto [2,3,4,5], Francisco Vale [6], Manuel Marques Ferreira [2,3,7], Anabela Paula [1,2,3] and Eunice Carrilho [1,2,3,*]

1. Faculty of Medicine, Institute of Integrated Clinical Practice, University of Coimbra, 3000-075 Coimbra, Portugal; marianammanaia@gmail.com (M.M.); larajesus1996@gmail.com (L.R.); ze-93@hotmail.com (J.S.); anasofiacoelho@gmail.com (A.C.); ines.amaros@hotmail.com (I.A.); anabelabppaula@sapo.pt (A.P.)
2. Area of Environment Genetics and Oncobiology (CIMAGO), Faculty of Medicine, Coimbra Institute for Clinical and Biomedical Research (iCBR), University of Coimbra, 3000-548 Coimbra, Portugal; cmiguel.marto@uc.pt (C.M.M.); m.mferreira@netcabo.pt (M.M.F.)
3. Clinical Academic Center of Coimbra (CACC), 3004-561 Coimbra, Portugal
4. Faculty of Medicine, Institute of Biophysics, University of Coimbra, 3004-548 Coimbra, Portugal
5. Faculty of Medicine, Institute of Experimental Pathology, University of Coimbra, 3004-548 Coimbra, Portugal
6. Faculty of Medicine, Institute of Orthodontics, University of Coimbra, 3000-075 Coimbra, Portugal; franciscofvale@gmail.com
7. Faculty of Medicine, Institute of Endodontics, University of Coimbra, 3000-075 Coimbra, Portugal
* Correspondence: eunicecarrilho@gmail.com

Abstract: Pre-eruptive enamel lesions occur during tooth formation and include fluorosis, traumatic hypomineralization, and molar incisor hypomineralization. Minimally invasive treatment approaches, such as microabrasion, should be considered for these cases. This article presents a case series of three patients with pre-eruptive enamel defects in esthetically compromised tooth regions which were treated with the microabrasion technique: two fluorosis cases, moderate and advanced, and one hypomineralization case of traumatic etiology. In Cases 1 and 3, there was a significant improvement in esthetics with a total resolution of the enamel defects. However, a slight yellowish coloration may be detected at close observation. In Case 2 (advanced fluorosis), although there was no full resolution of the white spots, there was a clear improvement in esthetics. Microabrasion is a safe and effective, minimally invasive treatment for pre-eruptive enamel lesions. It does not require local anesthesia, it is less destructive than restorative interventions, and allows good esthetic outcomes with no significant postoperative sensitivity. Its efficacy is directly related to the lesions' severity and depth. Although there are some limitations, further improvement can be achieved with dental bleaching. More invasive treatments might be considered if results are still unsatisfactory.

Keywords: enamel; fluorosis; hypomineralization; microabrasion; minimally invasive

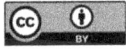

1. Introduction

Smile esthetics is a constant concern for patients, especially for the young generations. Enamel defects involving color alteration, mainly those in the anterior region, often compromise the esthetic appearance of teeth [1]. White enamel lesions are an example of a clinical condition corresponding to an enamel hypomineralization, which translates into a porous enamel surface that can, depending on the severity of each particular case, affect patients' lives and wellbeing [1–3]. These white defects can be classified as pre- or post-eruptive lesions [1].

Post-eruptive white enamel lesions correspond to the early stages of the carious disease which we refer to as white spot lesions (WSLs) [1]. WSLs occur due to the accumulation of organic acids produced by bacteria, which compromise the balance of the demineralization and remineralization process [4]. As such, they develop in sites prone to plaque accumulation such as the labial cervical third or around orthodontic appliances. They are chalky-white and most present well-defined outlines and a continuous enamel surface with a slight roughness [1,4]. On the other hand, pre-eruptive lesions occur during tooth formation and include fluorosis, traumatic hypomineralization, and molar incisor hypomineralization, among others [1]. Dental fluorosis results from the excessive fluoride incorporation during amelogenesis. Clinically, it translates as symmetrical lesions of homologous teeth and affects several teeth at once [1]. Horowitz et al. [5] proposed a classification for fluorosis—the Tooth Surface Index of Fluorosis (TSIF)—by which the teeth are classified from 0 to 7 based on the extent of coronal involvement and clinical appearance. In milder cases (TSIF 1–3) there is a progression of the affected tooth surface area by white enamel defects. At more advanced stages (TSIF > 4) the enamel presents alterations in surface texture, such as pits and fissures, and/or color changes [1,5]. Another example of pre-eruptive white enamel lesions, traumatic hypomineralization, results from periodontal trauma of the deciduous preceding teeth or periapical infections during the maturation stage of the ameloblasts [1]. Clinically, lesions may present with different shapes, outlines, localization, and color, but they mostly appear as punctiform lesions on the incisal third of only one tooth, usually a maxillary anterior tooth, in a unilateral pattern. The opponent mandibular tooth may also be affected [1]. Regarding molar incisor hypomineralization (MIH), it is characterized by the appearance of well-defined white, yellowish, or brownish opacities limited to the occlusal half of at least one of the first permanent molars associated, or not, with lesions of permanent incisors [1]. It may also affect, although less commonly, canine cusps and second permanent molars. Unlike WSLs, fluorosis, and traumatic hypomineralization, the lesions are not located at a subsurface level. Instead, MIH begins at the dentin–enamel junction and progresses outward [1]. Differential diagnosis might be difficult sometimes, but it is essential for the treatment success and improvement in esthetics.

Before considering a more invasive restorative approach for these enamel defects, minimally invasive procedures must be considered in an attempt to improve esthetics with minimal tooth structure loss. Depending on the depth of the enamel lesions, clinicians might be able to considerably solve or soften the appearance using these methods. Treatment options vary between remineralization with casein phosphopeptide-amorphous calcium phosphate (CPP-ACP) or products containing fluorides, infiltrative resins, such as ICON® (DMG, Hamburg, Germany), dental bleaching, and microabrasion [1].

The microabrasion procedure allows for the removal of superficial and intrinsic defects from teeth with minimal enamel loss. A smooth, regular, and lustrous enamel surface is obtained through a combined effect of abrasion and erosion—the "abrasion effect" [6–9]. It was first described by Croll and Cavanaugh [8,9], in which they proposed using hydrochloric acid at 18% and pumice to improve brown spots in the enamel and it has been modified throughout the years. Nowadays, several safe microabrasion slurries have been developed with different combinations of acids and abrasive particles [10].

The aim of this article is to describe the microabrasion technique for the management of pre-eruptive enamel lesions, describing the clinical protocol and the immediate esthetic outcomes.

2. Materials and Methods

2.1. Cases' Selection and Description

This article presents a case series of three patients who reported to the Dentistry Department of the Faculty of Medicine (University of Coimbra) presenting enamel defects in esthetically compromised tooth regions. A complete assessment of all patients' medical history was performed, as well as an intraoral examination to determine the etiology of the discolorations.

Case 1 (Figure 1) was diagnosed with a moderate case of fluorosis (TSIF 4). Case 2 (Figure 2) was diagnosed with an advanced case of fluorosis (TSIF 5). Case 3 (Figure 3) was diagnosed with traumatic hypomineralization, due to trauma of the preceding primary teeth. All treatment options were presented and discussed along with each patient. Written informed consent was obtained from each patient, and after careful evaluation, the microabrasion technique was selected.

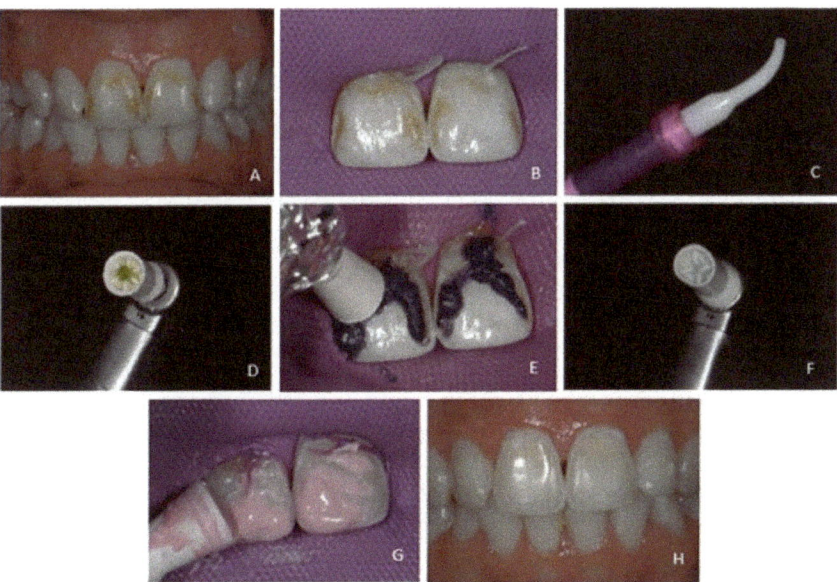

Figure 1. Case 1 with a moderate case of fluorosis diagnosis (TSIF 4). (**A**): Preoperative photograph showing enamel defects on teeth 11 and 21. (**B**): Rubber dam isolation with floss ligatures. (**C**): Opalustre® (Ultradent Products, Inc., South Jordan, UT, USA). (**D**): OpalCups™ Bristle (Ultradent Products, Inc., South Jordan, UT, USA). (**E**): Application of a 1 mm thick layer of the microabrasive product (Opalustre® over the enamel defects. (**F**): OpalCups™ Finishing (Ultradent Products, Inc., South Jordan, UT, USA). (**G**): Final polishing with a fluoride paste. (**H**): Immediate postoperative photograph.

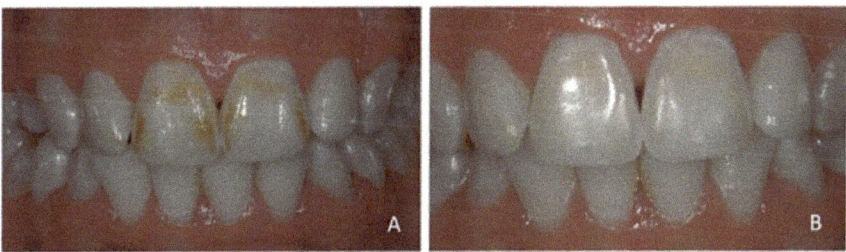

Figure 2. Case 1 with a moderate case of fluorosis diagnosis (TSIF 4). (**A**): Preoperative photograph showing enamel defects on teeth 11 and 21. (**B**): Immediate postoperative photograph.

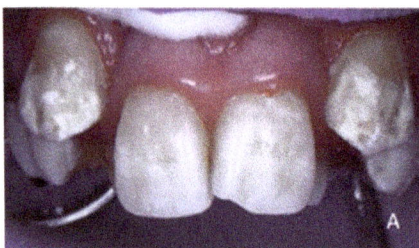 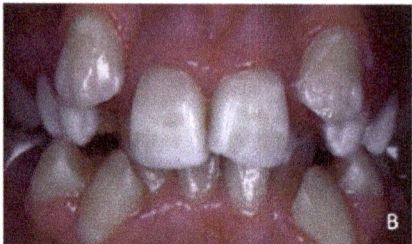

Figure 3. Case 2 with an advanced case of fluorosis diagnosis (TSIF 5). (**A**): Preoperative photograph with rubber dam isolation showing enamel defects on teeth 13, 11, 21 and 23. (**B**): Immediate postoperative photograph.

2.2. Microabrasion Procedure

The procedure was similar in all of the reported cases. Firstly, a preoperative intraoral photograph was taken for future reference (Figure 1A) using an adequate camera (Canon 80D) and lens (macro 100 mm, L series, Canon), and the appropriate parameters for intraoral photography (F25, shutter speed 1/125, and ISO 100). In all the cases, teeth were cleaned with water and a prophy brush and the operative field was isolated with a rubber dam (Figure 1B). Petroleum jelly was applied around the cervical portion of the teeth to prevent leakage of the hydrochloric acid or damage to the gingiva. Once the teeth were cleaned and isolated, the microabrasion product, a 6.6% hydrochloric acid slurry (Opalustre®, Ultradent Products, Inc., South Jordan, UT, USA) (Figure 1C), was applied in a 1 mm thick layer over the enamel defects and the product was spread over the lesions using a specially designed rubber cup (OpalCups™ Bristle, Ultradent Products, Inc., South Jordan, UT, USA) (Figure 1D,E) in a low-speed handpiece (500 rpm according to the manufacturer's instructions) under light pressure for 10–12 s. Between applications, the teeth were rinsed with water. The procedure was repeated 10 times in each tooth, which was deemed the maximum times the product could be applied without losing too much enamel. In the end, a 700 ppm fluoride polishing paste (CleanJoy, VOCO, Germany) was applied with a specially designed rubber cup (OpalCups™ Finishing, Ultradent Products, Inc., South Jordan, UT, USA) (Figure 1F) in a low-speed handpiece (2000 rpm according to the manufacturer's instructions) to polish and remineralize the enamel (Figure 1G). The rubber dam was then removed, and a postoperative intraoral photograph was taken (Figure 1H). Patients were also evaluated for postoperative hypersensitivity immediately after treatment and then again after one week and one month.

3. Results

Regarding Case 1 (Figure 2), the immediate postoperative photograph shows a significant improvement in esthetics with a total resolution of the brown defects. However, a slight yellowish coloration may be detected at close observation. The same applies to Case 3 (Figure 4), in which the white enamel defect on tooth 11 was solved but an underlying yellowish coloration was revealed. As for Case 2 (Figure 3), the teeth were affected by a more advanced case of fluorosis, with pitting in teeth 13 and 23. Even though there was no total resolution of the white spots, there was a clear improvement in esthetics as the microabrasion procedure was able to provide more uniformity, smoothness, and luster to the enamel. As for postoperative hypersensitivity, all three patients reported no effects either immediately or in the follow-up evaluations.

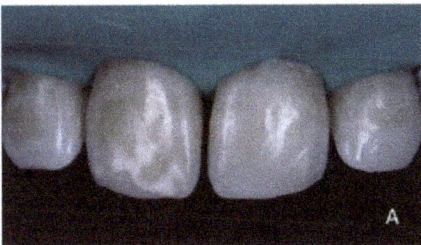 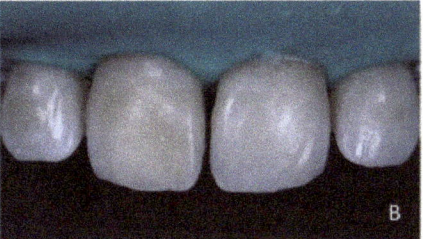

Figure 4. Case 3 diagnosed with traumatic hypomineralization. (**A**): Preoperative photograph with rubber isolation with floss ligatures showing a white enamel defect on tooth 11. (**B**): Immediate postoperative photograph.

4. Discussion

One of the biggest challenges dental clinicians face is the resolution of unesthetic enamel defects, which may vary in etiology, color, extension, and depth. Hypomineralization is the common feature to all white enamel defects, which include white spot carious lesions, dental fluorosis, traumatic hypomineralization, and molar incisor hypomineralization, and different treatment approaches might be used to improve the esthetic appearance of these lesions [1], which is of utter importance since these enamel defects present an optical problem due to their higher pore volume [2,3]. It is important to have a proper differential diagnosis based on clinical appearance, localization, and extension of lesions, and a detailed medical and dental history to select the best treatment for each case.

For WSLs, post-eruptive enamel defects, the recommended treatments are remineralization [1,4,11,12], microabrasion [6,11,13–15], and/or resin infiltration [1,4,6,11,12,14,16]. These are all valid treatment approaches; however, remineralizing agents, such as fluorides, suffer from very superficial effects and high pH-dependency [17]. When it comes to fluorosis and traumatic hypomineralization lesions, even though they differ in clinical aspects, the treatment approaches are similar since they include microabrasion associated, or not, with dental bleaching [1,6,15], and resin infiltration may also be a possibility [1,6]. Molar–incisor hypomineralization, however, unlike other enamel defects, starts from the dental–enamel junction and not the enamel subsurface [1]. In severe cases, microabrasion or resin infiltration may be attempted to attenuate the appearance [1,6], but in mild cases, no treatment is recommended since microabrasion and other techniques would require the removal of two thirds of sound enamel [1].

Microabrasion is a safe, practical, and quick technique and is used nowadays by a great number of clinicians to manage enamel defects. It is a minimally invasive treatment approach, it does not require local anesthesia, and it allows good esthetic results with no significant postoperative sensitivity [15]. This technique has evolved throughout the years and several studies have shown the importance of the combined use of abrasive and erosive actions. Not only is the abrasive component important to neutralize the erosive action of the acids, but the use of pumice alone is insufficient to remove the outer enamel layer [7]. Opalustre® (Ultradent Products, Inc.), which was used in the all the clinical cases, is a premixed slurry of 6.6% hydrochloric acid and silicon carbide microparticles. Its main advantage over other products is that, being a premixed slurry, it is more easily applied. According to some authors, other alternatives include using phosphoric acid at 35–37.5% and pumice, individually or by mixing them before application [7,15]. Due to the caustic and toxic effects of the hydrochloric acid component of the Opalustre® product (Ultradent Products, Inc.) [18], it is important to assure proper isolation, which was why in all the cases a rubber dam was used. However, with the use of the rubber dam, teeth become much more dry, and will need time to rehydrate, since the air that replaces the organic fluids when teeth become drier has a lower refractive index ($RI_{air} \approx 1 < RI_{organic\ fluids} = 1.33$), and the difference between healthy enamel ($RI_{hydroxyapatite} = 1.62$) and the enamel defects becomes more obvious, which is why it is necessary to reevaluate the results at a second appointment [1].

The good esthetic outcomes achieved through the microabrasion technique are due to the fact that the mineralized tissue in the enamel surface is compacted within the organic area, and the outer layer of prism-rich enamel is replaced with a densely compacted prism free layer, creating a fluorapatite-rich surface layer [6,7,10,15]. This prism-free layer of enamel will refract and reflect the light differently, which translates to a clinically smooth, shiny, and lustrous enamel, and camouflages any mild color imperfections in the underlying enamel—the "abrasion effect" [6,10,15]. Since the enamel surface becomes smoother, plaque adhesion is reduced, which is also a great advantage [15]. However, there are also some drawbacks when using microabrasion since the dental surface may acquire a yellowish appearance due to the fact that there is a reduction in enamel thickness, and the underlying dentin may become more visible [6,10], which is noticeable in the final photographs of Case 1 and 3. Nevertheless, if the Opalustre product is correctly used according to manufacturer's instructions, only approximately 10–200 μm of the outer enamel layer is removed, which is considered as clinically acceptable [19]. Moreover, Yetkiner et al. [11] showed that even though microabrasion had a favorable outcome initially, this might not be resistant to discoloration by smoking, consumption of tannin-rich foods, and long-term use of cationic agents. The efficacy of the microabrasion procedure is also directly related to the severity and depth of the lesions [7], which can be confirmed by Case 2 where, even though it was not possible to achieve full resolution of the lesions due to the severity of the case, it was still possible to improve esthetics significantly. The microabrasion technique is recommended for stains or defects that are no deeper than a few tenths of a millimeter in enamel [20], which is why proper evaluation with a photopolymerizer's light might be useful to decide between this technique and resin infiltration. By using the photopolymerizer and allowing the light to go through the tooth, it is possible to distinguish between deeper lesions, which appear darker, and more superficial lesions, which appear in a lighter shade. As for contraindications, this technique should not be carried out in uncooperative patients, patients with a history of sensitivity to hot, cold, or acidic foods, and patients with dentinogenesis or amelogenesis imperfecta [15].

When necessary, the microabrasion technique may be combined with other treatment approaches in order to improve the final esthetic result. Treatments such as dental bleaching may be useful to whiten the yellowish part of the tooth when there is a great enamel reduction and reduce contrast with the rest of the surface [6,10,18,21]. If, afterwards, there is still a need to further improve results, a resin-infiltration technique may be attempted and later, if necessary, a direct composite restoration. Some authors suggest the use of macro reduction prior to the microabrasion procedure in cases of advanced fluorosis with pitting [6,10]. Sunfeld et al. [6,10] showed how the use of a high-speed tapered fine diamond bur and copious irrigation to remove the superficial layer of the stained enamel was able to drastically improve the final results in severe cases of fluorosis. However, this procedure is more invasive and should therefore be, as much as possible, used only in cases where microabrasion and resin-infiltration techniques were attempted and proved insufficient.

5. Conclusions

Microabrasion is a safe and effective minimally invasive treatment for patients with enamel defects, namely pre-eruptive lesions. It is less destructive than restorative interventions and allows good esthetic outcomes with no significant postoperative sensitivity. Although there are some limitations to this technique, further improvements can be achieved if necessary when combining this procedure with other treatment approaches.

Author Contributions: Conceptualization, A.C., I.A., C.M.M., F.V., A.P. and E.C.; methodology, M.M. L.R., J.S. and A.P.; photography, J.S.; writing—original draft preparation, M.M., L.R., J.S., I.A. and A.P.; writing—review and editing, A.C., I.A., C.M.M. and A.P.; supervision, F.V., M.M.F. and E.C. A authors have read and agreed to the published version of the manuscript.

Funding: This research received no external funding.

Institutional Review Board Statement: Not applicable.

Informed Consent Statement: Written informed consent has been obtained from the patients to publish this paper if applicable.

Conflicts of Interest: The authors declare no conflict of interest.

References

1. Denis, M.; Atlan, A.; Vennat, E.; Tirlet, G.; Attal, J.P. White defects on enamel: Diagnosis and anatomopathology: Two essential factors for proper treatment (part 1). *Int. Orthod.* **2013**, *11*, 139–165. [CrossRef]
2. Krämer, N.; Bui Khac, N.N.; Lücker, S.; Stachniss, V.; Frankenberger, R. Bonding strategies for MIH-affected enamel and dentin. *Dent. Mater.* **2018**, *34*, 331–340. [CrossRef] [PubMed]
3. Bronckers, A.L.; Lyaruu, D.M.; DenBesten, P.K. The impact of fluoride on ameloblasts and the mechanisms of enamel fluorosis. *J. Dent Res.* **2009**, *88*, 877–893. [CrossRef] [PubMed]
4. Chen, M.; Li, J.Z.; Zuo, Q.L.; Liu, C.; Jiang, H.; Du, M.Q. Accelerated aging effects on color, microhardness and microstructure of ICON resin infiltration. *Eur. Rev. Med. Pharmacol. Sci.* **2019**, *23*, 7722–7731. [PubMed]
5. Horowitz, H.S.; Driscoll, W.S.; Meyers, R.J.; Heifetz, S.B.; Kingman, A. A new method for assessing the prevalence of dental fluorosis–the Tooth Surface Index of Fluorosis. *J. Am. Dent. Assoc.* **1984**, *109*, 37–41. [CrossRef]
6. Sundfeld, D.; Pavani, C.C.; Pini, N.I.P.; Machado, L.S.; Schott, T.C.; Sundfeld, R.H. Enamel microabrasion and dental bleaching on teeth presenting severe-pitted enamel fluorosis: A case report. *Oper. Dent.* **2019**, *44*, 566–573. [CrossRef]
7. Pini, N.I.P.; Lima, D.A.N.L.; Ambrosano, G.M.B.; da Silva, W.J.; Aguiar, F.H.B.; Lovadino, J.R. Effects of acids used in the microabrasion technique: Microhardness and confocal microscopy analysis. *J. Clin. Exp. Dent.* **2015**, *7*, e506–e512. [CrossRef]
8. Croll, T.P.; Cavanaugh, R.R. Enamel color modification by controlled hydrochloric acid-pumice abrasion. I. technique and examples. *Quintessence Int.* **1986**, *17*, 81–87.
9. Croll, T.P.; Cavanaugh, R.R. Enamel color modification by controlled hydrochloric acid-pumice abrasion. II. Further examples. *Quintessence Int.* **1986**, *17*, 157–164.
10. Sundfeld, R.H.; Franco, L.M.; Gonçalves, R.S.; de Alexandre, R.S.; Machado, L.S.; Neto, D.S. Accomplishing esthetics using enamel microabrasion and bleaching—A case report. *Oper. Dent.* **2014**, *39*, 223–227. [CrossRef]
11. Yetkiner, E.; Wegehaupt, F.; Wiegand, A.; Attin, R.; Attin, T. Colour improvement and stability of white spot lesions following infiltration, micro-abrasion, or fluoride treatments in vitro. *Eur. J. Orthod.* **2014**, *36*, 595–602. [CrossRef] [PubMed]
12. Abdullah, Z.; John, J. Minimally Invasive Treatment of White Spot Lesions -A Systematic Review. *Oral. Health Prev. Dent.* **2016**, *14*, 197–205.
13. Pliska, B.T.; Warner, G.A.; Tantbirojn, D.; Larson, B.E. Treatment of white spot lesions with ACP paste and microabrasion. *Angle. Orthod.* **2012**, *82*, 765–769. [CrossRef] [PubMed]
14. Paula, A.B.P.; Fernandes, A.R.; Coelho, A.S.; Marto, C.M.; Ferreira, M.M.; Caramelo, F.; do Vale, F.; Carrilho, E. Therapies for White Spot Lesions—A Systematic Review. *J. Evid. Based Dent. Pract.* **2017**, *17*, 23–38. [CrossRef] [PubMed]
15. Ashfaq, N.M.; Grindrod, M.; Barry, S. A discoloured anterior tooth: Enamel microabrasion. *Br. Dent. J.* **2019**, *226*, 486–489. [CrossRef]
16. Hallgren, K.; Akyalcin, S.; English, J.; Tufekci, E.; Paravina, R.D. Color Properties of Demineralized Enamel Surfaces Treated with a Resin Infiltration System. *J. Esthet. Restor. Dent.* **2016**, *28*, 339–346. [CrossRef]
17. Scholz, K.J.; Federlin, M.; Hiller, K.A.; Ebensberger, H.; Ferstl, G.; Buchalla, W. EDX-analysis of fluoride precipitation on human enamel. *Sci. Rep.* **2019**, *9*, 13442. [CrossRef]
18. Romero, M.F.; Babb, C.S.; Delash, J.; Brackett, W.W. Minimally invasive esthetic improvement in a patient with dental fluorosis by using microabrasion and bleaching: A clinical report. *J. Prosthet. Dent.* **2018**, *120*, 323–326. [CrossRef]
19. Sundfeld, R.H.; Croll, T.P.; Briso, A.L.; Alexandre, R.S.; Neto, D.S. Considerations about enamel microabrasion after 18 years. *Am. J. Dent.* **2007**, *20*, 67–72.
20. Zenouz, G.A.; Ezoji, F.; Enderami, S.A.; Khafri, S. Effect of Fluoride, Casein Phosphopeptide-Amorphous Calcium Phosphate and Casein Phosphopeptide-Amorphous Calcium Phosphate Fluoride on Enamel Surface Microhardness After Microabrasion: An in Vitro Study. *J. Dent.* **2015**, *12*, 705–711.
21. Vasconcelos, M.Q.S.B.; Vieira, K.A.; Salgueiro, M.C.C.; Alfaya, T.A.; Ferreira, C.S.; Bussadori, S.K. Microabrasion: A treatment option for white spots. *J. Clin. Pediatr. Dent.* **2014**, *39*, 27–29. [CrossRef] [PubMed]

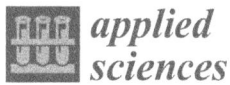

Article

Accuracy of the Fluorescence-Aided Identification Technique (FIT) for Detecting Residual Composite Remnants after Trauma Splint Removal—A Laboratory Study

Eva Magni [1,†], Wadim Leontiev [1,†], Sebastian Soliman [2], Christian Dettwiler [1], Christian Klein [3,4], Gabriel Krastl [2], Roland Weiger [1] and Thomas Connert [1,*]

[1] Department of Periodontology, Endodontology and Cariology, University Center for Dental Medicine UZB, University of Basel, 4075 Basel, Switzerland
[2] Department of Conservative Dentistry and Periodontology, Center of Dental Traumatology, University Hospital of Würzburg, 97080 Würzburg, Germany
[3] Department of Restorative Dentistry, Periodontology, Endodontology and Pediatric Dentistry, School of Dental Medicine, Eberhard Karls University, 72074 Tübingen, Germany
[4] Private Practice Meller Zahngesundheit, 71332 Waiblingen, Germany
* Correspondence: thomas.connert@unibas.ch
† These authors contributed equally to this work.

Abstract: Distinguishing composite remnants from tooth structure after trauma splint removal can be challenging. This study aimed to compare the Fluorescence-aided Identification Technique (FIT) with conventional light illumination (CONV) in terms of accuracy and time required for the detection of composite remnants after trauma splint removal. Ten bovine tooth models containing anterior teeth from 12 to 22 with composite remnants after trauma splint removal were used. These models were examined by 10 students and 10 general dentists. Each examiner assessed the 10 models using CONV or FIT three times with an interval of 2 weeks each using a prototype fluorescence-inducing headlamp with a spectral bandwidth of (405 ± 7) nm for FIT and a dental unit lamp for CONV. The examiners charted the location of identified composite remnants, and the procedure time needed for each method was recorded. Statistical analysis was performed with R 3.2.2 software with a significance level of $\alpha = 5\%$. FIT was more accurate and less time-consuming than CONV ($p < 0.001$). There were no significant differences between dentists and students concerning accuracy (CONV: $p = 0.26$; FIT: $p = 0.73$). Students performed FIT significantly faster than the dentists ($p < 0.001$). FIT is a quick and reliable method of identifying composite remnants after trauma splint removal.

Keywords: composite detection; fluorescence-aided identification technique; titanium trauma splint (TTS) removal

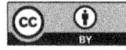

1. Introduction

Traumatic dental injuries are common in children and young adolescents [1]. Permanent teeth with root fractures and luxations require careful repositioning or replantation, followed by splinting [2]. The period of splinting varies depending on the type of injury. The splint is removed after one to four weeks in most cases (avulsion, subluxation and lateral, intrusive and extrusive luxation injuries), but may be left in place for as long as 12 weeks after certain injuries, such as root fractures [2]. The Titanium Trauma Splint (TTS, Medartis AG, Basel, Switzerland) was designed for this application. The TTS is a simple appliance that meets contemporary esthetic standards [3,4]. It is bendable and can therefore be adapted to the dental arch. The matt-silver TTS consists of intersecting rhombuses with gaps for the application of composite resin materials (CRM) to bond the splint to the teeth. Tooth-colored composite makes the TTS inconspicuous but is also difficult to differentiate from tooth enamel during splint removal [5].

Modern tooth-colored composite restorations can nearly perfectly imitate the visual appearance of the tooth structure [6]. Fluorescent materials, such as rare earth oxides, are added to the glass fillers of CRM to match the fluorescence properties of the enamel and dentine [7–9]. Nevertheless, the fluorescence emissions of these restorative materials differ from those of natural tooth structure when illuminated at different wavelengths of light [9]. The maximum fluorescence of composite resin materials occurs at a wavelength of (398 ± 5) nm [9]. The Fluorescence-aided Identification Technique (FIT) takes advantage of the different fluorescence properties of CRM and makes CRM appear brighter than natural tooth structure when illuminated with fluorescent light [10].

Several studies have shown that, compared to conventional illumination, fluorescence illumination improves the identification of composite fillings and selective composite removal on teeth in general and in posterior teeth [10–18]. FIT is a straightforward, fast, non-invasive diagnostic tool with good reliability and operator agreement [10]. Furthermore, FIT facilitates orthodontic bracket debonding [19–21] and the detection of composite restorations in forensics [13,22,23].

Dettwiler et al. showed the use of FIT to be beneficial during the removal of composite bonded trauma splints [5]. Compared to conventional dental lighting, using FIT resulted in significantly fewer composite remnants and less iatrogenic defects [5].

The potential consequences of composite remnants include esthetic impairment due to discoloration of composite margins and plaque retention spots that may result in demineralization of the enamel over time [24,25]. Furthermore, composite remnants may impair the bond strength of later adhesive restorations, which are often required after dental trauma [26–30].

The detection of composite remnants after trauma splint removal by a dentist or dental student who did not remove the splint initially has not been investigated to date. Therefore, the aim of this study was to compare the FIT versus conventional method (CONV) of detecting composite remnants after trauma splint removal in terms of the accuracy and procedure time, as well as with respect to the professional experience and gender of the examiner.

2. Materials and Methods

2.1. Tooth Model Fabrication and Digitalization

Intact extracted bovine incisors that had been cleaned and stored in 0.5% chloramine-T solution at room temperature directly after extraction until further processing were used to fabricate 10 upper jaw models ($n = 10$) of anterior bovine teeth 13 to 23 from ProBase polymethyl methacrylate resin (Ivoclar Vivadent AG, Schaan, Liechtenstein). Preoperative surface scans of the teeth were acquired using a CEREC Omnicam and CEREC SW 4.5.1 software (Dentsply Sirona, York, PA, USA). All scans of teeth with unimpaired surfaces were exported to OraCheck 2.13 (Cyfex AG, Zurich, Switzerland) for later superimposition and analysis, according to the study protocol.

2.2. Splint Application

A TTS splint (Medartis AG, Basel, Switzerland) was adhesively bonded to teeth 12 to 22 of each bovine model, following a standardized protocol. Briefly, the bonding surfaces were determined using a customized perforated silicon template. Due to the size of the bovine teeth, two bonding sites were placed in the middle third of the crown of each tooth (site diameter: 3 mm). Each bonding site was etched with Ultra-Etch (Ultradent Products Inc., South Jordan, UT, USA) for 30 s; Heliobond (Ivoclar Vivadent AG, Schaan, Lichtenstein) was applied and light-cured for 30 s with a Bluephase 20i light curing unit (Ivoclar Vivadent AG, Schaan, Lichtenstein) at an output intensity of 1200 mW/cm^2. Tetric EvoFlow A2 (Ivoclar Vivadent AG, Schaan, Lichtenstein) was applied using the aforementioned silicon template and light cured, as described above. The TTS splint was placed on the applied composite and covered with the same flowable composite while ensuring that the specified size of the bonding site was respected and not exceeded. The tooth models were stored at room temperature in Ringer solution (B Braun AG, Melsungen, Germany) until further processing.

2.3. Splint Removal

The removal of the TTS splints was performed by two dentists with 2 12 tw1elve years of professional experience, respectively. To simulate clinical conditions, the upper jaw model was inserted in the mouth of a dental mannequin (Frasaco GmbH, Tettnang, Germany), which was seated and secured in an Teneo dental chair (Dentsply Sirona, York, PA, USA). Splint removal was performed under standardized lighting conditions using the LEDview dental unit lamp (Sirona, York, PA, USA). The following instruments could be used in splint removal: dental mirrors, a curved dental explorer, a three-way triple air-water syringe, a high-speed contra-angle hand piece (1:5, KaVo Master Series, Biberach, Germany), cylindrical diamond burs (FG 4038, Intensiv SA, Montagnola, Switzerland), and carbide burs (Bonding Resin Remover, H22ALGK 016, Komet Dental, Lemgo, Germany). Postoperative surface scans of the teeth were performed using a CEREC Omnicam with CEREC SW 4.5.1 software (Dentsply Sirona, York, PA, USA). Following splint removal, all scans were exported to OraCheck 2.13 (Cyfex AG, Zurich, Switzerland) for superimposition and further analysis according to the study protocol. The models were stored in Ringer solution (B Braun AG, Melsungen, Germany) at room temperature until further processing.

2.4. Composite Remnant Identification

The tooth models were examined for composite remnants by 10 general dentists with 3 to 24 years of professional experience and by 10 dental undergraduate students. The inclusion criteria for participants were normal visual acuity and the absence of color blindness assessed by an Ishihara test [31]. For undergraduate students, the criteria were active participation in the first- or second-year master's degree program in dentistry and an average grade of B or better. Accordingly, exclusion criteria were visual impairment, color blindness, and missing clinical activity. The examiners were instructed to identify and chart all composite remnants using a dental mirror, a curved dental explorer, and a three-way triple air-water syringe by the respective illumination method. All examinations were carried out under standardized lighting conditions in a darkened room illuminated only by artificial light. The tooth surfaces were illuminated with an LEDview dental unit lamp (Sirona, York, PA, USA) for CONV and with a prototype fluorescence-inducing headlamp with a spectral bandwidth of (405 ± 7) nm (Karl Storz GmbH & Co. KG, Tuttlingen, Germany) for FIT (Figure 1). Each model was assessed in triplicate by each examiner with a break of 14 days in between, so that the participants could not remember previous findings. The investigators additionally recorded the procedure time required for each model. The experiments were performed as follows:

- Examination 1: Evaluation of all 10 models by CONV.
- Examination 2 (14 days later): Evaluation of five models by CONV and five models by FIT.
- Examination 3 (14 days later): Evaluation of all 10 models by FIT.
- All examinations were performed in the same room under the same ambient light conditions (examinations at the same day time with no direct solar irradiation, 500–800 Lux) at the University Center for Dental Medicine Basel, Switzerland.

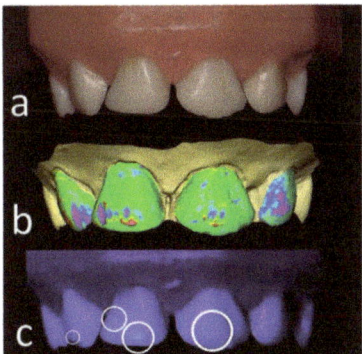

Figure 1. Representative model (**a**) illuminated by the conventional illumination (**b**) with visualized surface changes in the OraCheck software (**c**), illuminated by the fluorescence-inducing light source.

2.5. Data Analysis

Two experienced dentists (S.S. and T.C.) not involved in the identification of composite remnants evaluated the dental charting results on the basis of volumetric change calculation. Briefly, the pre- and postoperative scans were superimposed using the best-fit method [32]. All splinting sites on the teeth were overlapped independently for more accurate superimposition. Teeth 13 and 23 were not included in splinting to facilitate the registration of the scans. The OraCheck software color-coded the results for clear visualization of surface changes between scans. Green was used to indicate unchanged sites, blue and violet for substance loss, and yellow, red, and pink for excess material (Figure 1). The visualized areas were then analyzed with the OraCheck linear and volumetric measurement tool. The results were used to make a transparent solution template for each model that could be superimposed over the dental charts for grading purposes.

Each dentist evaluated the correctness of identification of composite remnants (COI) for each tooth on a scale of 1 to 7 (Table 1), where the score 1 represented "correct" identification and the scores 2 to 7 were classified as "false" identification for dichotomous analysis. If the two dentists disagreed on a site, it was jointly re-evaluated by both dentists until a consensus was reached. The 10 models with four teeth each were assessed for composite remnants by 20 examiners (10 dentists and 10 students), yielding a total of 800 assessments.

Table 1. Correctness of identification of the composite remnants (COI) scoring system.

1: FD	Fully correct detection
2: PD	Partly detected
3: ND	Not detected
4: FP	False positive entirely (no composite in situ)
5: FD+	FD + false positive
6: PD+	PD + false positive
7: ND+	ND + false positive

2.6. Statistical Analysis

As descriptive measures for categorical (years of professional experience) and binary parameters (CONV vs. FIT; dentist vs. student; male vs. female examiner), count and relative frequencies were used. For continuous measures (recorded time for examination), mean values, standard deviation, median, minimum, and maximum were calculated (Table 2) and normality was checked with quantile-quantile-plots (normality-plots, q-q-plots).

Table 2. Distribution of correctness of identification (COI) grades 1–7 and their dichotomous categorization as "correct" (score 1) and "false" (score 2–7) for examination 1 (CONV), 2 (CONV and FIT), and 3 (FIT).

		Examination		
	COI Score	1	2	3
CONV	1	209	95	/
	2	93	87	/
	3	147	92	/
	4	105	31	/
	5	58	34	/
	6	45	18	/
	7	143	43	/
	Correct	209	95	/
	False	591	305	/
FIT	1	/	354	714
	2	/	5	27
	3	/	15	22
	4	/	10	12
	5	/	13	20
	6	/	0	1
	7	/	3	4
	Correct	/	354	714
	False	/	46	86

For inter-rater-reliability and retest-reliability, Cohens Kappa with 95%-confidence interval (CI) was calculated.

Comparison of the binary outcome ("correct" (rating 1) vs. "false" (rating 2–7)) between examination 1 and examination 3 was calculated with the McNemar test and with Fisher's Exact test for examination 2, respectively.

For comparison of the binary outcome "correct" (grading 1) vs. "false" (grading 2–7) between students vs. dentist, male vs. female examiners, and examiners with a variable professional experience, the Fisher's Exact test was utilized, excluding data from examination 2 due to a small sample size.

The recorded time was compared for CONV and FIT using the nonparametric Wilcoxon test, comparing examination 1 and examination 3 and the measured values within examination 2. Likewise, the time needed for examination was compared for dentists vs. students for CONV (examination 1) and FIT (examination 3), using the Wilcoxon test.

The level of significance was set at $\alpha = 5\%$ in all analyses, which were performed utilizing the software R version 3.2.2.

3. Results

3.1. Correctness of Identification of Composite Remnants

Overall differences in the correctness of identification of composite remnants between CONV vs. FIT were significant ($p < 0.001$) in examinations 1 and 3, as well as in examination 2 ($p < 0.001$). The distributions of COI grades 1–7 and their dichotomous categorization as correct vs. false identification in examinations 1, 2, and 3 are presented in Table 2. There were no significant differences in COI between dentists vs. students ($p = 0.26$ for CONV; $p = 0.73$ for FIT), male vs. female examiners ($p = 0.42$ for CONV; $p = 0.25$ for FIT), or years of examiner experience ($p = 0.74$ for CONV and $p = 0.46$ for FIT). The relative frequencies of correct identification of composite remnants in the various groups are presented in Figure 2.

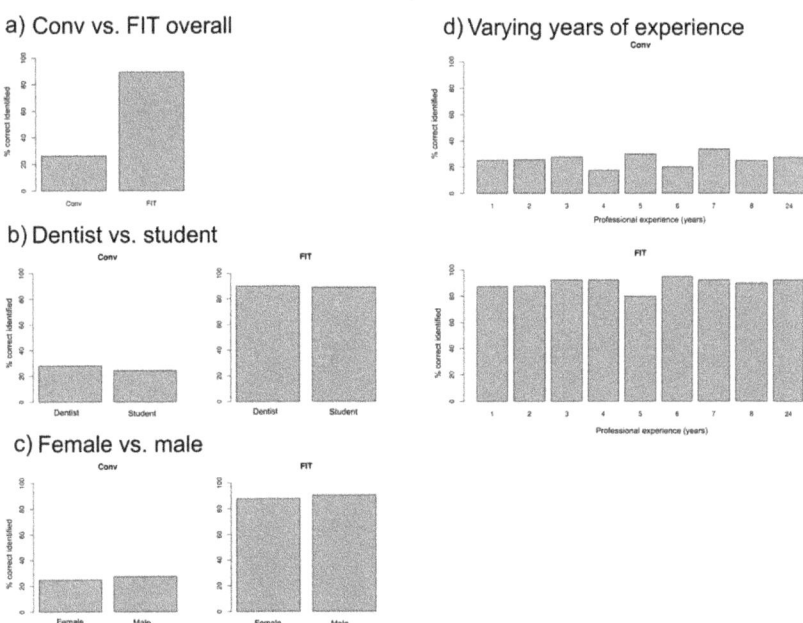

Figure 2. Relative frequencies of correctness of identification (COI) grade 1 ("correct") for (**a**) CONV vs. FIT overall, (**b**) dentists vs. students for CONV and FIT, (**c**) female vs. male examiners for CONV and FIT, and (**d**) years of dental experience for FIT and CONV.

3.2. Procedure Time

Differences in the procedure times for CONV vs. FIT were significant ($p < 0.001$ for examination 1 vs. 3; $p < 0.001$ for examination 2). There were no significant differences in procedure time between dentist and students for CONV ($p = 0.17$). However, the procedure time for the identification of composite remnants by FIT was significantly shorter for students compared to dentists (22 s vs. 25 s per tooth; $p < 0.001$). The measured procedure times are detailed in Table 3.

Table 3. Procedure time required for the identification of composite remnants by CONV vs. FIT.

Examination		n	Mean ± Standard Deviation [s]	Median [s]	Min [s]	Max [s]
1	CONV	800	117 ± 9	120	70	120
	FIT		No assessment			
2	CONV	400	118 ± 5	120	90	120
	FIT	400	23 ± 5	22	10	38
3	CONV		No assessment			
	FIT	800	24 ± 5	24	10	38

3.3. Inter-Rater-Reliability

Inter-rater-reliability was high ($\kappa = 0.98$, 95%—CI 0.98–0.99). For retest-reliability, the agreement was fair for CONV ($\kappa = 0.34$, 95%—CI 0.28–0.40) and moderate for FIT ($\kappa = 0.43$, 95%—CI 0.30–0.56).

4. Discussion

The main objective of this study was to compare the accuracy and procedure time of the Fluorescence-aided Identification Technique (FIT) and the conventional illumination method (CONV) of detecting composite remnants after trauma splint removal when performed by dentists and students. CEREC surface scanning of the teeth before and after splint removal was used as the gold standard for remnant identification. Additional data on the impact of examiner experience and gender on the accuracy and procedure time, as well as the inter-rater-reliability and retest-reliability of the two methods were also collected. The detection of composite remnants after trauma splint removal by a dentist other than the operator who removed the splint initially is a clinically relevant situation that has not been investigated yet.

The detection of composite remnants after trauma splint removal was more accurate and faster with FIT compared to conventional illumination. This is in line with the results of previous studies where FIT was superior to the conventional method of composite remnant identification with regard to accuracy and procedure time [10,13,15–18]. Contrary to expectations, the dental students in this study performed the FIT method faster than the dentists. Although the difference in procedure time was statistically significant, it most probably is not clinically relevant. Furthermore, the inter-rater-reliability results showed good consensus between the examiners. Conversely, the retest reliability was low. Moreover, examiner experience did not have an impact on the results. The gender of the examiner is known to influence color shade matching quality [33] but did not have an impact on the results of the study.

A bovine incisor model was used in the present study due to difficulties in acquiring enough suitable human front teeth. Most extracted human anterior teeth are inappropriate for this type of study because of the presence of coronal restorations or carious defects. The use of bovine teeth enabled a standardized study protocol. However, the use of non-human teeth differs significantly from the clinical situation, which may have influenced the results. All teeth were extracted on the same day and cleaned and stored in the same manner.

The template used to evaluate the results of composite remnants charting was generated by superimposing the intraoral scans with the OraCheck software. Intraoral scanners have a deviation tolerance of 20 μm for single teeth, 35 μm for quadrants, and 50 to 80 μm for full-arch scans [34–36]. To achieve precise superimposition, we used teeth 13 and 23 as unchanging reference points and kept the accuracy setting for superimpositions very high in light of the very small changes observed in this study (level "0.00 mm < distance $\leq$ 0.1 mm" over 95%) [5].

The fluorescence of the resin composite material used in this study was noticeably greater than that of natural tooth substance. However, some resin composites have even stronger fluorescence [9]. The choice of composite might have influenced the results of this study. While different composite resin products fluoresce at different intensities, the FIT method is suitable for identification of most of the commercially available composites [9,37]. The clinician should take the fluorescence properties of the composite used for trauma splint fixation into account in regard to the application of the FIT method.

Several studies have shown that different composite resins are subject to aging processes and a related decrease in fluorescence properties [38–41]. Any effects of aging in the present study were most likely negligible due to the short storage time in particular and the short period of time that splints remain in the mouth in general. The composite identification experiments in the current study were performed shortly after the precursor study by Dettwiler et al. [5].

FIT was performed using a prototype headlamp. A recent study showed that various light sources with a wavelength of approximately 400 nm are suitable fluorescence-inducing devices, which are superior to the conventional method [18]. FIT can be performed by affordable and easy to handle devices, such as headlamps that illuminate the whole oral cavity.

The present study was designed to simulate clinical conditions as closely as possible to increase the reliability of the results. Moreover, a template to mark the sites of application of adhesive composite resin in order to standardize the trauma splint bonding procedure was used. This might have influenced the results of the study as bonding composites are more randomly placed on the teeth in routine clinical practice. All examinations were performed under standardized lighting conditions, in a darkened room to obtain reliable data.

Accurate differentiation of dental composite materials from natural tooth substance enables the minimally invasive and nearly complete removal of composite remnants. This is clinically relevant since composite remnants may lead to impaired esthetics and plaque accumulation. Furthermore, no drying of the teeth is necessary with the FIT method, whereas frequent drying of the teeth is needed during the removal of composite remnants by the conventional method. This has important clinical implications since constant drilling and drying significantly increases the procedure time. Moreover, when using high-speed rotary instruments, continuous water cooling is crucial to maintaining the integrity of the pulpal tissues, particularly in traumatized teeth [42–44].

5. Conclusions

FIT is a fast and reliable method for detecting composite remnants after trauma splint removal. Moreover, the accuracy and procedure time of FIT is not dependent on the level of professional experience of the dentist.

Author Contributions: Conceptualization, T.C., G.K. and C.D.; methodology, T.C. and R.W.; formal analysis, R.W.; investigation, C.D. and S.S.; resources, C.K.; data curation, E.M. and W.L.; writing—original draft preparation, E.M. and W.L.; writing—review and editing, E.M., W.L., S.S., C.D., C.K., G.K., R.W. and T.C.; visualization, W.L. and C.D.; supervision, T.C.; project administration, T.C.; funding acquisition, T.C. and C.D. All authors have read and agreed to the published version of the manuscript.

Funding: This research was funded by the Swiss Dental Association (SSO), grant number 292-16.

Institutional Review Board Statement: This investigation was conducted in conformity with the principles set for the WMA's Statement on Animal Use in Biomedical Research.

Informed Consent Statement: Not applicable.

Acknowledgments: The authors would like to thank Daniela Keller for the help with the statistical analysis. The authors also like to thank the Swiss Dental Association (SSO) for funding this work through SSO Research Grant 292-16.

Conflicts of Interest: The authors declare no conflict of interest.

References

1. Glendor, U. Epidemiology of traumatic dental injuries—A 12 year review of the literature. *Dent. Traumatol.* **2008**, *24*, 603–611. [CrossRef] [PubMed]
2. Day, P.F.; Flores, M.T.; O'Connell, A.C.; Abbott, P.V.; Tsilingaridis, G.; Fouad, A.F.; Cohenca, N.; Lauridsen, E.; Bourguignon, C.; Hicks, L.; et al. International Association of Dental Traumatology guidelines for the management of traumatic dental injuries: 3. Injuries in the primary dentition. *Dent. Traumatol.* **2020**, *36*, 343–359. [CrossRef] [PubMed]
3. Von Arx, T.; Filippi, A.; Buser, D. Splinting of traumatized teeth with a new device: TTS (Titanium Trauma Splint). *Dent. Traumatol.* **2001**, *17*, 180–184. [CrossRef]
4. Meier, A.; Connert, T.; Dagassan-Berndt, D.; Filippi, A. Dental trauma splint color preference of adults. *Swiss Dent. J.* **2020**, *131*, 320–325.
5. Dettwiler, C.; Meller, C.; Eggmann, F.; Saccardin, F.; Kühl, S.; Filippi, A.; Krastl, G.; Weiger, R.; Connert, T. Evaluation of a Fluorescence-aided Identification Technique (FIT) for removal of composite bonded trauma splints. *Dent. Traumatol.* **2018**, *34*, 353–359. [CrossRef] [PubMed]
6. Dietschi, D. Free-hand composite resin restorations: A key to anterior aesthetics. *Pract. Periodontics Aesthet. Dent.* **1995**, *7*, 15–25.
7. Uo, M.; Okamoto, M.; Watari, F.; Tani, K.; Morita, M.; Shintani, A. Rare earth oxide-containing fluorescent glass filler for composite resin. *Dent. Mater. J.* **2005**, *24*, 49–52. [CrossRef]
8. Fondriest, J. Shade matching in restorative dentistry: The science and strategies. *Int. J. Periodontics Restor. Dent.* **2003**, *23*, 467–479. [CrossRef]
9. Meller, C.; Klein, C. Fluorescence properties of commercial composite resin restorative materials in dentistry. *Dent. Mater. J.* **2012**, *31*, 916–923. [CrossRef]
10. Meller, C.; Connert, T.; Löst, C.; ElAyouti, A. Reliability of a Fluorescence-aided Identification Technique (FIT) for detecting tooth-colored restorations: An ex vivo comparative study. *Clin. Oral Investig.* **2017**, *21*, 347–355. [CrossRef]

11. Klein, C.; Babai, A.; von Ohle, C.; Herz, M.; Wolff, D.; Meller, C. Minimally invasive removal of tooth-colored restorations: Evaluation of a novel handpiece using the fluorescence-aided identification technique (FIT). *Clin. Oral Investig.* **2020**, *24*, 2735–2743. [CrossRef] [PubMed]
12. Dettwiler, C.; Eggmann, F.; Matthisson, L.; Meller, C.; Weiger, R.; Connert, T. Fluorescence-aided Composite Removal in Directly Restored Permanent Posterior Teeth. *Oper. Dent.* **2020**, *45*, 62–70. [CrossRef] [PubMed]
13. Kiran, R.; Chapman, J.; Tennant, M.; Forrest, A.; Walsh, L.J. Detection of Tooth-Colored Restorative Materials for Forensic Purposes Based on Their Optical Properties: An In Vitro Comparative Study. *J. Forensic Sci.* **2019**, *64*, 254–259. [CrossRef] [PubMed]
14. Kiran, R.; Chapman, J.; Tennant, M.; Forrest, A.; Walsh, L.J. Fluorescence-aided selective removal of resin-based composite restorative materials: An in vitro comparative study. *J. Esthet. Restor. Dent.* **2020**, *32*, 310–316. [CrossRef]
15. Hermanson, A.S.; Bush, M.A.; Miller, R.G.; Bush, P.J. Ultraviolet illumination as an adjunctive aid in dental inspection. *J. Forensic Sci.* **2008**, *53*, 408–411. [CrossRef] [PubMed]
16. Tani, K.; Watari, F.; Uo, M.; Morita, M. Discrimination between composite resin and teeth using fluorescence properties. *Dent. Mater. J.* **2003**, *22*, 569–580. [CrossRef]
17. Carson, D.O.; Orihara, Y.; Sorbie, J.L.; Pounder, D.J. Detection of white restorative dental materials using an alternative light source. *Forensic Sci. Int.* **1997**, *88*, 163–168. [CrossRef]
18. Leontiev, W.; Magni, E.; Dettwiler, C.; Meller, C.; Weiger, R.; Connert, T. Accuracy of the fluorescence-aided identification technique (FIT) for detecting tooth-colored restorations utilizing different fluorescence-inducing devices: An ex vivo comparative study. *Clin. Oral Investig.* **2021**, *25*, 5189–5196. [CrossRef]
19. Ribeiro, A.A.; Almeida, L.F.; Martins, L.P.; Martins, R.P. Assessing adhesive remnant removal and enamel damage with ultraviolet light: An in-vitro study. *Am. J. Orthod. Dentofac. Orthop.* **2017**, *151*, 292–296. [CrossRef]
20. Stadler, O.; Dettwiler, C.; Meller, C.; Dalstra, M.; Verna, C.; Connert, T. Evaluation of a Fluorescence-aided Identification Technique (FIT) to assist clean-up after orthodontic bracket debonding. *Angle Orthod.* **2019**, *89*, 876–882. [CrossRef]
21. Schott, T.C.; Meller, C. A new Fluorescence-aided Identification Technique (FIT) for optimal removal of resin-based bracket bonding remnants after orthodontic debracketing. *Quintessence Int.* **2018**, *49*, 809–813. [PubMed]
22. Kiran, R.; Walsh, L.J.; Forrest, A.; Tennant, M.; Chapman, J. Forensic applications: Fluorescence properties of tooth-coloured restorative materials using a fluorescence DSLR camera. *Forensic Sci. Int.* **2017**, *273*, 20–28. [CrossRef] [PubMed]
23. Pretty, I.A.; Smith, P.W.; Edgar, W.M.; Higham, S.M. The use of quantitative light-induced fluorescence (QLF) to identify composite restorations in forensic examinations. *J. Forensic Sci.* **2002**, *47*, 831–836. [CrossRef] [PubMed]
24. Eliades, T.; Gioka, C.; Heim, M.; Eliades, G.; Makou, M. Color stability of orthodontic adhesive resins. *Angle Orthod.* **2004**, *74*, 391–393.
25. Quirynen, M.; Marechal, M.; Busscher, H.J.; Weerkamp, A.H.; Darius, P.L.; van Steenberghe, D. The influence of surface free energy and surface roughness on early plaque formation. An in vivo study in man. *J. Clin. Periodontol.* **1990**, *17*, 138–144. [CrossRef]
26. Crumpler, D.C.; Bayne, S.C.; Sockwell, S.; Brunson, D.; Roberson, T.M. Bonding to resurfaced posterior composites. *Dent. Mater.* **1989**, *5*, 417–424. [CrossRef]
27. Kupiec, K.A.; Barkmeier, W.W. Laboratory evaluation of surface treatments for composite repair. *Oper. Dent.* **1996**, *21*, 59–62.
28. Lucena-Martín, C.; González-López, S.; Navajas-Rodríguez de Mondelo, J.M. The effect of various surface treatments and bonding agents on the repaired strength of heat-treated composites. *J. Prosthet. Dent.* **2001**, *86*, 481–488. [CrossRef]
29. Bonstein, T.; Garlapo, D.; Donarummo, J.; Bush, P.J. Evaluation of varied repair protocols applied to aged composite resin. *J. Adhes. Dent.* **2005**, *7*, 41–49.
30. Hannig, C.; Laubach, S.; Hahn, P.; Attin, T. Shear bond strength of repaired adhesive filling materials using different repair procedures. *J. Adhes. Dent.* **2006**, *8*, 35–40.
31. Ishihara, S. *Tests for Colour Blindness*; Handaya Hongo Harukich: Tokyo, Japan, 1917.
32. Mehl, A.; Gloger, W.; Kunzelmann, K.H.; Hickel, R. A new optical 3-D device for the detection of wear. *J. Dent. Res.* **1997**, *76*, 1799–1807. [CrossRef] [PubMed]
33. Haddad, H.J.; Jakstat, H.A.; Arnetzl, G.; Borbely, J.; Vichi, A.; Dumfahrt, H.; Renault, P.; Corcodel, N.; Pohlen, B.; Marada, G.; et al. Does gender and experience influence shade matching quality? *J. Dent.* **2009**, *37*, 40–44. [CrossRef] [PubMed]
34. Ender, A.; Mehl, A. Full arch scans: Conventional versus digital impressions—An in-vitro study. *Int. J. Comput. Dent.* **2011**, *14*, 11–21.
35. Patzelt, S.B.; Emmanouilidi, A.; Stampf, S.; Strub, J.R.; Att, W. Accuracy of full-arch scans using intraoral scanners. *Clin. Oral Investig.* **2014**, *18*, 1687–1694. [CrossRef] [PubMed]
36. Ender, A.; Mehl, A. In-vitro evaluation of the accuracy of conventional and digital methods of obtaining full-arch dental impressions. *Quintessence Int.* **2015**, *46*, 9–17.
37. Meller, C.; Klein, C. Fluorescence of composite resins: A comparison among properties of commercial shades. *Dent. Mater. J.* **2015**, *34*, 754–765. [CrossRef] [PubMed]
38. Takahashi, M.K.; Vieira, S.; Rached, R.N.; de Almeida, J.B.; Aguiar, M.; de Souza, E.M. Fluorescence intensity of resin composites and dental tissues before and after accelerated aging: A comparative study. *Oper. Dent.* **2008**, *33*, 189–195. [CrossRef] [PubMed]
39. Klein, C.; Wolff, D.; Ohle, C.V.; Meller, C. The fluorescence of resin-based composites: An analysis after ten years of aging. *Dent. Mater. J.* **2021**, *40*, 94–100. [CrossRef]

40. Lee, Y.K.; Lu, H.; Powers, J.M. Changes in opalescence and fluorescence properties of resin composites after accelerated aging. *Dent. Mater.* **2006**, *22*, 653–660. [CrossRef]
41. Lee, Y.K.; Lu, H.; Powers, J.M. Optical properties of four esthetic restorative materials after accelerated aging. *Am. J. Dent.* **2006**, *19*, 155–158.
42. Jonke, E.; Weiland, F.; Freudenthaler, J.W.; Bantleon, H.P. Heat generated by residual adhesive removal after debonding of brackets. *World J. Orthod.* **2006**, *7*, 357–360. [PubMed]
43. Baysal, A.; Uysal, T.; Usumez, S. Temperature rise in the pulp chamber during different stripping procedures. *Angle Orthod.* **2007**, *77*, 478–482. [CrossRef]
44. Kley, P.; Frentzen, M.; Küpper, K.; Braun, A.; Kecsmar, S.; Jäger, A.; Wolf, M. Thermotransduction and heat stress in dental structures during orthodontic debonding: Effectiveness of various cooling strategies. *J. Orofac. Orthop.* **2016**, *77*, 185–193. [CrossRef] [PubMed]

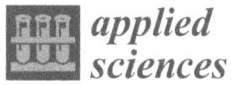

Article

Clinical Outcomes of the Double Lateral Sliding Bridge Flap Technique with Simultaneous Connective Tissue Graft in Sextant V Recessions: Three-Year Follow-Up Study

Norberto Quispe-López [1,*], Antonio Castaño-Séiquer [2], Beatriz Pardal-Peláez [1], Pablo Garrido-Martínez [3], Cristina Gómez-Polo [1], Jesús Mena-Álvarez [3] and Javier Montero-Martín [4]

1. Department of Surgery, Faculty of Medicine, Dental Clinic, University of Salamanca, 37007 Salamanca, Spain; bpardal@usal.es (B.P.-P.); crisgodent@usal.es (C.G.-P.)
2. Tenured Lecturer in Preventive Dentistry, Faculty of Dentistry, University of Seville, 41009 Sevilla, Spain; acastano@us.es
3. Department of Dentistry, Faculty of Health Sciences, Alfonso X El Sabio University, 28691 Madrid, Spain; Pablogarrido86@hotmail.com (P.G.-M.); jmenaalvarez@gmail.com (J.M.-Á.)
4. Faculty of Medicine, Dental Clinic, University of Salamanca, 37007 Salamanca, Spain; javimont@usal.es
* Correspondence: norberto_quispe@usal.es

Abstract: The presence of isolated or multiple gingival recessions in the mandibular anterior region is a challenge for the clinician, as they may be associated with a shallow vestibule, high frenum insertion and/or little or no attached gingiva. Only limited evidence is available on the use of the double lateral sliding bridge flap technique with connective tissue graft (CTG) technique for treating gingival recessions in the mandibular anterior region. The aim of this study was to describe and evaluate the clinical and esthetic outcomes of the double lateral sliding bridge flap technique with CTG on isolated and multiple gingival recessions at the level of the mandibular incisors. Nine patients required treatment of gingival recessions in the mandibular incisors at the University of Salamanca (Spain) (seven females, two males; mean age: 27.9 ± 6.9) with a total of 14 isolated (42.9%) and multiple (57.1%) Miller class II and III gingival recessions. After a mean follow-up of 36 months, the mean percentage of root coverage was 80.5% for all treated recessions. Statistically significant differences ($p < 0.05$), were observed for reduction in recession depth, increased width of keratinized tissue and increased gingival thickness, this being dependent on the Miller class. The esthetic outcome was acceptable, with a final mean esthetic score of 7.4 out of 10. The double lateral sliding bridge flap surgical technique with CTG is an effective procedure for the coverage of isolated and multiple gingival recessions in the anterior mandibular region, as it offers satisfactory esthetic results.

Keywords: gingival recession; connective tissue graft; root-coverage esthetic score; bridge flap technique; multiple gingival recession; localized gingival recession

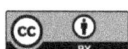

1. Introduction

Gingival recession (GR) is defined as the apical displacement of the gingival margin in relation to the cementoenamel junction (CEJ), which exposes the root surfaces to the oral environment and is associated with attachment loss [1]. It occurs frequently in adults and increases with age [2], regardless of the level of oral hygiene [3].

It is a common clinical problem and can affect the root surface of one or several teeth, being more frequent on the vestibular surface of single-rooted teeth [1]. While in most cases gingival recessions are symptomless, the patient may see them as an esthetic problem [4] that sometimes hinders or prevents good oral hygiene and may increase the risk of root hypersensitivity [5], caries, and non-carious cervical lesions [6].

In recent decades, it has been shown that complete root coverage in single and multiple recessions can be predictably achieved with different techniques [7,8]. Of these procedures, the coronally advanced flap with connective tissue graft (CTG) is the most effective treatment of recession with or without clinical interproximal attachment loss [9–11]. Most clinical trials tend to focus on maxillary gingival recessions (esthetic zone), while little information is available on treatment of mandibular defects [12]. There are various anatomical and mucogingival conditions in the mandibular anterior region, especially sextant V, that make treatment of an isolated or multiple GR in that region different to that performed in other sextants. Consequently, clinicians may encounter aberrant frenums with a very coronal insertion, high muscle attachment, a larger avascular surface area, malpositioned teeth that impede effective decision-making and surgical outcomes [1], shallow vestibules, and/or the presence of a thin phenotype [13]. The onset or progression of GR during or after orthodontic treatment is also more common in this region [14]. It is also important to remember that orthodontics has a vital role in managing and resolving periodontal problems [15].

In these situations, the choice of technique will depend on the characteristics of the recession and whether it is single or multiple. Several surgical techniques have been described for treating single and multiple gingival recessions in the anterior mandibular zone, including the free gingival graft technique [16], subepithelial connective tissue graft, as well as several flap designs: the envelope flap [17], coronally advanced flap [18], lateral sliding flap [19], double pedicle flap [20] and laterally closed tunnel flap [21]. For multiple gingival recessions in sextant V, the most well-tested and predictable techniques are the bilaminar approaches such as the tunnel technique [22] and the coronally advanced flap technique [23]. However, most of these surgical techniques lead to further collapse of the vestibule, compromise the vascular supply and fail to produce predictable results in terms of complete root coverage while, in the case of the free gingival graft technique, the outcome is rather unesthetic (dissatisfaction with color matching and soft tissue texture, as well as misalignment of the mucogingival junction) [24,25].

An esthetic gingival recession scoring system (RES) has been developed to evaluate the esthetic outcome of root coverage (RC) procedures [26]. This score is based on the evaluation of five variables: the gingival margin level, gingival contour, soft tissue texture, mucogingival junction alignment, and gingival color. Sixty percent of the RES value is attributed to the level of the gingival margin, since one of the main goals of the treatment is complete root coverage (CRC), and 40% is attributed to the other four variables. The sum of the five variables produces an RES score, ranging from 0 (final recession equal or apical to the initial recession) to 10 (the best esthetic result).

Therefore, the purpose of this case series was to evaluate the efficacy of the double lateral sliding bridge flap technique with connective tissue graft in mucogingival surgery for treating isolated and multiple recessions in mandibular incisors after a mean follow-up of 36 months. The esthetic outcome was also analyzed using the RES index.

2. Materials and Methods

This study was approved by the Bioethics Committee of the University of Salamanca (Spain) (registration number 483, date of approval: 22 June 2020). The clinical study included nine patients (two males and seven females) with 36.0 ± 22.1 months of mean follow-up, who had a mean age of 27.9 ± 6.9, and had isolated or multiple Miller [27] class II and III gingival recessions located in the mandibular anterior region. Patients were selected from subjects who needed mucogingival surgery treatment using the double lateral sliding bridge flap technique with CTG between September 2014 and January 2020. Cases were chosen according to the following inclusion criteria. Patients were to: (1) be of legal age (>18 years) and provide signed informed consent; (2) have isolated or multiple (adjacent) Miller class I, II or III recessions affecting mandibular anterior teeth; (3) have a plaque index <20%; (4) have no restorations or caries in the area to be treated; (5) have had no previous periodontal surgeries at the experimental sites; (6) have a detectable cementoenamel junction and lack of a cervical step. The following exclusion criteria were also applied, omitting: (1) smokers of more than 10 cigarettes per day; (2) patients with a systemic disease (diabetes, intake of drugs causing gingival enlargement, or any contraindication for mucogingival surgery).

2.1. Surgical Protocol

Two weeks prior to surgical treatment, dental prophylaxis and instructions on proper oral hygiene were given to the patient (Figure 1A).

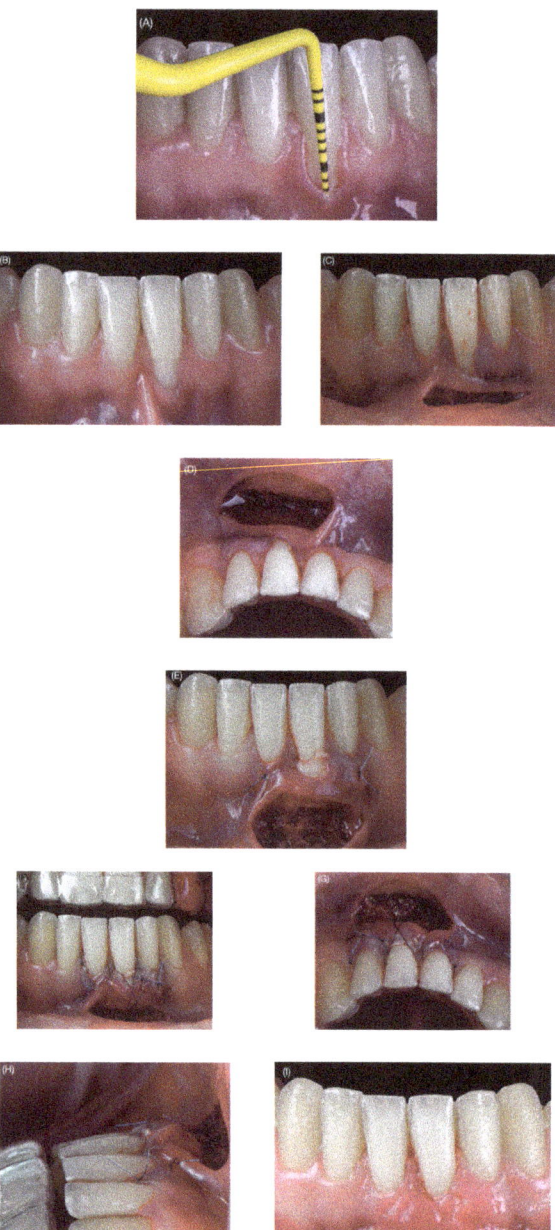

Figure 1. (**A**) Man with recession at the mandibular left central incisor, before the prophylaxis appointment. (**B**) Preoperative view, 2 weeks after prophylaxis appointment. (**C**) Apical horizontal

incision at a distance (2GR + 2 mm) from the gingival margin with recession. (**D**) Occlusal view. Horizontal incision made at partial thickness extending from mesial of the right central incisor to distal of the left lateral incisor. (**E**) Connective tissue graft sutured at the level of the CEJ using two horizontal mattress sutures. (**F**) Note the coronally repositioned flap and the palatal protection plate. (**G**) Occlusal view. Crossed horizontal mattress suture anchored in the periosteum. No suture was placed along the horizontal incision, to allow healing by second intention. (**H**) Lateral view. The flap, made predominantly of alveolar mucosa, was advanced coronally to completely cover the connective tissue graft. (**I**) After 1 month of follow-up.

All surgeries were performed by the same experienced periodontist (NQ), using the bridge flap technique with CTG. Prior to surgery, patients were required to rinse their mouths for 1 min with 0.12% chlorhexidine mouthwash +0.05% CPC (Perio-Aid, Dentaid, Barcelona, Spain). After local anesthesia, the surgical technique began with preparation of the recipient area: a partial-thickness sulcular incision was made at the level of each recession/s using a micro-scalpel (Spoon Blade, MJK instruments, Marseille, France), dissecting apically beyond the mucogingival junction and laterally under each papilla without cutting it, extending 3 to 5 mm from each recession/s. Subsequently, a horizontal incision was made using a 15C scalpel blade (Swann-Morton, Sheffield, UK) in the alveolar mucosa of the bottom of the vestibule, leaving a bridge of tissue that was to serve later for a double blood supply to the CTG. The horizontal incision extended one tooth on either side of the tooth/teeth with recession/s and was made at a minimum distance of 8 mm from the gingival margin of the tooth with recession (Figure 1B–D).

To calculate the distance at which the horizontal incision should be made, the formula proposed by Romanos et al. [28] ($2 \times GR + 2$ mm) was used as a reference. The tissue coronal to the horizontal incision was subsequently repositioned apico-coronally, maintaining the marginal integrity of the tissue. The root surface was then mechanically decontaminated using Gracey curettes, treating only the exposed root surfaces with clinical attachment loss.

Once the recipient bed had been created, a CTG of 1.5 mm thickness was extracted from the palatal masticatory mucosa, from the upper canine to the mesial surface of the first molar. Immediate closure of the donor site was performed with horizontal mattress sutures and single stitches (Seralene® 5-0, Serag-Wiessner Iberia, Madrid, Spain). Patients also received a palatal plate for protection.

The CTG was introduced through the horizontal incision and repositioned at the level of the CEJ by means of two horizontal mattress stitches using 5-0 non-absorbable suture (Seralene®, Serag-Wiessner Iberia, Madrid, Spain): one located mesially and the other distally (Figure 1E).

To reposition the tissue coronally and achieve greater adaptation and stabilization of the flap and papillae, suspensory stitches were placed, including the papilla and graft, using non-absorbable 5-0 suture. Additionally, tooth-suspended sutures were placed, anchored in the periosteum, apical to the graft and suspended around the lingual side of the tooth with the recession, using 5-0 resorbable suture (SERAFAST®, Serag Wiessner iberia, Madrid, Spain). The area of the horizontal incision was left to heal by secondary intention (Figure 1F–H).

A check-up was performed 1 week after the intervention and, after 15 days, we removed the sutures and observed revascularization of the graft and epithelialization of the raw area resulting from the horizontal incision. Photographic assessment and follow-up were performed at 1 month, 3 months and upon the final review in December 2020 (Figures 2A–C and 3A–E).

After surgery, patients received anti-inflammatory medication (25 mg of Dexketoprofen [Enantyum, Menarini, Barcelona, Spain] three times a day for 5 days) and antibiotics (1 g of Amoxicillin [Amoxicillin, Cinfa, Toledo, Spain] twice a day for 7 days). Patients were not allowed to brush the surgical sites for 14 days after surgery and were recommended to use a 0.12% + CPC 0.05% chlorhexidine spray (Perio-Aid, Dentaid, Barcelona, Spain) three times a day. Patients resumed tooth brushing 4 weeks after surgery, using the roll technique with a soft toothbrush. Patients were instructed not to pull on their lower lip and to follow a soft and liquid diet for the first days after surgery. Sutures at the donor site were removed at 7 days and sutures near the treated teeth were removed at 14 days after surgery.

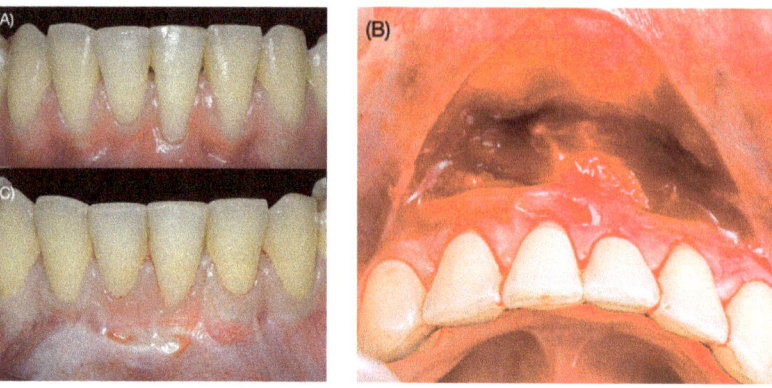

Figure 2. (**A**) Preoperative view, woman with multiple gingival recessions on the facial aspect from the right lateral incisor to the left lateral incisor. (**B**) The flap, made predominantly of alveolar mucosa, was advanced coronally to completely cover the connective tissue graft. (**C**) Post-treatment follow-up at 24 months. Only partial root coverage is shown on the lower left central incisor.

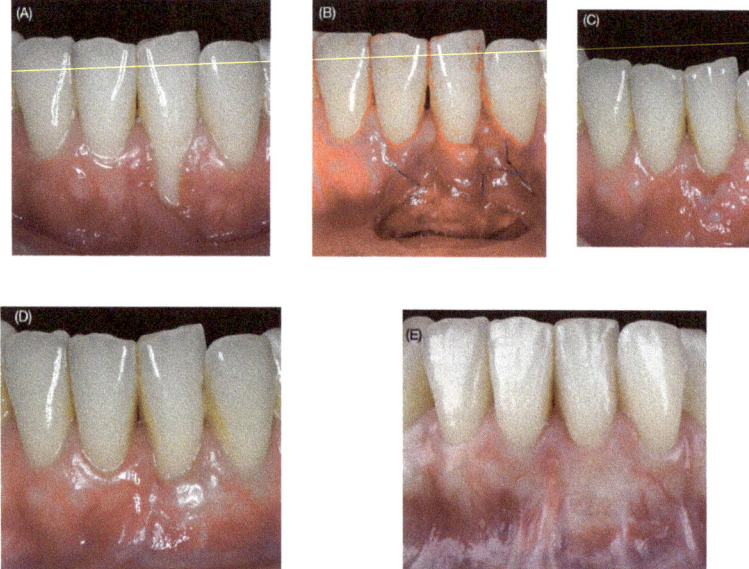

Figure 3. (**A**) Pre-surgery, gingival recession defect on the left central incisor. Note the narrow band of keratinized tissue and coronal frenum insertion. (**B**) Connective tissue graft sutured at the level of the CEJ using two horizontal mattress sutures. In this case, the graft was exposed 2 mm. (**C**) Fifteen days postoperative evaluation. (**D**) Healing 3 months after surgery. Note the increased keratinized tissue width but the incomplete root coverage. (**E**) Check-up 3 years after surgery showing complete root coverage. There was spontaneous coronal migration of gingival marginal tissue, due to the phenomenon of creeping attachment.

2.2. Baseline Clinical Assessment

The following clinical parameters were assessed, both at baseline and at the final postoperative evaluation, using a table corresponding to each clinical case to collect the data. All initial measurements were taken on the day of surgery using a millimetric periodontal probe by adjusting the measurement in multiples of half a millimeter (Colorvue UNC 12, Hu-friedy, Chicago, IL, USA), on the buccal midface of the teeth under study:

- Recession type (RT): the Miller [27] classification was used.
- Gingival recession depth (GRD), recorded in millimeters from the cementoenamel junction to the most apical point of the gingival margin.
- Probing depth (PD), recorded in millimeters from the gingival margin to the bottom of the gingival sulcus.
- Clinical attachment level (CAL): algebraic sum of the PD and GRD.
- Keratinized tissue width (KTW), measured in millimeters from the most apical point of the gingival margin to the mucogingival junction (MGJ).
- Gingival thickness (GT), measured in millimeters at 2 mm from the new gingival margin using a K#10 endodontic file with rubber stop (transgingival probing) [29].
- The percentage of root coverage (RC) was calculated according to the following formula: ([preoperative REC—postoperative REC]/preoperative REC) ×100.

To evaluate the esthetic treatment outcome using the RES index, 28 photographs were taken with a Canon EOS 700D camera, Canon EF 100 mm f/2.8 L Macro lens (Canon, Tokyo, Japan) and two 60 × 60 cm softboxes with studio flash (Neewer, Shenzhen, China). The patient was positioned lying on the dental chair, completely parallel to the floor, and we placed ourselves at 12 o'clock, at a distance of 0.49 m, and with an f 20 diaphragm placing the camera lens perpendicular to the longitudinal axis of the experimental tooth. Intra-examiner reproducibility was determined by measuring PD and GRD in five different patients on two occasions, 48 h apart. Calibration was accepted if 90% of the recordings could be reproduced to within 1 mm. A calibrated examiner (JM) initially examined and evaluated the images taken before and after three years of follow-up in all nine patients (intraclass correlation coefficient = 0.98; $p < 0.01$). This examiner (JM) was a dentist with over 20 years of experience in clinical assessments of periodontal health, although he was not familiar with the characteristics of each patient. All preoperative and postoperative images from each clinical case were imported and matched on a Keynote 2020 slide for evaluation and presentation. For each photograph, calibration was performed using parameterized digital rulers, inspired by the ABFO (American Board of Forensic Odontology) system.

2.3. Statistical Analysis

Variables reporting quantitative results were expressed as mean ± SD, median, and interquartile range. Variables reporting categorical outcomes were expressed as frequency distributions. Since most of the data did not follow a normal distribution, non-parametric tests such as the Wilcoxon signed rank test were used to evaluate differences between baseline and 36-month follow-up values for probing depth, gingival recession depth, clinical attachment level, keratinized tissue width, and gingival thickness.

Statistical analysis was performed using a statistical software program (SPSS Statistics, version 20.0, IBM). All tests were considered statistically significant when the p-value was < 0.05.

3. Results

Nine patients with 14 isolated (42.9%) and multiple (57.1%) recessions in mandibular incisors were treated, of whom three (21.4%) were classified as Miller class II and 11 (78.6%) as Miller class III defects. Healing was uneventful in most patients. Only one patient experienced partial detachment of the connective tissue graft at 10 days. After 4 weeks, all grafts were fully integrated and completely re-epithelialized.

All clinical parameters had changed significantly between the baseline and the final examination at 36 months, as shown in Tables 1 and 2.

Table 1. Descriptive statistics at baseline and 36-month follow-up.

Patient (n)	Age	Tooth (FDI)	RT	PD (mm)	GRD (mm)	CAL (mm)	KTW (mm)	CEJ (A/B)	Step (+/−)	PD (mm)	GRD (mm)	CAL Gain (mm)	KTW (mm)	GT (mm)
						Baseline						3 Years		
1	29	31	II	2	3	5	0	A	-	4	0	4	3	1.1
2	27	41	II	1.5	2.5	4	0.5	A	-	2	0	2	3	1
3	41	41	III	2	6	8	0.5	A	-	5	1.5	6.5	5	1.7
4	37	41	III	2	1.5	3.5	4	A	-	2.5	0.5	3	4	1.7
4	37	31	III	2	3.5	5.5	1	A	-	2	0.5	2.5	5	1.2
5	38	31	III	1	6	7	0	A	-	3	0	3	5	1.3
6	31	31	II	2	4	6	1	A	-	2	0.5	2.5	3	1.1
7	22	42	III	2	1.5	3.5	0	A	-	2	0	2	1	1
7	22	41	III	2	1	3	0.5	A	-	4	0	4	1	1.5
7	22	31	III	1	4	5	0	A	-	1.5	1	2.5	1	1.1
7	22	32	III	2	2	4	0	A	-	2.5	0	2.5	2	1.1
8	28	31	III	2	4	6	0	A	-	3	2.5	5.5	1	1.5
9	38	41	III	1	3	4	1	A	-	3	1	4	1	1.4
9	38	31	III	1	3	4	1	A	-	2	2	4	1.5	2

RT: recession type; PD: probing depth; GRD: gingival recession depth; CAL: clinical attachment level; KTW: keratinized tissue width; CEJ: cementoenamel junction (A = detectable CEJ, B = undetectable CEJ); STEP: + = presence of a cervical step > 0.5 mm, − = absence of a cervical step; GT: gingival thickness.

Table 2. Clinical parameters at baseline and 36-month follow-up.

Parameters	N	Mean ± SD	Range	p
		Baseline and 36-Month Follow-Up		
GRD (mm)	14			
Baseline	14	3.2 ± 1.5	1–6	
36 months	14	0.7 ± 0.8	0–2.5	
Difference	14	2.5 ± 1.5	1–6	<0.01
PD (mm)	14			
Baseline	14	1.7 ± 0.5	1–2	
36 months	14	2.7 ± 1	1.5–5	
Difference	14	1.1 ± 1.0	0–6	<0.01
CAL (mm)	14			
Baseline	14	4.9 ± 1.5	3–8	
36 months	14	3.4 ± 1.3	2.0–6.5	
Difference	14	1.5 ± 1.4	(−1)–4	<0.01
KTW (mm)	14			
Baseline	14	0.7 ± 1	0–4	
36 months	14	2.6 ± 1.6	1–5	
Difference	14	1.9 ± 1.7	0–5	<0.01
GT (mm)	14			
Baseline	14	0.0 ± 0.0	0–0	
36 months	14	1.3 ± 0.3	1–2	
Difference	14	1.3 ± 0.3	1–2	<0.01

GRD: gingival recession depth; PD: probing depth; CAL: clinical attachment level; KTW: keratinized tissue width; GT: gingival thickness; SD: standard deviation.

On average, the GRD was 3.2 ± 1.5 mm (ranging from 1 to 6 mm) at baseline, with a CAL of 4.9 ± 1.5 mm (bounded in a range of 3 to 8 mm). The KTW was 0.7 ± 1 mm (ranging from 0 to 4 mm). After surgical treatment and a 36-month follow-up, the GRD was, on average, 0.7 ± 0.8 mm (range 0 to 2.5 mm), representing 80.5% ± 23% RC. Similarly, the CAL at the end of the evaluation period averaged 3.4 ± 1.3 mm (range 2.0 to 6.5 mm). The final mean KTW was 2.6 ± 1.6 (range 1 to 5 mm), and the mean GT gain was 1.3 ± 0.3 (range 1 to 2 mm). All of these changes were found to be statistically significant ($p < 0.05$) after a comparison with the Wilcoxon signed-rank test (non-parametric test for paired data). The non-parametric comparison of the degree of root coverage (RC) and GT gain, according to the Miller class (II and III), showed statistically significant differences ($p < 0.05$). Specifically, RC gain was significantly higher in Miller class II (95.8 ± 7.2%) vs. Miller class III (76.4 ± 24.2%). However, GT gain was significantly ($p < 0.01$) higher in Miller class III (1.4 ± 0.3 mm) compared to Miller class II (1.1 ± 0.1 mm).

Finally, as shown in Table 3, the change in the final esthetic outcome score averaged 7.4 ± 2.7 points out of 10, with a median of 8.5 and an interquartile range of 4. Given that all patients had scores of zero on the RES scale at the beginning of the study, these results imply that there was a 74% improvement in esthetic terms. Esthetic changes were mainly observed in the following areas: the level of the gingival margin, complete RC (undetectable CEJ) having been achieved for 64.3% of recessions; the gingival contour, an adequate marginal contour with the MGJ aligned with that of adjacent teeth having been obtained for 71.4% of recessions; and gingival color, with 78.6% of recessions having a normal color that matched the adjacent tissues. However, in 57.1% of the cases there were apical scars, compared to 42.9% in which no scars were observed.

Table 3. Detailed description of the preoperative and final recession scoring system (RES), according to Cairo et al. [26].

Parameter	Level of Gingival Margin *			Marginal Tissue Contour **		Soft Tissue Texture ***		Mucogingival Junction ****		Gingival Color *****	
TF											
Score	0	3	6	0	1	0	1	0	1	0	1
n. (%)	1 (7.1)	4 (28.6)	9 (64.3)	4 (28.6)	10 (71.4)	8 (57.1)	6 (42.9)	4 (28.6)	10 (71.4)	3 (21.4)	11 (78.6)
Total Score Average Mean (SD)						7.4 (2.7)					
Median (IQR)						8.5 (4)					

* score 0: gingival margin apical or equal to the baseline recession; score 3: partial root coverage; score 6: complete root coverage with undetectable CEJ. ** score 0: irregular gingival margin; score 1: proper marginal contour. *** score 0: presence of scar formation and/or keloid-like appearance, score 1: absence of scar or keloid formation. **** score 0: mucogingival junction (MGJ) not aligned with MGJ on adjacent teeth, score 1: MGJ aligned with MGJ on adjacent teeth. ***** score 0: color of tissue differs from gingival color on adjacent teeth, score 1: normal color and integration with the adjacent soft tissues. TF: mean follow-up of 36 months. Nine patients (14 sites) were evaluated at TF.

4. Discussion

The present study was carried out to evaluate the clinical and esthetic efficacy of treating recessions in mandibular incisors by performing the double lateral sliding bridge flap technique with CTG. This traditional technique was specifically designed to cover isolated and multiple gingival recessions at both the maxillary and mandibular levels [30]. Originally, clinicians did not use the CTG, but simply manipulated the flap by moving it coronally to achieve their root coverage goal [30]. The results obtained in the present study prove that a CTG together with the double lateral sliding bridge flap technique is a valid treatment option for the coverage of gingival recessions in the mandibular anterior region. Predictable techniques, such as pedicled flaps (positioned either laterally or coronally) covering the denuded root surface, with or without the use of a CTG, are available to reconstruct the soft tissues over the recession [9,18,19]. Systematic reviews have evaluated the efficacy of these procedures to establish root coverage percentages ranging from 35% to 97%, and conclude that subepithelial connective tissue grafting (obtained from the palatal mucosa) is the surgical treatment producing the best results [31,32].

As we expected to fully correct all the recessions treated with this technique, we did not estimate the sample size at baseline, although we knew that a previous clinical trial in which this technique had been used evaluated 15 recessions in seven patients and found significant pre-post differences [33]. Currently, based on the data dispersion for gingival recession depth after 36 months of follow up (2.5 ± 1.5 mm), we can estimate that the recommended sample size for this pre-post comparison is seven recessions, with a power of 80% and an alpha error of 0.05. Since a control/placebo group may not be ethically viable, we used baseline data as controls to legitimate pre-post comparisons.

For the treatment of isolated mandibular gingival recessions, several surgical techniques have been proposed, including the use of a free gingival graft (FGG) [16] or CTG combined with various flap designs, such as the envelope flap [17], coronally advanced flap [18], laterally sliding flap [19], double pedicle flap [20], or laterally closed tunnel technique [21]. However, the scant literature we have found on the treatment of isolated and multiple recessions in sextant V using the bridge flap technique is limited to case series [28,30,33]. Furthermore, treating multiple recessions at the mandibular anterior level is more challenging, as there may be anatomical variants that affect the prognosis [1]. Graziani et al. [10] performed a systematic review and meta-analysis in which they evaluated the efficacy of the following techniques: coronally advanced flap, modified coronally advanced flap, and modified coronally advanced tunnel, in multiple recessions at both the level of the fifth sextant and the upper maxilla. Their findings suggest that the various surgical treatments are associated with moderate to high levels of clinical efficacy, obtaining more than 80% RC for Miller class I, II, and III recessions. However, none of them has become the gold standard technique. Essentially, we can currently choose between the tunnel technique and the coronally advanced flap technique with CTG [22,23] to address multiple recessions in sextant V, with few studies [28,30,33] analyzing combined techniques such as that tested here. It was Marggraft [30] who proposed the double lateral bridging flap technique as a procedure for covering gingival recessions in 1985. This same technique, with certain modifications, was described by Edlan-Mejchar [34] for deepening the vestibule.

Romanos et al. [28] are among the few authors who have presented results on the double lateral bridging flap [30] technique with a follow-up of 5–8 years: in their 1993 study, complete root coverage was observed in 24% of the 75 gingival recessions treated in 18 patients. However, Romanos et al. [28] did not classify the severity of gingival recessions based on any standardized criteria (such as the Miller classification), meaning that their efficacy cannot be properly evaluated. Subsequently, Azzi et al. [35] described a modification of the Marggraft technique [30] in a clinical case in the maxilla. This variation of the technique involved adding a connective tissue graft, in addition to the incision in the bottom of the vestibule, as well as mobilizing the flap coronally to cover multiple gingival recessions and to reconstruct the papilla in Miller class IV recessions. Another analysis of this technique was published by Bethaz et al. [33] in 2014, based on findings derived from 15 recessions in seven subjects with a follow-up of up to 2 years. Both isolated and multiple recessions were treated in the mandibular anterior area, classified as Miller class I and II; bicuspids and canines were also included. This technique is similar to that used in the present study, i.e., a bilaminar technique with only one horizontal incision in the bottom of the vestibule. These researchers achieved complete RC in 11/15 recessions (73.3%) at 24 months; the mean RC was $90.6\% \pm 16.8\%$ and they obtained a mean KTW gain of 1.4 ± 0.8 mm.

Compared to the outcomes achieved by Bethaz et al. [33], our results showed a slightly lower mean RC (80.5% vs. 90.6%), but this difference may be due to the fact that, unlike that research, the present study also included Miller class III defects in most of the treated cases. Moreover, further analysis of our data showed a mean RC of 95.8% when only Miller class II defects were included in the analysis, so our results appear to have high efficacy. Similarly, the observed KTW gain in our study was slightly higher (1.9 mm) than that reported in Bethaz and colleagues' research (1.4 mm) [33]. It should be noted that we chose to analyze the gingival thickness parameter in our study, since recent literature [1] recommends evaluating the gingival biotype, due to the higher risk of development or progression of gingival recession in cases with periodontal biotypes of <1 mm. Based on the above, we have observed that recessions did not recur after 36 months of follow-up, reaching a medium-term gingival stability that could be accountable to the average GT gain having been greater than 1 mm (1.3 ± 0.3 mm); therefore, statistically significant differences were found. Finally, in the study by Bethaz et al. [33], a fine white scar located apically in the bottom of the vestibule, which was undetectable without intraoral inspection, was also observed in 71.4% of patients, whereas in our study this occurred in 57.1% of patients (Table 3). Therefore, in just over half the cases, this surgical technique involves an esthetic limitation: the formation of a small scar that is undetectable, given its location at the bottom of the vestibule. Nevertheless, the proposed treatment is a recommendable therapeutic option for patients with a shallow vestibule, coronal frenum insertion or mandibular incisors with a lack of keratinized tissue.

Regarding the efficacy of other techniques to treat mandibular anterior recessions, it is worth highlighting the work of Aroca et al. [11], who observed complete RC in 38% of patients (8/20 patients) after treating Miller class III recessions with the modified tunnel technique combined with an enamel matrix derivative and CTG. While the coverage efficiency was low, the fact that their technique addressed the challenge of Miller class III recessions should be noted. Nart et al. [36] also treated a total of 14 isolated Miller class II and III recessions in mandibular incisors in 10 patients using a coronally advanced flap (CAF) and CTG. At 11.7 months after surgery, the mean RC was $90.22\% \pm 12.36\%$ for all recessions treated. In Miller class II defects, the mean RC was $94.04\% \pm 10.45\%$, while a complete RC was reached in five (71.42%) out of seven defects. In class III recessions, the mean RC amounted to $86.41\% \pm 13.70\%$ and a complete RC was obtained in three out (42.85%) of seven defects. Statistical analysis revealed no differences between the two groups. In the present study, if we limit the analysis to the results for Miller class III defects, a mean RC of $76.4\% \pm 24.2\%$ was obtained, which is lower than the values reported in the study by Nart and colleagues [36] (around 86%) and higher than the results of the study by Aroca et al. [11] (around 40%).

A recent systematic review [37] included 18 articles with 399 Miller class I and II isolated gingival recessions that were treated using the CAF technique. In this review, 43 gingival recessions affected mandibular central incisors and 26 affected mandibular lateral incisors; the mean root coverage obtained ranged from 86.28% to 91.04%, and complete root coverage varied from 53.8% to 75%. The high variability in the percentage of complete root coverage may be explained by the challenging anatomical conditions present in the mandibular anterior region.

The results obtained with the double lateral sliding bridge flap technique with CTG in Miller class II and III defects are promising for the treatment of isolated and multiple mandibular recessions located in the anterior region. However, it should be noted that the results are highly dependent on a careful selection of patients: in particular, whether heavy smokers are included or not [38], and the level of oral hygiene [6]. Therefore, the importance of prescribing chlorhexidine spray after the operation should be stressed, due to its bactericide and bacteriostatic properties, as well as its vital role in reducing gingival inflammation and in soft-tissue healing [39].

Recently, Parween et al. [40] performed a randomized clinical trial comparing the outcome of the modified tunnel technique with CTG with and without recombinant human platelet-derived growth factor (rhPDGF-BB) in 24 Miller class I and III mandibular multiple recessions. At 6 months, the mean reduction in recession depth was greater in the test group (2.08 ± 0.90 mm) than in the control group (1.83 ± 0.93 mm) and the mean RC was 82.6% ± 23.69% in the test group and 56.3% ± 28.55% in the control group. A mean KTW gain of 0.58 and 0.75 mm was observed for the control and test groups, respectively. In the present study, similar results to those of Parween [40] were observed in terms of recession depth reduction (2.5 mm vs. 2.1 mm in Test and 1.8 mm in the control). Our findings on root coverage were also comparable (80.5% ± 23%) to those observed by Parween and colleagues (82.6% ± 23.69%) in the test group. This evidence suggests that although plasma improves healing, comparable results can be obtained with the technique described here.

To analyze the esthetic results after root coverage surgery, the RES index proposed by Cairo et al. [26] was used. In our study, a mean score of 7.4 was observed, which is higher than that observed by Pini Prato et al. [41] (6.8) for the treatment of multiple maxillary and mandibular recessions. After a 6-month follow-up, Parween et al. [40] obtained a mean score of 7.6 for the control group and 8.8 for the test group in multiple mandibular recessions, which is higher than our values (Table 3). Unfortunately, we have not found any studies analyzing RES after using the double lateral sliding bridge flap technique with CTG. Therefore, it is highly recommendable for future studies to use standardized measures of esthetics to facilitate the comparison of results. In addition to the significant changes to the clinical parameters analyzed with this technique, we have been able to conclude that it is an efficient surgical procedure in mucogingival surgery in the mandibular anterior region, especially when anatomical anomalies such as aberrant frenums and shallow vestibules are present.

5. Conclusions

The double lateral sliding bridge flap technique with CTG appears to be a satisfactory technique for the treatment of isolated and multiple Miller class II and III recessions in the mandibular anterior region, with statistically significant gains in gingival thickness (1.3 ± 0.3), keratinized tissue width (1.9 ± 1.7) and recession depth reduction (1.1 ± 1.0). The mean percentage of root coverage was 80.5% in general and 95% in Miller type II recessions. An improvement in esthetics was also obtained, ranging from 42.9% in gingival texture to 78% in gingival color. The RES index reports good esthetic results for the double lateral sliding bridge flap technique with CTG, despite the probable appearance of scars, which are imperceptible to the patient due to their apical location.

Author Contributions: All the authors contributed to the research, supervision, writing, review, and editing of the study. Conceptualization, N.Q.-L. and J.M.-M.; methodology, N.Q.-L. and J.M.-M.; validation N.Q.-L. and J.M.-Á.; writing—original draft preparation, N.Q.-L., P.G.-M., B.P.-P.; writing—review and editing, N.Q.-L., A.C.-S., C.G.-P., J.M.-Á. and J.M.-M. All authors have read and agreed to the published version of the manuscript.

Funding: This research received no external funding.

Institutional Review Board Statement: The study was conducted according to the guidelines of the Declaration of Helsinki, and approved by the Ethics Committee of the University of Salamanca (protocol code 483, 22 June 2020).

Informed Consent Statement: Written informed consent has been obtained from the patient(s) to publish this paper.

Data Availability Statement: The datasets used and/or analyzed during the current study are available from the corresponding author on reasonable request.

Acknowledgments: The study was conducted within the Research Group "Avances en Salud Oral" (Advances in Oral Health) of the University of Salamanca. https://avancessaludoral.usal.es (accessed on 23 November 2021). The authors would like to thank Elena P. Hernández Rivero (SCI-Language Centre, USAL) for translation and linguistic support.

Conflicts of Interest: The authors declare no conflict of interest.

Abbreviations

CEJ	cementoenamel junction
CTG	connective tissue graft
GR	gingival recession
RT	recession type
GRD	gingival recession depth
PD	probing depth
CAL	clinical attachment level
KTW	keratinized tissue width
GT	gingival thickness
MGJ	mucogingival junction
RC	root coverage
CRC	complete root coverage
CAF	coronally advanced flap

References

1. Cortellini, P.; Bissada, N.F. Mucogingival conditions in the natural dentition: Narrative review, case definitions, and diagnostic considerations. *J. Periodontol.* **2018**, *89* (Suppl. 1), S204–S213. [CrossRef] [PubMed]
2. Hugoson, A.; Sjödin, B.; Norderyd, O. Trends over 30 years, 1973–2003, in the prevalence and severity of periodontal disease. *J. Clin. Periodontol.* **2008**, *35*, 405–414. [CrossRef]
3. Matas, F.; Sentís, J.; Mendieta, C. Ten-year longitudinal study of gingival recession in dentists. *J. Clin. Periodontol.* **2011**, *38*, 1091–1098. [CrossRef]
4. Nieri, M.; Pini Prato, G.P.; Giani, M.; Magnani, N.; Pagliaro, U.; Rotundo, R. Patient perceptions of buccal gingival recessions and requests for treatment. *J. Clin. Periodontol.* **2013**, *40*, 707–712. [CrossRef]
5. Douglas de Oliveira, D.W.; Oliveira-Ferreira, F.; Flecha, O.D.; Gonçalves, P.F. Is surgical root coverage effective for the treatment of cervical dentin hypersensitivity? A systematic review. *J. Periodontol.* **2013**, *84*, 295–306. [CrossRef] [PubMed]
6. Merijohn, G.K. Management and prevention of gingival recession. *Periodontol. 2000* **2016**, *71*, 228–242. [CrossRef]
7. Cairo, F.; Pagliaro, U.; Nieri, M. Treatment of gingival recession with coronally advanced flap procedures: A systematic review. *J. Clin. Periodontol.* **2008**, *35*, 136–162. [CrossRef]
8. Cairo, F.; Nieri, M.; Pagliaro, U. Efficacy of periodontal plastic surgery procedures in the treatment of localized facial gingival recessions. A systematic review. *J. Clin. Periodontol.* **2014**, *41* (Suppl. 15), s44–s62. [CrossRef]
9. Cairo, F.; Cortellini, P.; Tonetti, M.; Nieri, M.; Mervelt, J.; Cincinelli, S.; Pini-Prato, G. Coronally advanced flap with and without connective tissue graft for the treatment of single maxillary gingival recession with loss of inter-dental attachment. A randomized controlled clinical trial. *J. Clin. Periodontol.* **2012**, *39*, 760–768. [CrossRef]
10. Graziani, F.; Gennai, S.; Roldan, S.; Discepoli, N.; Buti, J.; Madianos, P.; Herrera, D. Efficacy of periodontal plastic procedures in the treatment of multiple gingival recessions. *J. Clin. Periodontol.* **2014**, *41*, s63–s76. [CrossRef] [PubMed]
11. Aroca, S.; Keglevich, T.; Nikolidakis, D.; Gera, I.; Nagy, K.; Azzi, R.; Etienne, D. Treatment of class III multiple gingival recessions: A randomized-clinical trial. *J. Clin. Periodontol.* **2010**, *37*, 88–97. [CrossRef]
12. Tonetti, M.S.; Jepsen, S.; Working Group 2 of the European Workshop on Periodontology. Clinical efficacy of periodontal plastic surgery procedures: Consensus report of Group 2 of the 10th European Workshop on Periodontology. *J. Clin. Periodontol.* **2014**, *41* (Suppl. 15), S36–S43. [CrossRef] [PubMed]
13. Müller, H.P.; Könönen, E. Variance components of gingival thickness. *J. Periodontal. Res.* **2005**, *40*, 239–244. [CrossRef] [PubMed]
14. Gebistorf, M.; Mijuskovic, M.; Pandis, N.; Fudalej, P.-S.; Katsaros, C. Gingival recession in orthodontic patients 10 to 15 years posttreatment: A retrospective cohort study. *Am. J. Orthod. Dentofacial. Orthop.* **2018**, *153*, 645–655. [CrossRef] [PubMed]
15. Kaitsas, R.; Kaitsas, F.; Paolone, G.; Paolone, M.-G. Ortho-Perio Risk Assessment and timing flowchart for lingual orthodontics in an interdisciplinary adult ortho-perio patient: A case report of "Perio-Guided" Orthodontic treatment. *Int. Orthod.* **2021**, S1761–7227, 00143–1. [CrossRef]
16. Cortellini, P.; Tonetti, M.; Prato, G.-P. The partly epithelialized free gingival graft (pe-fgg) at lower incisors. A pilot study with implications for alignment of the mucogingival junction. *J. Clin. Periodontol.* **2012**, *39*, 674–680. [CrossRef] [PubMed]
17. Nart, J.; Valles, C. Subepithelial Connective Tissue Graft in Combination with a Tunnel Technique for the Treatment of Miller Class II and III Gingival Recessions in Mandibular Incisors: Clinical and Esthetic Results. *Int. J. Periodontics Restor. Dent.* **2016**, *36*, 591–598. [CrossRef]
18. Zucchelli, G.; Marzadori, M.; Mounssif, I.; Mazzotti, C.; Stefanini, M. Coronally advanced flap + connective tissue graft techniques for the treatment of deep gingival recession in the lower incisors. A controlled randomized clinical trial. *J. Clin. Periodontol.* **2014**, *41*, 806–813. [CrossRef]
19. De Angelis, N.; Yumang, C.; Benedicenti, S. Efficacy of the lateral advanced flap in root-coverage procedures for mandibular central incisors: A 5-year clinical study. *Int. J. Periodontics Restor. Dent.* **2015**, *35*, e9–e13. [CrossRef]

20. Harris, R.J. The connective tissue and partial thickness double pedicle graft: A predictable method of obtaining root coverage. *J. Periodontol.* **1992**, *63*, 477–486. [CrossRef] [PubMed]
21. Sculean, A.; Allen, E.-P. The Laterally Closed Tunnel for the Treatment of Deep Isolated Mandibular Recessions: Surgical Technique and a Report of 24 Cases. *Int. J. Periodontics Restor. Dent.* **2018**, *38*, 479–487. [CrossRef] [PubMed]
22. Zabalegui, I.; Sicilia, A.; Cambra, J.; Gil, J.; Sanz, M. Treatment of multiple adjacent gingival recessions with the tunnel subepithelial connective tissue graft: A clinical report. *Int. J. Periodontics Restor. Dent.* **1999**, *19*, 199–206.
23. Stefanini, M.; Zucchelli, G.; Marzadori, M.; de Sanctis, M. Coronally Advanced Flap with Site-Specific Application of Connective Tissue Graft for the Treatment of Multiple Adjacent Gingival Recessions: A 3-Year Follow-Up Case Series. *Int. J. Periodontics Restor. Dent.* **2018**, *38*, 25–33. [CrossRef] [PubMed]
24. Harris, R.J.; Miller, L.H.; Harris, C.R.; Miller, R.J. A comparison of three techniques to obtain root coverage on mandibular incisors. *J. Periodontol.* **2005**, *76*, 1758–1767. [CrossRef]
25. Kerner, S.; Sarfati, A.; Katsahian, S.; Jaumet, V.; Micheau, C.; Mora, F.; Monnet-Corti, V.; Bouchard, P. Qualitative cosmetic evaluation after root-coverage procedures. *J. Periodontol.* **2009**, *80*, 41–47. [CrossRef]
26. Cairo, F.; Nieri, M.; Cattabriga, M.; Cortellini, P.; De Paoli, S.; De Sanctis, M.; Fonzar, A.; Francetti, L.; Merli, M.; Rasperini, G.; et al. Root coverage esthetic score after treatment of gingival recession: An interrater agreement multicenter study. *J. Periodontol.* **2010**, *81*, 1752–1758. [CrossRef]
27. Miller, P.D., Jr. A classification of marginal tissue recession. *Int. J. Periodontics Restor. Dent.* **1985**, *5*, 8–13.
28. Romanos, G.E.; Bernimoulin, J.P.; Marggraf, E. The double lateral bridging flap for coverage of denuded root surface: Longitudinal study and clinical evaluation after 5 to 8 years. *J. Periodontol.* **1993**, *64*, 683–688. [CrossRef]
29. Ronay, V.; Sahrmann, P.; Bindl, A.; Attin, T.; Schmidlin, P.-R. Current status and perspectives of mucogingival soft tissue measurement methods. *J. Esthet. Restor. Dent.* **2011**, *23*, 146–156. [CrossRef]
30. Marggraf, E. A direct technique with a double lateral bridging flap for coverage of denuded root surface and gingiva extension. Clinical evaluation after 2 years. *J. Clin. Periodontol.* **1985**, *12*, 69–76. [CrossRef]
31. Chambrone, L.; Sukekava, F.; Araújo, M.-G.; Pustiglioni, F.-E.; Chambrone, L.-A.; Lima, L.-A. Root-coverage procedures for the treatment of localized recession-type defects: A Cochrane systematic review. *J Periodontol.* **2010**, *81*, 452–478. [CrossRef]
32. Tatakis, D.-N.; Chambrone, L.; Allen, E.-P.; Langer, B.; McGuire, M.-K.; Richardson, C. Periodontal soft tissue root coverage procedures: A consensus report from the AAP Regeneration Workshop. *J. Periodontol.* **2015**, *86* (Suppl. S2), S52–S55. [CrossRef]
33. Bethaz, N.; Romano, F.; Ferrarotti, F.; Mariani, G.-M.; Aimetti, M. A mucogingival technique for the treatment of multiple recession defects in the mandibular anterior region: A case series with a 2-year follow-up. *Int. J. Periodontics Restor. Dent.* **2014**, *34*, 345–352. [CrossRef] [PubMed]
34. Edlan, A.; Mejchar, B. Plastic surgery of the vestibulum in periodontal therapy. *Int. Dent. J.* **1963**, *13*, 593–596.
35. Azzi, R.; Etienne, D.; Sauvan, J.L.; Miller, P.D. Root coverage and papilla reconstruction in Class IV recession: A case report. *Int. J. Periodontics Restor. Dent.* **1999**, *19*, 449–455.
36. Nart, J.; Valles, C.; Mareque, S.; Santos, A.; Sanz-Moliner, J.; Pascual, A. Subepithelial connective tissue graft in combination with a coronally advanced flap for the treatment of Miller Class II and III gingival recessions in mandibular incisors: A case series. *Int. J. Periodontics Restor. Dent.* **2012**, *32*, 647–654.
37. Zucchelli, G.; Tavelli, L.; Ravidà, A.; Stefanini, M.; Suárez-López Del Amo, F.; Wang, H.-L. Influence of tooth location on coronally advanced flap procedures for root coverage. *J. Periodontol.* **2018**, *89*, 1428–1441. [CrossRef]
38. Chambrone, L.; Chambrone, D.; Pustiglioni, F.-E.; Chambrone, L.-A.; Lima, L.-A. The influence of tobacco smoking on the outcomes achieved by root-coverage procedures: A systematic review. *J. Am. Dent. Assoc.* **2009**, *140*, 294–306. [CrossRef]
39. Polizzi, E.; Tetà, G.; Bova, F.; Pantaleo, G.; Gastaldi, G.; Capparà, P.; Gherlone, E. Antibacterial properties and side effects of chlorhexidine-based mouthwashes. A prospective, randomized clinical study. *J. Osseointegr.* **2019**, *12*, 2–7. [CrossRef]
40. Parween, S.; George, J.-P.; Prabhuji, M. Treatment of Multiple Mandibular Gingival Recession Defects Using MCAT Technique and SCTG With and Without rhPDGF-BB: A Randomized Controlled Clinical Trial. *Int. J. Periodontics Restor. Dent.* **2020**, *40*, e43–e51. [CrossRef]
41. Pini-Prato, G.; Cairo, F.; Nieri, M.; Rotundo, R.; Franceschi, D. Esthetic evaluation of root coverage outcomes: A case series study. *Int. J. Periodontics Restor. Dent.* **2011**, *31*, 603–610.

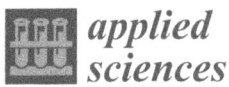

Article

The Effect of Feldspathic Thickness on Fluorescence of a Variety of Resin Cements and Flowable Composites

Joana Santos de Cunha Pereira [1,2,*], José Alexandre Reis [1,3], Francisco Martins [1,3], Paulo Maurício [1,3] and M. Victoria Fuentes [4]

[1] Oral Rehabilitation Department, Instituto Universitário Egas Moniz, Monte de Caparica, 2829-511 Almada, Portugal; jreis@egasmoniz.edu.pt (J.A.R.); fmartins@egasmoniz.edu.pt (F.M.); pmauricio@egasmoniz.edu.pt (P.M.)
[2] Faculty of Health Sciences, Rey Juan Carlos University, 28922 Madrid, Spain
[3] CiiEM, Instituto Universitário Egas Moniz, Monte de Caparica, 2829-511 Almada, Portugal
[4] Idibo Research Group, Area of Stomatology, Faculty of Health Sciences, Rey Juan Carlos University, 28922 Madrid, Spain; victoria.fuentes@urjc.es
* Correspondence: jpereira@egasmoniz.edu.pt; Tel.: +351-9-1629-0724

Abstract: (1) Background: The shade of resin-based materials and ceramic thickness influence the optical color of laminate restorations. The purpose of this study is to evaluate—in vitro—the effect of resin-based cement shade and ceramic thickness on fluorescence of feldspathic laminate veneers; (2) Methods: 180 samples of feldspathic ceramic A2 shade with two different thicknesses (0.5 and 0.8 mm) were obtained. The samples were cemented to composite resin substrates with one of the following materials in different shades (n = 10): resin cement (Variolink Esthetic in Light, Neutral and Warm shades; or RelyX Veneer in B0.5 /white, Translucent and A3 Opaque/yellow opaque shades); flowable composite resin (G-aenial Flo in A2 and A3 shades) or a pre-heated composite resin (Filtek Supreme XTE, A3 body shade). The fluorescence spectra were obtained by means of a spectrofluorometer. Two-way ANOVA, Tukey, and Student's t-tests were performed ($\alpha = 0.05$); (3) Results: Fluorescence values were significantly influenced by the resin-based agent tested ($p < 0.001$), the thickness of ceramic ($p < 0.001$), and their interaction ($p < 0.001$). The lowest fluorescence values were achieved by RelyX Veneer resin cement regardless its shade and the ceramic thickness; (4) Conclusions: both the shade of resin-based agent and the feldspathic ceramic thickness influenced the fluorescence of laminate restorations.

Keywords: feldspathic ceramic; resin cement; flowable resin; fluorescence; thickness

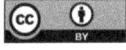

1. Introduction

Nowadays, ceramic laminate veneers are one of the main choices to perform a highly aesthetic oral rehabilitation [1–3]. Feldspathic porcelain, the first type of ceramic used in dentistry, is a suitable clinical solution for fabricating veneers, due to excellent esthetic and biocompatibility properties and long-lasting performance [1–4]. Long-term success of ceramic veneers depends partly on the adhesive cementation [4,5]. Once adhesively cemented, ceramic laminate veneers exhibit an increased fracture strength and propitious success rates [6–8].

The restoration's aesthetic goal should reproduce the optical characteristics of the natural tooth. Several factors—such as ceramic thickness, cement, and abutment color—influence the final color of the restored tooth [9–14]. Translucency, opalescence, and fluorescence are other optical properties that alter the overall appearance of the restoration [15].

Fluorescence of the natural teeth occurs when their surface absorbs ultraviolet light (UV) (350–400 nm) and emits light with a longer wavelength, creating a bluish-white color [16–21]. This property is mostly determined by dentin because of the greater amount of organic material, which contains fluorescence-releasing amino acids—such as tryptophan, providing three times more fluorescence than enamel [11,20,22–24]. Fluorescence can be classified as distinctive clinical optical property that not only makes teeth appear whiter but also brighter by emitting more blue radiation due to fluorescence, which converts UV radiation (invisible to the eye) to blue radiation (visible to the eye). Thus, to provide better integration, it is mandatory that teeth restored with ceramic veneers have a fluorescence emission similar to that of the natural teeth [19].

The type and composition of the ceramic will influence the intensity of fluorescence [19]. Some luminescent additives—such as europium and other rare-earth elements that exhibit visible fluorescence—are included in composition of ceramics and resin cements to obtain fluorescence properties similar to the tooth structure [19,25–28]. To date, few studies have evaluated the fluorescence of ceramic restorations. Rafael et al. [27] evaluated the impact of tooth substrate shade on color differences, transmittance, and fluorescence of CAD-CAM (Computer Aided Design and Computer Aided Design Manufacturer) leucite based ceramics. The association of ceramic samples with darker substrates decreased fluorescence intensity. Silami et al. [28] showed that the apparent fluorescence of laminate veneers was influenced by the combination of two different ceramic veneers and the cement (light-cured or self-adhesive dual resin cements). Other authors also showed that high-fluorescence resin-based cement may interfere with the final esthetic result of thin restorations [20].

Light-cure resin cements are indicated when luting relatively thin and translucent restorations, as it allows light irradiance to activate the photo-initiators [29]. This type of resin cement exhibits clinical advantages such as long period of working time, setting on demand, and better color stability [30]. Recently, there has been an increasing trend to use flowable composite resins as light-cure cements for adhesive luting [29] in order to benefit from their physical properties (more filler-loaded than resin cements), as well as an improved cost–benefit compared to resin cements [31].

Several devices and methods for analysis of fluorescence in aesthetic materials have been employed in previous papers. Fluorometers or spectrofluorometers are commonly used because they provide quantitative results without the limitations of photography methods [19,27]. These devices measure fluorescence parameters, such as intensity and distribution, at various wavelengths. An emission spectrum corresponds to the wavelength intensity distribution of the emitted fluorescence at a constant excitation wavelength [19].

Due to higher translucency of feldspathic ceramic, the brand and shade of material used for the cementation may interfere with the fluorescence of the restoration. Therefore, the aim of this in vitro study was to evaluate the effect of light-cure resin cement and flowable composite resins in different shades on fluorescence of CAD-CAM feldspathic veneer restorations in two thicknesses. Our research hypothesis was that the emission intensity of fluorescence of feldspathic ceramics restorations is not influenced by the shade of resin-based material, nor by the thickness of feldspathic veneer.

2. Materials and Methods

The materials used in the present study are listed in Table 1.

Five CAD-CAM feldspathic ceramic (CEREC Blocs; Denstply Sirona, PA, USA), A2 shade, were used for the present study (10 × 12 mm). The ceramic blocks were cut into slices with thicknesses of 0.5 and 0.8 mm (ninety slices for each thickness) with a water-cooled diamond saw (Isomet 1000; Buehler, Lake Bluff, IL, USA) at a speed of 450 rpm. To ensure a uniform surface roughness, both sides of the samples were polished with a sequence of 400-, 600-, and 1200-grit SiC paper for 15 s at a constant speed of 100 rpm using a grinding machine (LaboIPol-4; Struers, Madrid, Spain) under water cooling. To ensure a uniform thickness of the samples (± 0.05 mm), we employed a precision digital caliper (Heavyware Tools) at three different points. The samples were then randomly assigned to the following experimental groups according to the resin-based luting agent and its shade (n = 10): two resin cements Variolink Esthetic in Light, Neutral, and Warm shades (Ivoclar Vivadent, Schaan, Liechtenstein) and RelyX Veneer, in B0.5/white, Translucent and A3

Opaque/yellow opaque shades (3M Oral Care, Seefeld, Germany); a flowable composite resin (G-aenial Flo in A2 and A3 shades (GC Europe, Leuven, Belgium); and a preheated composite resin (Filtek Supreme XTE, A3 Body shade (3M Oral Care, St. Paul, MN, USA)). The latter composite resin was used for the control group.

Table 1. Manufacturer and composition of ceramic, resin-based material and composite resin tested.

Material and Manufacturer	Composition	Batch Number
Cerec® Blocs C/PC VITA Shade: A2 CAD-CAM feldspathic ceramic	SiO_2 (56–64%), Al_2O_3 (20–23%), Na_2O (6–9%), K_2 (6–8%), CaO (0.3–0.8%), TiO_2 (0.0–0.1%), pigments <0.1%.	66301
RelyX Veneer 3M Oral Care Shade: B0.5, A3 and Translucent Resin cement	Bis-GMA, TEGDMA, Zirconia/silica, modified silica. Particle loading approximately 66% by weight, particle size approximately 0.6 mm, photoinitiator.	N862421 N816236 N843828
Variolink Esthetic LCIvoclar Vivadent Shade: Light, Neutral and Warm Resin cement	Dimethacrylate, methacrylate monomers, inorganic particles Ytterbium trifluoride and spheroid oxide mixed. primers, stabilizers and pigments. Particle size is from 0.04 to 0.2 μm. Inorganic charge is approximately 38%.	v48653 w05218 w06171
G-aenial Universal GC Corporation Shade: Flo A2 and A3Flowable composite resin	Urethanedimetrylate, Bis-MEPP, TEGDMA (31%). Silicon dioxide (16 nm), Strontium glass (200 nm), pigments (69%), photoinitiator.	161202
Filtek Supreme XTE3M Oral Care Shade: A3 Body Nanofilled composite resin	UDMA, Bis-GMA, Bis-EMA, Silica (20 nm) Zirconia (4–10 nm). Size of the particles together 0.6 to 10 μm. Inorganic particles represent 72.5% of the total charge.	N859611

Composite resin discs (Filtek Supreme XTE (3M Oral Care, St. Paul, MN, USA,)) (n = 180) with a thickness of 1 mm (± 0.05 mm) were used as substrate. The composite discs were prepared using a resin former (sample ref. 7015 Smile Line Porcelain, St-Imier, Switzerland) and light-cured with a LED unit (Elipar S10; 3M Oral Care, Seefeld, Germany) for 40 s at high intensity (1000 mW/cm^2) according to the manufacturer's instructions. Resin discs were also calibrated using a digital caliper (Heavyware Tools). The ceramic samples were randomly paired with the resin disks to make 18 groups with 10 samples per group.

Surface treatment of the ceramic was carried out according to the manufacturer's instructions. Firstly, application of 9.6% hydrofluoric acid (PulpDent Corporation, Watertown, MA, USA) for 90 s, then rinsed for 60 s and followed by application of 37% phosphoric acid (R&S Supraetch; R&S, Paris, France) making vigorous circular movements for 60 s and using a microbrush. The ceramic samples were washed with distilled water, followed by an ultrasonic bath for 4 min. The surfaces were dried with 96% alcohol, and a silane coupling agent (Ultradent, South Jordan, UT, USA) was applied for 20 s and evaporated for 60 s. Finally, an adhesive system (Optibond™ FL; Kerr Dental, Orange, CA, USA) was applied without curing.

Each ceramic sample was cemented maintaining a constant force of 50 Newtons for 60 s [32] to standardize the luting agent thickness. In the control group, the composite resin used for luting (Filtek Supreme XTE, A3 Body shade) was previously heated in a resin oven (55 °C) (Micerium, Avegno, Italy) before its application.

Photopolymerization was carried out with the same LED unit for 40 s in the center of each sample. The intensity of the light was checked regularly with a Demetron radiometer (Kerr). After polymerization, the bonded samples were stored for 24 h in a dry environment and protected from light.

Fluorescence spectra of each sample was obtained on a spectrofluorometer (SPEX Fluorolog 212I; Horiba, Kyoto, Japan) at a wavelength of 380 nm and at room temperature. The area under each curve was integrated and used as a reference for each sample. For each group, a single spectrum was averaged.

The results of the fluorescence were statistically analyzed by a two-way ANOVA was performed to analyze the effect of the resin-based luting agent and the thickness of feldspathic ceramic (0.5 or 0.8 mm). Post-hoc comparisons were performed using Tukey and the Student's t-tests. All statistical tests were performed with a statistical software program (IBM SPSS v22; IBM Corp., New York, NY, USA) ($\alpha = 0.05$).

3. Results

The fluorescence spectrum of all tested materials showed similar pattern with a fluorescence peak around 450 nm and slowly decreased to 700 nm. In Figures 1 and 2 each color represents the average group pattern. Lower fluorescence emission intensity peaks were detected around 542 nm. The resin-based materials tested had different intensities of fluorescence emission.

Table 2 and Figure 3 show the mean fluorescence values (standard deviation, SD) for each experimental group. The two-way ANOVA revealed that fluorescence values were significantly influenced by the resin-based agent tested ($p < 0.001$), the ceramic thickness ($p < 0.001$), and the interaction between these factors ($p < 0.001$).

For feldspathic ceramic thickness of 0.5 mm (Table 2 and Figure 1), samples luting with flowable composite resin G-aenial Flo A3 obtained the highest fluorescence values although statistically similar to those luting with the same brand in A2 shade, Variolink Neutral and with the group cemented with preheated composite (reference group). The samples cemented with Variolink Esthetic, regardless the shade, obtained similar values of fluorescence and also similar to reference group. The lowest values of fluorescence were obtained for the three groups cemented with RelyX Veneer, regardless of the shade.

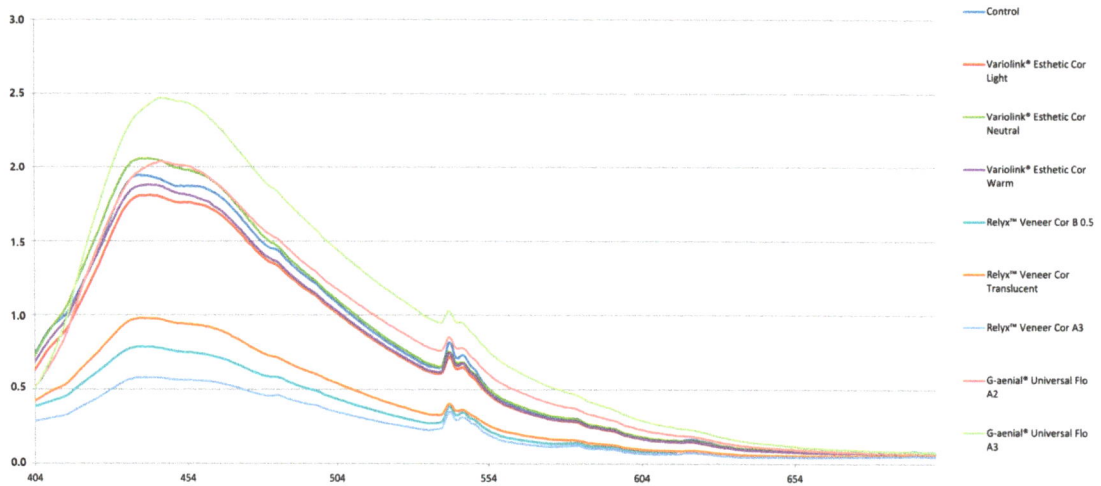

Figure 1. Fluorescence emission spectra different groups according to resin-based material used for luting feldspathic veneers (0.5 mm thickness). Graph values are in millions of a.u.

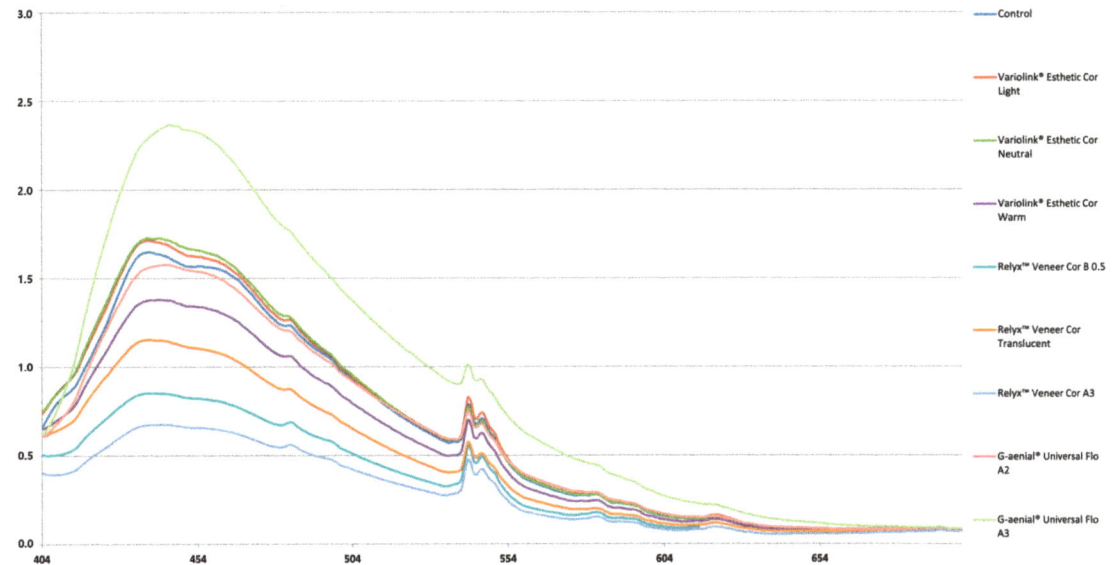

Figure 2. Fluorescence emission spectra different groups according to resin-based material used for luting feldspathic veneers (0.8 mm thickness). Graph values are in millions of a.u.

For the thickness of 0.8 mm (Table 2 and Figure 2), the highest fluorescence level was obtained for G-aenial Flo A3 group, followed by Variolink Esthetic Light and Neutral, G-aenial Flo A2, and the reference groups. The fluorescence of Variolink Warm group were lower than the groups luted with Light and Neutral from the same brand, and statistically similar to G-aenial Flo A2, RelyX Translucent, and the reference group. RelyX Veneer B0.5 and A3 groups yielded the lowest values, demonstrating that the latter group showed statistically lower fluorescence than RelyX Translucent.

Student's *t*-test did not show significant differences in fluorescence intensities between 0.5 and 0.8 mm thickness, except for Variolink Neutral and Warm, and G-aenial Flo A2 groups, in which the values decreased with veneer thickness of 0.8 mm.

Table 2. Mean fluorescence values (arbitrary unit, a.u.) and standard deviation (SD) obtained for bonded ceramic samples according to the resin-based luting agent and the feldspathic ceramic thickness (n = 10). For each column, different letters indicate significantly different fluorescence mean values among luting agents used for each feldspathic ceramic thickness.

| Resin-Based Material | Ceramic Thickness | | 0.5 mm vs. 0.8 mm (*p*-Value) |
	0.5 mm Mean ± SD	0.8 mm Mean ± SD	
Variolink Light	$1.81 \times 10^6 \pm (3 \times 10^5)$ ^{B}	$1.71 \times 10^6 \pm (1 \times 10^5)$ ^{E}	0.361
Variolink Neutral	$2.06 \times 10^6 \pm (2 \times 10^5)$ ^{BC}	$1.73 \times 10^6 \pm (1 \times 10^5)$ ^{E}	0.005
Variolink Warm	$1.88 \times 10^6 \pm (2 \times 10^5)$ ^{B}	$1.38 \times 10^6 \pm (1 \times 10^5)$ ^{CD}	<0.001
RelyX Veneer B0.5	$8.01 \times 10^5 \pm (2 \times 10^5)$ ^{A}	$8.99 \times 10^5 \pm (1 \times 10^5)$ ^{AB}	0.296
RelyX Veneer Translucent	$9.78 \times 10^5 \pm (2 \times 10^5)$ ^{A}	$1.15 \times 10^6 \pm (1 \times 10^5)$ ^{BC}	0.072
RelyX Veneer A3	$6.53 \times 10^5 \pm (4 \times 10^5)$ ^{A}	$7.78 \times 10^5 \pm (1 \times 10^5)$ ^{A}	0.442
G-aenial Flo A2	$2.04 \times 10^6 \pm (3 \times 10^5)$ ^{AC}	$1.58 \times 10^6 \pm (2 \times 10^5)$ ^{DE}	0.003
G-aenial Flo A3	$2.47 \times 10^6 \pm (6 \times 10^5)$ ^{C}	$2.36 \times 10^6 \pm (2 \times 10^5)$ ^{F}	0.630
F Supreme XTE A3 (preheated)	$2.02 \times 10^6 \pm (2 \times 10^5)$ ^{BC}	$1.65 \times 10^6 \pm (2 \times 10^5)$ ^{DE}	0.05

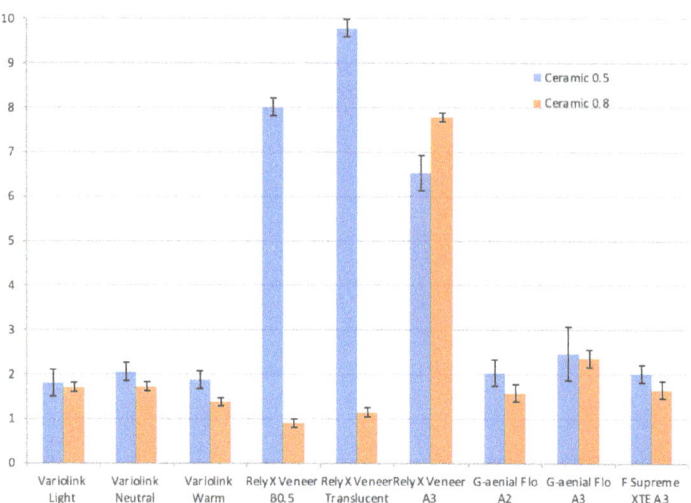

Figure 3. Mean fluorescence values (millions of arbitrary unit, a.u.) and standard deviation bars obtained for bonded ceramic samples according to the resin-based luting agent and the feldspathic ceramic thickness (n = 10).

4. Discussion

According to the results of the present study, the research hypothesis was rejected because the emission intensity of fluorescence of feldspathic ceramic restorations is influenced by the shade of resin-based material, as well as by the thickness of feldspathic veneer.

In order to achieve a natural looking restoration, the restorative materials should imitate the optical properties of the natural tooth, including fluorescence [15]. The wavelength of the excitation beam was 360 nm, which is the wavelength that causes a peak emission fluorescence intensity of the tooth. Ceramic veneers are usually fabricated as thin layers; therefore, the type and color of the cementing agent could influence the fluorescence of the restoration, as well as the final result [27].

Different levels of fluorescence were detected among groups tested. It is evident that the high translucency of the feldspathic ceramic allows the fluorescence of the luting agent to influence the final fluorescence of the restoration. Hence, the fluorescence values of restorations are the result of combination of the fluorescence of feldspathic ceramic and the underlying cement filtered by the ceramic [32].

In the present study, only one type of ceramic has been evaluated. Although fluorescence of dental ceramics have been previously reported [18,21,27,32–35], literature about this optical property in current ceramics is scarce [21,27] and, as far as we know, there are no data about the ceramic (CEREC Blocs) used in this study. Feldspathic ceramic is characterized as an extremely aesthetic material, indicated to mimic the dental structure [36]. The ceramic used in this study was a CAD-CAM feldspathic ceramic, available for digital manufacturing, and sintered by optimized industrial procedures, which results in blocks with fewer flaws and pores, and better mechanical properties than the traditional or hand-built ceramic [37,38].

Basic components of ceramics and dental resins are not able to produce fluorescence, so this can be achieved by incorporating rare-earth oxides—such as europium, terbium, and cerium—which have a strong fluorescence when exposed to UV light [17,19,33,39]. Other procedures, such as the application of an external fluorescent glaze layer on a pressed lithium disilicate ceramic, have been recently reported [21]. Regarding composite resin, manufacturers do not disclose the exact composition of these materials, although it is known that some luminescent species—such as rare-earth oxides, terbium coordination polymers of PEMA, or aromatic complex—have frequently been used [19,22,24].

Despite the fact that fluorescence is one of the optical properties of natural teeth that has attracted the attention of dental professionals in recent years [19], papers on this subject are limited. Silami et al. [28] also quantified the fluorescence of two different ceramic veneers (lithium disilicate glass-ceramic and fluorapatite glass-ceramic) and two types of resin cements (light-curing versus self-adhesive resin cements). However, the difference in materials and methodology does not allow a direct comparison of the results.

With ceramic veneers of 0.5 mm thickness, the groups in which Variolink Veneer and the flowable composite resin G-aenial were used, exhibited similar fluorescence values to the group used as reference (preheated Filtek Supreme XTE). In contrast, the fluorescence intensities were the lowest when RelyX Veener resin cements were used. These results might be explained by the luminophore content of the cements evaluated. In the case of Variolink Veneer, it contains ytterbium trifluoride, a compound that provides fluorescence [40]. It was previously reported that the light-cured resin cement Variolink II (Ivoclar Vivadent), also includes ytterbium trifluoride, and improved the fluorescence level of the e.max Press ceramic restoration [28]. On the other hand, the manufacturer of RelyX Veneer cement does not report luminophores in its composition. This may possibly explain why the fluorescence level was lower than in the other groups.

In the groups with ceramic thickness of 0.8 mm, a greater influence of the shade of the cement was appreciated between cements of the same brand. Darker shades within the same brand obtained a lower emission of the final fluorescence of the restoration. Thus, for example, veneers cemented with RelyX Veneer A3 had lower fluorescence values than RelyX Veneer Translucent. The same was observed with G-aenial Flo A3 compared to A2, and Variolink Veneer Warm compared to Light and Neutral. This trend was also confirmed in a recent paper in which the authors investigated the fluorescence behavior of different shades of selected contemporary tooth-colored restorative materials and concluded that—within any one brand of material—fluorescence emissions differed according to shade, with the lightest shades giving the strongest emissions [41].

According to the results, the fluorescence values emitted with thicker veneers showed a decrease with respect to 0.5 mm thickness significant for G-aenial A2, and Variolink Neutral and Warm groups. This decrease can be due to the fluorescence emitted mainly by the ceramic, since the luting material does not have constituents with the capacity to overcome the emission of fluorescence by the ceramic itself. RelyX Veneer cement, regardless of its shade, maintained the lowest fluorescence values.

In the present study, the composite resin Filtek Supreme XTE was used as a substrate instead natural tooth in order to avoid biological variability [27]. It is known that fluorescence in natural teeth is a multifactorial phenomenon based on multiple organic and inorganic components, age, and biotype [19,42]. Furthermore, fluorescence is lost after extraction unless fixation procedures are performed [42]. Thus, to replicate this optical property artificially, Filtek Supreme XTE was selected due to previous papers revealing an optimal fluorescence similar to the natural tooth [42–44].

Fluorescence makes the teeth look brighter and whiter in daylight [45]. Therefore, fluorescence appears in UV light above all, but ambient light is also relevant, because it influences the color of restorations. In our study, UV light has been used, but ambient light can also induce a certain degree of fluorescence, and that is why it has been evaluated in different studies [17,18,27,32–35].

The peak of fluorescence emission intensity was determined to be around 450 nm. In the visible light spectrum, this wavelength corresponds to the blue color. The blue complement given by the fluorescence present in the cements should be taken into account not only by the restorative dentist, but also by the laboratory technician. Thus, the communication between the dental office and the laboratory should also indicate the type of cement that is going to be used.

Natural teeth have fluorescence intensity peaks that are located at wavelengths of 350, 360, 405, 410, and 440 nm [46], which is in agreement with the obtained results, where the materials under this study present two peaks of fluorescence emission intensity around

450 nm and at 542 nm, and according to previous reports [22,47–50]. This indicates that the materials used in the present study may contain similar elements with fluorescence emission capacity, but in different percentages.

Limitations of the present study include the use of only one ceramic and specific brands of resin cement, so the behavior may vary with other materials. Further studies are recommended to assess the change of the emission of fluorescence with other ceramics and resin cements.

5. Conclusions

Based on the results obtained in this in vitro investigation, it is possible to conclude that:

- The fluorescence of feldspathic ceramic veneer restorations (CEREC Blocs) can be influenced by the shade and brand of resin-based materials used for luting;
- Thicker feldspathic veneers show less fluorescence emission intensity when they are cemented with resin cements or flowable composite resins in darker shades.

Author Contributions: Conceptualization, J.S.d.C.P. and J.A.R.; Data curation, F.M.; Formal analysis, F.M.; Investigation, J.S.d.C.P.; Methodology, J.A.R.; Project administration, P.M. and M.V.F.; Resources, J.S.d.C.P.; Software, F.M.; Supervision, P.M. and M.V.F.; Validation, J.A.R., F.M., P.M. and M.V.F.; Visualization, J.A.R.; Writing—original draft, J.S.d.C.P.; Writing—review and editing, J.A.R. and M.V.F. All authors have read and agreed to the published version of the manuscript.

Funding: This research received no external funding.

Institutional Review Board Statement: Not applicable.

Informed Consent Statement: Not applicable.

Data Availability Statement: The data presented in this study are available on request from the corresponding author.

Conflicts of Interest: The authors declare no conflict of interest.

References

1. Beier, U.S.; Dumfahrt, H. Clinical performance of porcelain laminate veneers for up to 20 years. *J. Prosthet. Dent.* **2012**, *107*, 157. [CrossRef]
2. Mauro, F.; Marco, R.; Marcantonio, C. Porcelain laminate veneers: 6- to 12-year clinical evaluation—A retrospective study. *Int. J. Periodontics Restor. Dent.* **2005**, *25*, 9–17.
3. Faus-Matoses, V.; Ruiz-Bell, E.; Faus-Matoses, I.; Özcan, M.; Salvatore, S.; Faus-Llácer, V.J. An 8-year prospective clinical investigation on the survival rate of feldspathic veneers: Influence of occlusal splint in patients with bruxism. *J. Dent.* **2020**, *99*, 103352. [CrossRef] [PubMed]
4. Hong, N.; Yang, H.; Li, J.; Wu, S.; Li, Y. Effect of preparation designs on the prognosis of porcelain laminate veneers: A systematic review and meta-analysis. *Oper. Dent.* **2017**, *42*, E197–E213. [CrossRef]
5. Morimoto, S.; Albanesi, R.; Sesma, N.; Agra, C.; Braga, M. Main Clinical Outcomes of Feldspathic Porcelain and Glass-Ceramic Laminate Veneers: A Systematic Review and Meta-Analysis of Survival and Complication Rates. *Int. J. Prosthodont.* **2016**, *29*, 38–49. [CrossRef] [PubMed]
6. D'Arcangelo, C.; Vanini, L.; Rondoni, G.D.; De Angelis, F. Wear properties of dental ceramics and porcelains compared with human enamel. *J. Prosthet. Dent.* **2016**, *115*, 350–355. [CrossRef]
7. Ghazal, M.; Kern, M. Wear of human enamel and nano-filled composite resin denture teeth under different loading forces. *J. Oral Rehabil.* **2009**, *36*, 58–64. [CrossRef] [PubMed]
8. D'Arcangelo, C.; De Angelis, F.; Vadini, M.; D'Amario, M.; Caputi, S. Fracture Resistance and Deflection of Pulpless Anterior Teeth Restored with Composite or Porcelain Veneers. *J. Endod.* **2010**, *36*, 153–156. [CrossRef]
9. Dozić, A.; Kleverlaan, C.J.; Meegdes, M.; Van Der Zel, J.; Feilzer, A.J. The influence of porcelain layer thickness on the final shade of ceramic restorations. *J. Prosthet. Dent.* **2003**, *90*, 563–570. [CrossRef]
10. Pissaia, J.F.; Guanaes, B.K.A.; Kintopp, C.C.A.; Correr, G.M.; da Cunha, L.F.; Gonzaga, C.C. Color stability of ceramic veneers as a function of resin cement curing mode and shade: 3-year follow-up. *PLoS ONE* **2019**, *14*, e0219183. [CrossRef]
11. Silami, F.D.J.; Tonani, R.; Alandia-Román, C.C.; Pires-De-Souza, F.C.P. Influence of different types of resin luting agents on color stability of ceramic laminate veneers subjected to accelerated artificial aging. *Braz. Dent. J.* **2016**, *27*, 95–100. [CrossRef] [PubMed]
12. Vichi, A.; Ferrari, M.; Davidson, C.L. Influence of ceramic and cement thickness on the masking of various types of opaque posts. *J. Prosthet. Dent.* **2000**, *83*, 412–417. [CrossRef]

13. Volpato, C.A.M.; Monteiro, S.; de Andrada, M.C.; Fredel, M.C.; Petter, C.O. Optical influence of the type of illuminant, substrates and thickness of ceramic materials. *Dent. Mater. J.* **2009**, *25*, 87–93. [CrossRef] [PubMed]
14. Turgut, S.; Bagis, B. Effect of resin cement and ceramic thickness on final color of laminate veneers: An in vitro study. *J. Prosthet. Dent.* **2013**, *109*, 179–186. [CrossRef]
15. Joiner, A. Tooth colour: A review of the literature. *J. Dent.* **2004**, *32*, 3–12. [CrossRef]
16. Mclaren, E.A. Luminescent Veneers. *J. Esthet. Dent.* **1997**, *9*, 3–12. [CrossRef]
17. Baran, G.R.; O'brien, W.J.; Tien, T.Y. Colored Emission of Rare Earth Ions in a Potassium Feldspar Glass. *J. Dent. Res.* **1977**, *56*, 1323–1329. [CrossRef]
18. Wozniak, W.T.; Moore, B.K. Luminescence Spectra of Dental Porcelains. *J. Dent. Res.* **1978**, *57*, 971–974. [CrossRef]
19. Volpato, C.A.M.; Pereira, M.R.C.; Silva, F.S. Fluorescence of natural teeth and restorative materials, methods for analysis and quantification: A literature review. *J. Esthet. Restor. Dent.* **2018**, *30*, 397–407. [CrossRef]
20. Correia, A.M.O.; Borges, A.B.; Caneppele, T.M.F.; Torres, C.R.G. Influence of interim cements on the optical properties of interim restorations. *J. Prosthet. Dent.* **2019**, *121*, 821–827. [CrossRef]
21. Revilla-León, M.; Sorensen, J.A.; Nelson, L.Y.; Gamborena, I.; Yeh, Y.M.; Özcan, M. Effect of fluorescent and nonfluorescent glaze pastes on lithium disilicate pressed ceramic color at different thicknesses. *J. Prosthet. Dent.* **2020**, *125*, 932–939. [CrossRef] [PubMed]
22. Takahashi, M.K.; Vieira, S.; Rached, R.N.; De Almeida, J.B.; Aguiar, M.; De Souza, E.M. Fluorescence intensity of resin composites and dental tissues before and after accelerated aging: A comparative study. *Oper. Dent.* **2008**, *33*, 189–195. [CrossRef] [PubMed]
23. Ecker, G.A.; Moser, J.B.; Wozniak, W.T.; Brinsden, G.I. Effect of repeated firing on fluorescence of porcelain-fused-to-metal porcelains. *J. Prosthet. Dent.* **1985**, *54*, 207–214. [CrossRef]
24. Uo, M.; Okamoto, M.; Watari, F.; Tani, K.; Morita, M.; Shintani, A. Rare earth oxide-containing fluorescent glass filler for composite resin. *Dent. Mater. J.* **2005**, *24*, 49–52. [CrossRef]
25. Rüttermann, S.; Ritter, J.; Raab, W.H.M.; Bayer, R.; Janda, R. Laser-induced fluorescence to discriminate between a dental composite resin and tooth. *Dent. Mater.* **2007**, *23*, 1390–1396. [CrossRef]
26. Foreman, P.C. The excitation and emission spectra of fluorescent components of human dentine. *Arch. Oral Biol.* **1980**, *25*, 641–647. [CrossRef]
27. Rafael, C.F.; Güth, J.-F.; Kauling, A.E.C.; CesaR, P.F.; Volpato, C.A.M.; Liebermann, A. Impact of background on color, transmittance, and fluorescence of leucite based ceramics. *Dent. Mater. J.* **2017**, *36*, 394–401. [CrossRef]
28. Silami, F.D.J.; Pratavieira, S.; Nogueira, M.S.; Barrett, A.A.; Sinhoreti, M.A.C.; Geraldeli, S.; Pires-DE-Souza, F.C.P. Quantitative image of fluorescence of ceramic and resin-cement veneers. *Braz. Oral Res.* **2019**, *33*, 1–10. [CrossRef]
29. Lise, D.P.; Van Ende, A.; De Munck, J.; Yoshihara, K.; Nagaoka, N.; Cardoso Vieira, L.C.; Van Meerbeek, B. Light irradiance through novel CAD–CAM block materials and degree of conversion of composite cements. *Dent. Mater.* **2018**, *34*, 296–305. [CrossRef]
30. Pegoraro, T.A.; da Silva, N.R.F.A.; Carvalho, R.M. Cements for use in esthetic dentistry. *Dent. Clin. N. Am.* **2007**, *51*, 453–471. [CrossRef]
31. Archegas, L.R.P.; Freire, A.; Vieira, S.; Caldas, D.B.D.M.; Souza, E.M.H. Colour stability and opacity of resin cements and flowable composites for ceramic veneer luting after accelerated ageing. *J. Dent.* **2011**, *39*, 804–810. [CrossRef] [PubMed]
32. Monsénégo, G.; Burdairon, G.; Clerjaud, B. Fluorescence of dental porcelain. *J. Prosthet. Dent.* **1993**, *69*, 106–113. [CrossRef]
33. Peplinski, D.R.; Wozniak, W.T.; Moser, J.B. Spectral Studies of New Luminophors for Dental Porcelain. *J. Dent. Res.* **1980**, *59*, 1501–1506. [CrossRef] [PubMed]
34. Tani, K.; Watari, F.; Uo, M.; Morita, M. Fluorescent Properties of Porcelain-Restored Teeth and Their Discrimination. *Mater. Trans.* **2004**, *45*, 1010–1014. [CrossRef]
35. Gawriolek, M.; Sikorska, E.; Ferreira, L.F.V.; Costa, A.I.; Khmelinskii, I.; Krawczyk, A.; Sikorski, M.; Koczorowski, R. Color and Luminescence Stability of Selected Dental Materials In Vitro. *J. Prosthodont.* **2012**, *21*, 112–122. [CrossRef]
36. Conrad, H.J.; Seong, W.-J.; Pesun, I.J. Current ceramic materials and systems with clinical recommendations: A systematic review. *J. Prosthet. Dent.* **2007**, *98*, 389–404. [CrossRef]
37. Silva, L.H.; Lima, E.; Miranda, R.B.P.; Favero, S.S.; Lohbauer, U.; Cesar, P.F. Dental ceramics: A review of new materials and processing methods. *Braz. Oral Res.* **2017**, *31*, 133–146. [CrossRef]
38. Spitznagel, F.A.; Boldt, J.; Gierthmuehlen, P.C. CAD/CAM Ceramic Restorative Materials for Natural Teeth. *J. Dent. Res.* **2018**, *97*, 1082–1091. [CrossRef]
39. Mack, P.J. The recent history of radioactive fluorescers in dental porcelain. *Aust. Dent. J.* **1988**, *33*, 404–406. [CrossRef]
40. Lu, H.; Lee, Y.K.; Villalta, P.; Powers, J.M.; Garcia-Godoy, F. Influence of the amount of UV component in daylight simulator on the color of dental composite resins. *J. Prosthet. Dent.* **2006**, *96*, 322–327. [CrossRef]
41. Kiran, R.; Chapman, J.; Tennant, M.; Forrest, A.; Walsh, L. Direct tooth-colored restorative materials: A comparative analysis of the fluorescence properties among different shades. *Int. J. Esthet. Dent.* **2020**, *15*, 318–332. [PubMed]
42. Duro, F.R.; Andrade, J.S. Fluorescence: Clinical Evaluation of New Composite Resins. *Quintessence Dent. Technol.* **2012**, *35*, 145–157.
43. Ameer, Z.M.A.; Sc, M. In Vitro Evaluation of Fluorescence Stability of Different Composites and Dental Tissues before and after Accelerated Aging. *J. Med. Dent. Sci. Res.* **2015**, *3*, 1–6.

44. de Lima, L.M.; Abreu, J.D.; Cohen-Carneiro, F.; Regalado, D.F.; Pontes, D.G. A new methodology for fluorescence analysis of composite resins used in anterior direct restorations. *Gen. Dent.* **2015**, *63*, 66–69. [PubMed]
45. Magne, P.; Belser, U. *Bonded Porcelain Restorations in the Anterior Dentition: A Biomimetic Approach*; Quintessence Publishing Co, Inc.: Berlin, Germany, 2002; ISBN 0-86715-422-5.
46. Matsumoto, H.; Kitamura, S.; Araki, T. Applications of fluorescence microscopy to studies of dental hard tissue. *Front. Med. Biol. Eng.* **2001**, *10*, 269–284. [CrossRef]
47. Matsumoto, H.; Kitamura, S.; Araki, T. Autofluorescence in human dentine in relation to age, tooth type and temperature measured by nanosecond time-resolved fluorescence microscopy. *Arch. Oral Biol.* **1999**, *44*, 309–318. [CrossRef]
48. Tani, K.; Watari, F.; Uo, M.; Morita, M. Discrimination between composite resin and teeth using fluorescence properties. *Dent. Mater. J.* **2003**, *22*, 569–580. [CrossRef]
49. Caneppele, T.M.F.; Torres, C.R.G.; Bresciani, E. Analysis of the color and fluorescence alterations of enamel and dentin treated with hydrogen peroxide. *Braz. Dent. J.* **2015**, *26*, 514–518. [CrossRef]
50. Lee, Y.-K. Fluorescence properties of human teeth and dental calculus for clinical applications. *J. Biomed. Opt.* **2015**, *20*, 040901. [CrossRef]

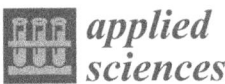

Article

Colour Changes of Acetal Resins (CAD-CAM) In Vivo

Cristina Gómez-Polo [1,*], Ana María Martín Casado [2], Norberto Quispe [1], Eva Rosel Gallardo [3] and Javier Montero [1]

[1] Department of Surgery, Faculty of Medicine, University of Salamanca, 37007 Salamanca, Spain
[2] Department of Statistics, Faculty of Medicine, University of Salamanca, 37007 Salamanca, Spain
[3] Department of Preventive and Community Dentistry, Faculty of Dentistry, University of Granada, 18011 Granada, Spain
* Correspondence: crisgodent@usal.es; Tel.: +34-923294500 (ext. 1996)

Abstract: To quantify the discolouration of the temporary acetal resins in vivo, based on the weeks of follow-up and the salivary pH in the three thirds of the tooth. To find out if the final CIELAB coordinates can be predicted from the initial colour coordinates, the salivary pH, the situation (in thirds) and the weeks of follow-up. Colour coordinates (L, C, and h) were recorded by spectrophotometry in 13 participants fitted with hybrid provisional complete dentures made of acetal resin. Colour recordings were made on the day of placement and after several weeks of follow-up (6 to 31 weeks). Salivary pH was also measured as a predictor variable for colour change. The ANOVA statistical test and regression models have been used. The highest colour difference according to ΔEab* was 27.46 units after 15 weeks of follow-up and the lowest was 7.34 units after 17 weeks of follow-up. Neither in the cervical nor in the middle third any regressor variable (initial L*, initial C*, initial h*, salivary pH and weeks of follow-up) was able to significantly predict any of the final colour coordinates ($p > 0.05$). The colour change of the temporary acetal resins used exceeds the threshold of clinical acceptability, and it is not acceptable to maintain satisfactory aesthetics. The weeks of follow-up and the salivary pH are not capable of satisfactorily predicting the final color coordinates of the acetal resins.

Keywords: acetal resins; spectrophotometer; CIELAB colour space; difference of colour formulae; interim dental restoration; dentistry; temporal resin

---

Citation: Gómez-Polo, C.; Martín Casado, A.M.; Quispe, N.; Gallardo, E.R.; Montero, J. Colour Changes of Acetal Resins (CAD-CAM) In Vivo. *Appl. Sci.* 2023, 13, 181. https://doi.org/10.3390/app13010181

Academic Editor: Andrea Scribante

Received: 1 December 2022
Revised: 15 December 2022
Accepted: 16 December 2022
Published: 23 December 2022

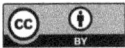

Copyright: © 2022 by the authors. Licensee MDPI, Basel, Switzerland. This article is an open access article distributed under the terms and conditions of the Creative Commons Attribution (CC BY) license (https://creativecommons.org/licenses/by/4.0/).

1. Introduction

Tooth colour affects the attractiveness of an individual's smile; if it is not pleasing, it can lead to rejection and discomfort on the part of the patient and their environment. People with bright teeth are associated with better personal, social and economic characteristics [1]. One of the factors influencing the perception of smile attractiveness is gender and dental symmetry [2]. Although the vast majority of research indicates that the most valued aesthetic factor is tooth colour [1,3,4]. The materials used to fabricate temporary prosthetic restorations are becoming increasingly important in the treatment plan, mainly because they are made more quickly and allow the patient to assess the shape, colour, position, and size of the teeth before the final dental prosthesis is made. All provisional materials must maintain acceptable aesthetics and resemble the natural tooth for an adequate period of time [5]. The success of dental prosthetic restorations includes patient satisfaction with aesthetics. The constant evolution of dental restorative materials has increased the selection options for the clinician. It is possible to use everything from classical metal alloys and ceramics, through zirconia, leucite, lithium disilicate, which have appeared more recently as definitive materials, to temporary materials derived from acrylic resins or hybrids [6]. Temporary dental prosthesis is defined as "a fixed or removable dental prosthesis, or maxillofacial prosthesis designed to enhance aesthetics, stabilization, and/or function for a limited period of time, after which it is to be replaced by a definitive dental or maxillofacial prosthesis; often such prostheses are used to assist in determination of the therapeutic effectiveness of a specific treatment plan or the form and function of the planned definitive prosthesis" [7]. The proper fabrication of a temporary fixed prosthesis plays a major role in the success or failure of definitive restorative treatment. Implant-supported fixed provisional dental restorations, especially in fully edentulous patients, serve as a mock-up to assess whether the more costly definitive fixed dental restorations fit the patient's aesthetic needs and preferences, providing a predictability factor. On the one hand, the patient "tries in" the provisional fixed prosthesis and can express their satisfaction or dissatisfaction. On the other hand, the clinician assesses the adaptability of the dental and/or gingival structures [8] and thus generates a more approximate judgement to modify the treatment plan if necessary, minimising costs. Nowadays, the high aesthetic demands and the reduction of waiting times to get patients' teeth in place have led to a remarkable improvement in the field of provisional restorations. Temporary restorations can be fabricated using conventional techniques (often self-curing polymeric materials) and by CAD/CAM (Computer-aided design/Computer-aided manufacturing) techniques [9,10]. The materials used for the fabrication of provisional prostheses need to fulfil certain characteristics: they must preserve the health of adjacent periodontal tissues, be biologically inert, resist masticatory functional loads, offer adjusted handling and working time, provide good occlusion, adequate phonetics, satisfactory aesthetics, colour stability, low cost, speed of fabrication, and ideally, offer the possibility of being repaired/modified [11,12]. Within the group of temporary materials derived from acrylic resins, one of the most widely used and studied is polymethylmethacrylate (PMMA) [9,13]. Acetal resins have recently been introduced for the purpose of making temporary dental prostheses by CAD-CAM, although their use is not yet widespread. Acetal resins are thermoplastic polymers derived from formaldehyde. They are usually coloured to more closely mimic tooth colour, as their natural colour is white. The homopolymer of acetal resin is called polyoxymethylene (POM) and its composition is a chain of methyl groups alternating with oxygen molecules [14]. In the surgical-medical field, acetal resins have already been frequently used to make hip prostheses and heart valves. In dentistry, they appeared as an alternative to the poor aesthetics of metal retainers in removable acrylic partial dentures [14,15] and as an alternative material for patients who are allergic to any of the components of chrome-cobalt alloys [16]. POM has favourable properties [14], such as resistance to deformation [16], wear [17] and water absorption [18]. Few studies have been published on the quality of POM as a temporary restorative material and on assessing its colour stability [9,11]. Depending on the results obtained on its colour behaviour, it might be possible to recommend its use for a longer period of time.

To quantify tooth colour, colourimeters and spectrophotometers [19,20] are used to provide colour results in coordinates in the CIELAB color space [21] system. The CIELAB color space consists of 3 coordinates: (1) L* (lightness) measures the amount of black and white, (2) a* coordinate (green-red axis) and (3) b* coordinate (blue-yellow axis)*. They are interpreted as follows: the higher the L* coordinate, the greater the amount of white, which gives a brighter tooth; the higher the a* coordinate, the greater the amount of red; the higher the numerical value of the b* coordinate, the greater the amount of yellow [22]. Subsequently, with the aim of each coordinate to represent one of the three dimensions of colour (Lightness, Chroma, and hue), the CIELCh color space appeared. In this nomenclature, the L* coordinate remains identical, representing the lightness*, the C* coordinate represents the chroma (amount of hue) and the angular coordinate h* represents the hue (circular axis; the units were in the form of degrees (or angles), ranging from $0°$ (red) through $90°$ (yellow), $180°$ (green), $270°$ (blue) [22]. In the dental field, two formulas have been used to calculate the difference between two colours: (1) Classical Euclidean Formula widely used in dentistry whose equation is $\Delta Eab^* = [(\Delta L^*)^2 + (\Delta a^*)^2 + (\Delta b^*)^2]^{1/2}$. ΔEab^* represented the magnitude of the colour difference [23] and (2) the CIEDE2000 formula

(ΔE00*) [23,24] which is closer to the threshold for colour discrimination than the formula ΔEab* and is better suited for interpreting clinical results [25].

$$\Delta E00 = \left[\left(\frac{\Delta L'}{K_L S_L} \right)^2 + \left(\frac{\Delta C'}{K_C S_C} \right)^2 + \left(\frac{\Delta H'}{K_H S_H} \right)^2 + R_T \left(\frac{\Delta C'}{K_C S_C} \right) \left(\frac{\Delta H'}{K_H S_H} \right) \right]^{1/2}$$

Several research studies have focused on the study of colour in the dental environment through the perceptibility and acceptability threshold (colour differences that can be perceived and accepted by 50% of the observers) [26,27], in order to categorise colour changes. Several factors are involved in the discolouration of temporary dental restorative materials, including: the composition of saliva (immunoglobulins, enzymes, nitrogenous products and mucins), salivary pH [28] ranging from 5.8 to 7.1 (slightly acidic) [29], and exogenous colouring substances [30,31].

The aim of the present research in vivo was:

1. To study whether the degree of discolouration or difference of color, of acetal resin (POM) used as a provisional material in complete upper hybrid prostheses, is significantly related to the weeks of follow-up and to salivary pH in the three thirds of the tooth (gingival third (area 1), middle third (area 2), and incisal third (area 3).
2. To find out if the final CIELAB coordinates can be predicted from the initial colour coordinates, the salivary pH, the situation (in thirds) and the weeks of follow-up.

The null hypothesis stated was (1) that there is no colour change (AEab*/ΔE00) in the implant-supported fixed provisional restorations made of acetal resins (POM) below the dental chromatic acceptance limit and (2) the final CIELAB coordinates can be predicted in thirds, from the initial colour coordinates, the salivary pH and the weeks of follow-up.

2. Materials and Methods

A total of 13 subjects were included in the study to undergo complete rehabilitation with temporary fixed tooth-supported hybrid prostheses with acetal resins in the upper jaw. All hybrid provisional complete prothesis made of acetal resin were designed with facebow and a semi-adjustable articulator. Inclusion criteria for this study were: being an adult, of full mental capacity, in good general health and with availability of time to attend check-ups. Subjects with severe bruxism and those with diagnosed gastric reflux were excluded. All patients signed the informed consent form. This research was conducted in accordance with the ethical principles of the World Medical Association Declaration of Helsinki. The experimental protocol was approved by the Bioethics Committee of the University (201500006834). Polyoxymethylene (POM, Definifit, GT Medical, Spain) was used as a temporary restorative material; POM is a resin intended for the fabrication of temporary dental prostheses, according to its manufacturer. The POM discs used in this study were machined with fine-grained tungsten carbide burs, following the manufacturer's instructions. For the fabrication of the POM hybrid prostheses, the concept proposed by Kapos et al. [32] of "Complete CAD/CAM Product" was used, which means that the final restoration has undergone a fully computerised design and fabrication process throughout; therefore, the prostheses used were fabricated from a pre-polymerised block of POM in its entirety, without interphases. All milled POM discs (CAM) had the same initial colour: A3, according to the Vita Classical guide. After completing the milling process, finishing, and polishing treatments were carried out on the provisional hybrid prostheses, following the manufacturer's instructions: non-aggressive pastes, (Acrypol, Bredent, Senden, Germany), without generating excessive heat and with silicone polishers. The milling and finishing process of all the prostheses was carried out in the same prosthetic laboratory with the same machinery (DWX-4,DGSHAPE, Barcelona, Spain) and by the same laboratory technician with 12 years of experience. Colour coordinates (L*, C*, h*, a*, and b*) were recorded by spectrophotometry (Spectroshade Micro, MHT Optic Research, Switzerland) in each of the three thirds of the upper right central incisor: cervical, middle, and incisal edge. Each third of the tooth was measured three times and arithmetic means were used for further statistical analysis. The tooth colour of the temporary hybrid restoration was measured at two time points: on the day of placement and after several weeks in the mouth (from 6 weeks to a maximum of 31 weeks) (Figure 1). In addition, Euclidian equation and CIEDE200 colour difference formulae were used to calculate the colour difference. In the present study, the reference values for interpreting the colour difference were those published by Douglas et al. with ΔEab* = 2.6 units as the threshold of perception and ΔEab* = 5.5 units as the threshold of clinical acceptability [27]. The software used for the descriptive and inferential statistical analysis of the results was IBM Corp. Released 2017. IBM SPSS Statistics for Windows, Version 25.0. Armonk, NY: IBM Corp. ANOVA test and linear regression analyses with R squared for indicate how well data fit a statistical model were used. Based on the sample size of similar studies [10,32,33] an initial sample size of 30 subjects was established for detecting clinical discolorations (ΔEab > 5.5 units) in the fixed provisional restorations made of acetal resins [26], but consecutive sampling was discontinued due to the severity of the colour discolorations.

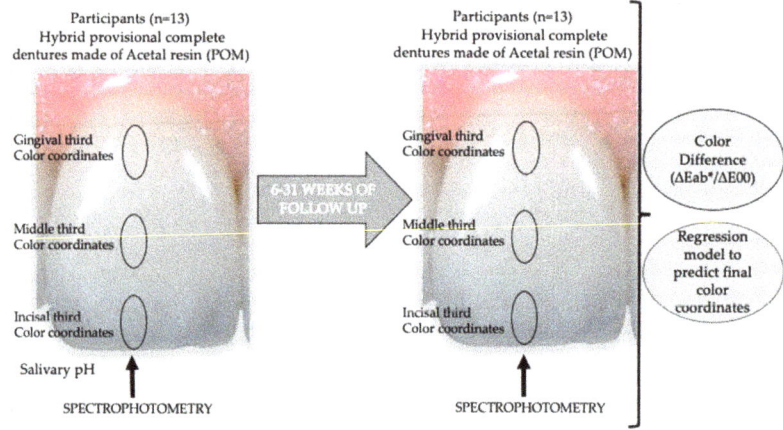

Figure 1. Scheme of the methodology.

3. Results

Table 1 shows the colour changes, according to the ΔEab* formula and the ΔE00* formula, between the day of placement of the provisional hybrid POM prosthesis and after the different weeks of follow-up in the three thirds of the tooth. The highest colour difference according to the ΔEab* formula was 27.46 units after 15 weeks of follow-up and occurred in the cervical third. On the other hand, the lowest shade difference was 7.34 units after 17 weeks of follow-up and took place in the incisal third. These colour differences exceeded the threshold of clinical acceptability (Figure 2) proposed by Douglas et al. [27] According to the ΔE00* formula, the lowest colour change was 5.23 units, and the highest colour change was 22.61 units (Figure 3). The pH range varied from 6 to 9 units and the follow-up weeks ranged from a minimum of 6. to a maximum of 31.

Table 1. Colour differences, according to the Euclidean and CIEDE2000 formulae, in the three thirds of the upper central incisor.

Participants	CIELAB (ΔEab*)			CIEDE2000 (ΔE00*)			pH	Weeks of Follow-Up
	Cervical ΔEab*	Middle ΔEab*	Incisal ΔEab*	Cervical ΔE00*	Middle ΔE00*	Incisal ΔE00*		
1	24.92	25.09	19.67	21.06	20.37	16.29	6	16
2	17.44	13.88	18.98	15.04	11.07	16.21	6.5	12
3	18.71	19.36	20.16	15.88	16.28	17.48	7	31
4	18.24	16.29	9.63	16.41	13.57	8.40	6	14
5	16.01	15.13	11.10	13.75	12.23	8.81	8	27
6	15.49	17.02	14.15	13.01	13.13	10.84	9	18
7	19.51	21.14	17.77	18.20	17.76	14.51	8.5	18
8	11.01	12.01	11.42	8.68	9.53	9.36	6.5	6
9	9.87	9.21	7.34	8.16	6.72	5.23	6	17
10	18.03	16.50	13.97	14.97	13.47	11.45	9	15
11	23.71	25.59	19.81	18.70	19.28	13.43	7.5	15
12	10.58	10.75	9.54	7.65	7.81	6.96	8	15
13	27.46	23.86	15.35	22.61	18.38	11.20	7.5	15

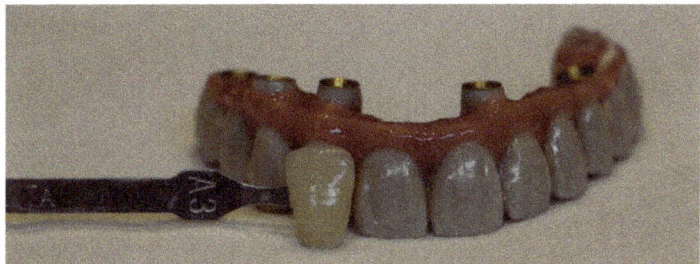

Figure 2. Color difference between A3 dental shade tab and hybrid provisional complete prothesis made of acetal resin.

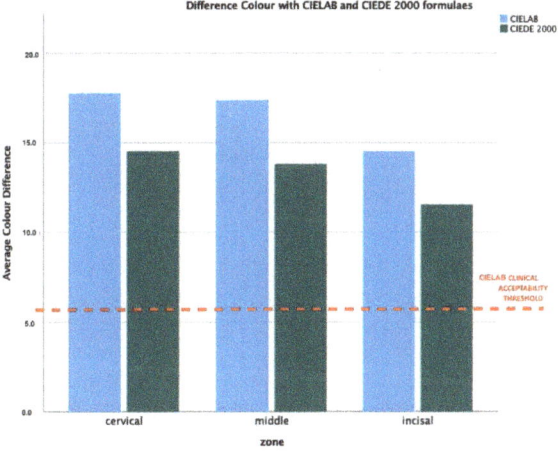

Figure 3. Colour differences (ΔEab* and ΔE00*) exceeded the threshold of clinical acceptability.

With both formulas, the ANOVA with one factor of variation (thirds of the tooth) in a randomised block design (subjects) revealed that the chromatic changes in the three areas differed significantly ($p = 0.002$). Subsequently, Duncan's test showed that discolourations in the cervical and middle areas did not differ significantly, but discolourations in the incisal area did, where colour changes were significantly smaller.

By using regression models, it was assessed whether the degree of discolouration was significantly related to the weeks of follow-up and to pH, according to the two colour formulae in each of the tooth thirds.

Euclidean formula (ΔEab^*):

$$\widehat{\text{Dif}}\text{cervical} = 16.379 - 0.034\text{pH} + 0.097 \text{ Weeks of follow up } (R^2 = 0.012)$$

$$\widehat{\text{Dif}}\text{middle} = 12.561 + 0.363\text{pH} + 0.127 \text{ Weeks of follow up } (R^2 = 0.032)$$

$$\widehat{\text{Dif}}\text{incisal} = 11.493 + 0.090\text{pH} + 0.141 \text{ Weeks of follow up } (R^2 = 0.041)$$

In all three areas, the coefficients of determination were small, which indicates that discolouration depends on explanatory variables other than pH and follow-up weeks. However, an increase in the coefficient of determination was observed from the cervical to the incisal area. No model was significant (tests for significance of regression with $p > 0.05$). It is noteworthy that the signs of the regression coefficients for 'pH' varied according to the area (negative in the cervical area, positive in the middle and incisal area), while the signs of the regression coefficients for the variable 'weeks of follow-up' were the same (positive) in all three areas.

CIEDE2000 formula ($\Delta E00^*$):

$$\widehat{\text{Dif}}\text{cervical} = 13.729 - 0.099\text{pH} + 0.115 \text{ Weeks of follow up } (R^2 = 0.022)$$

$$\widehat{\text{Dif}}\text{middle} = 9.938 + 0.206\text{pH} + 0.140 \text{ Weeks of follow up } (R^2 = 0.047)$$

$$\widehat{\text{Dif}}\text{incisal} = 10.467 - 0.211\text{pH} + 0.157 \text{ Weeks of follow up } (R^2 = 0.062)$$

In all three zones, the coefficients of determination were small (although larger than those of the models constructed with the Euclidean formula), which indicates that discolouration depends on more explanatory variables (apart from salivary pH and weeks of follow-up). Again, an increase in the coefficient of determination was observed from the cervical to the incisal area. No model was significant (tests for significance of regression at $p > 0.05$). The signs of the regression coefficients for 'pH' varied according to the area (negative in the cervical and incisal areas), while the signs of the regression coefficients for the variable 'Weeks of follow-up' were the same (positive) in all three areas.

It was studied whether the final colour coordinates, in each of the three thirds, could be predicted from the initial colour coordinates, pH, salivary and weeks of follow-up. In the cervical and middle third, no regressor variable (initial L^*, initial C^*, initial h^*, salivary pH and follow-up weeks) was able to significantly predict any of the three final colour coordinates: Final L^*, final C^*, and final h^* ($p > 0.05$). In the middle third, no regressor variable (initial L^*, initial C^*, initial h^*, salivary pH and weeks of follow-up) was able to significantly explain the dependent variables ($p > 0.05$). On the contrary, in the incisal third, the independent variable initial C^* had a predictive power of the final C^* coordinate and the model was significant ($p = 0.017$). Similarly, in the incisal third, the independent variable initial h^* had significant explanatory power over the dependent variable final h^* ($p = 0.006$). Thus, in the incisal third, the final intensity (final C^* coordinate) and the final shade (final h^* coordinate) can be explained by the corresponding initial colour coordinates of the acetal resins.

4. Discussion

The first null hypothesis was rejected because all the color differences were above the threshold of dental clinical acceptability ($\Delta Eab^* > 5.5$ units). The null's second hypothesis cannot be accepted either, since the predictive power of the initial color coordinates, salivary pH, and weeks of follow-up have small coefficients of determination.

Many works have studied provisional restorative materials in relation to marginal fit, hardness, roughness, fracture, and strength [9,10,34,35], but few have focused on acetal resins (POM). CAD-CAM technology has also made it possible to achieve an extraordinary improvement in quality based on mechanical strength [36,37], flexural strength [38], better marginal fit [39], fewer imperfections [40] and improved aesthetics [41,42]. There are contradictory results such as those published by Tieh et al. who claim that the colour stability of CAD-CAM in denture teeth is similar to that of traditional PMMA denture teeth [43]. In the same line, Stawarczyk et al. concluded, in in vitro studies, that resins manufactured by CAD-CAM display the same colour stability as glass-ceramic materials [40]. These differences could be due to the variation in the methodology of the studies and the diversity of Bis-acrylic resins on the market in terms of composition.

According to the manufacturer, Definitfit® acetal resins are sensitive to salivary pH below 4, and also if the material is heated excessively during the milling phase, if it is left in contact with carotenes for a long time and if polishing is not carried out properly. In none of the participants was the pH below 6. If the results obtained in in vivo studies on shade stability are favourable, acetal resins could be used as a material for long-term temporaries (more than 6 months) [44]. The main aesthetic disadvantage of interim restoration materials is that they undergo absorption and adsorption processes of liquids present in the oral environment, which can cause discolouration and reduce the degree of aesthetic satisfaction of the patient [5,44–46]. In vitro studies have concluded that factors such as type of diet, intake of certain medications and mouthwashes influence the degree of staining of different types of polymeric materials [40,47–49]; this is particularly true with the consumption of cofee, tea, and wine [5], which are the beverages most capable of creating discolourations [50] and the intensity of its action is difficult to quantify as it depends on its quality [5,17,51]. This could have explained better the color change of patient #9 that, although higher than clinical acceptable thresholds, showed a marked lower color-change in respect to other patients.

The main disadvantages of the present research may be that the diet and deleterious habits of the participants were not recorded, and these variables could also be responsible for the significant colour changes observed; on the other hand, salivary pH and weeks of follow-up have not been shown to be a determining factor in the colour changes. For this reason, future research would need to broaden the baseline variables (diet and habits) in order to quantify the independent effect on the intraoral discolouration of these materials. In this regard, due to the inherent difficulty of fully controlling the oral diet invivo there are still no published studies that quantify the effect of each food on tooth color. Most of the research had studies beverages (staining solutions) [30]. Also, it is necessary to take into account the different chromatic behavior of food and drinks in vivo than in vitro [30]. One of the disadvantages of in vivo studies is the difficulty of standardising intraoral conditions, because they depend on many factors; however, they bring us closer to the intraoral reality. A small number of in vivo studies of dental restorations made of polymeric materials [44,52–54] are available, most of them in the field of denture prosthetics. Depite the small sample size, the primary outcome (change discoloration) was found to be statistically significant between baseline and postoperative evaluations (Table 1), demonstrating that this sample size was enough potent to detect severe change discolorations.

The great variety of materials of this nature on the market as well as the wide range of fabrication techniques, the different methodologies, and the lack of standardisation in evaluation criteria and follow-up times make it difficult to compare their results. The in vivo study by Díez-Quijano et al. on implant-supported fixed temporary prosthesis with CAD-CAM acetal resin in posterior sectors, using a colourimeter for colour coordinate registration, revealed that at six months the mean colour change according to the ΔEab^* formula was 12.90 units. They also found that the h^*-coordinate (hue) and a^*-coordinate decreased significantly at six months compared with baseline ($p < 0.05$). They concluded that PMMA showed better colour behaviour than POM. [11] In the present work, colour was recorded spectrophotometrically on the surface of the upper incisors (which is less convex than the surface of the posterior sectors). The smallest colour change according to the ΔEab* formula was 7.34 units (after 15 weeks of follow-up) and the largest was 27.46 units (after 17 weeks of follow-up). These differences in results may be due to the composition of acetal resins, smoking habits, diet, and different electronic colour-recording devices. Spectrophotometers are known to record the amount of light reflected by an object, but they have the disadvantage of scattering, especially on convex surfaces. In these in vivo studies [15], the average colour change also exceeds the colour acceptability threshold (ΔEab* 5.5 units), which prevents the desired colour stability requirement from being met. Most authors publish results according to the Euclidean formula, although the CIEDE2000 formula is more in line with human visual perception [22,55]. In reference to the in vitro colour changes of POM resins not processed by CAD-CAM, we found ΔE* values lower than 5.4 units [9] after six weeks of immersion in different solutions. Another in vitro study along the same lines by Ozkan et al. [19] compared the colour stability of acetal resin and conventional PMMA subjected to a thermocycling process. Although significant differences in colour change were found at the initial and final time, both materials obtained clinically acceptable ΔE* values (1.33 units for PMMA and 1.13 units for acetal resin). Caution should be exercised when analysing these colour differences, as the composition of the acetal resin varies, as well as the manufacturing and processing process. It was not possible to predict the colour change that the POM resins will show, depending on the variables analysed, with statistical determination in this research. Only in the incisal third, the dependent variables final C^* and final h^* were found to be significant regressors of initial C^* and initial h^*, respectively. Another aspect to take into account is hygiene habits, which could also play an important role in the maintenance of the initial shade of the POM restoration [14]. Also, Alkhatib et al. [56] found that there is a significant difference between heavy smokers and non-smokers with regard to the presence of discolourations. With reference to saliva, there is an increasing need to study its involvement in discolourations and the influence of salivary enzymes on the degradation of temporary resin materials. [31] Additionally, more studies are needed in order to test also flexural [57] and hardness [58] test, as these variables have a significant influence on material choice. The results presented do not encourage the use of POM resins as a long-term temporary restorative material, as the colour changes observed exceeded the colour acceptance threshold, and this may lead to patient dissatisfaction.

5. Conclusions

With the limitations of this study, we can be affirm that the colour change of the acetal resins used is not acceptable to maintain satisfactory aesthetics (exceeds the threshold of clinical acceptability). The discolouration of acetal resins is not only dependent on pH and weeks of follow-up.

Author Contributions: Conceptualization, C.G.-P., N.Q., E.R.G. and J.M.; methodology, C.G.-P.; data analysis, J.M. and C.G.-P.; writing—original draft preparation, C.G.-P., E.R.G. and N.Q.; writing—review and editing, J.M. and C.G.-P. A.M.M.C. made the last revision of the manuscript. All authors have read and agreed to the published version of the manuscript.

Funding: This research received no external funding.

Institutional Review Board Statement: The study was conducted according to the guidelines of the Declaration of Helsinki, and approved by the Research Ethics Committee of the University of Salamanca, Spain (USAL/2017).

Informed Consent Statement: All participants were volunteers.

Data Availability Statement: Not applicable.

Acknowledgments: The study was conducted within the Research Group "Avances en Salud Oral" (Advances in Oral Health) of the University of Salamanca, led by the first author. https://avancessaludoral.usal.es (accessed on 10 December 2022). Thanks for the translation work of Elena H. Rivero (SCI-USAL).

Conflicts of Interest: The authors declare no conflict of interest.

References

1. Montero, J.; Gómez Polo, C.; Rosel, E.; Barrios, R.; Albaladejo, A.; López-Valverde, A. The role of personality traits in self-rated oral health and preferences for different types of flawed smiles. *J. Oral Rehabil.* **2016**, *43*, 39–50. [CrossRef] [PubMed]
2. Chrapla, P.; Paradowska-Stolarz, A.; Skoskiewicz-Malinowska, K. Subjective and Objective Evaluation of the Symmetry of Maxillary Incisors among Residents of Southwest Poland. *Symmetry* **2022**, *14*, 1257. [CrossRef]
3. Newton, J.T.; Subramanian, S.S.; Westland, S.; Gupta, A.K.; Luo, W.; Joiner, A. The impact of tooth colour on the perceptions of age and social judgements. *J. Dent.* **2021**, *112*, 103771. [CrossRef] [PubMed]
4. Polyzois, G.; Niarchou, A.; Ntala, P.; Pantopoulos, A.; Frangou, M. The effect of immersion cleansers on gloss, colour and sorption of acetal denture base material. *Gerodontology* **2013**, *30*, 150–156. [CrossRef]
5. Paolone, G.; Formiga, S.; De Palma, F.; Abbruzzese, L.; Chirico, L.; Scolavino, S.; Goracci, C.; Cantatore, G.; Vichi, A. Color stability of resin-based composites: Staining procedures with liquids-A narrative review. *J. Esthet. Restor. Dent.* **2022**, *34*, 865–887. [CrossRef] [PubMed]
6. Saeed, F.; Muhammad, N.; Khan, A.S.; Sharif, F.; Rahim, A.; Ahmad, P.; Irfan, M. Prosthodontics dental materials: From conventional to unconventional. *Mater. Sci. Eng. C Mater. Biol. Appl.* **2020**, *106*, 110167. [CrossRef]
7. The glossary of prosthodontic terms. *J. Prosthet. Dent.* **2005**, *94*, 10–92. [CrossRef]
8. Proussaefs, P. Immediate provisionalization with a CAD/CAM interim abutment and crown: A guided soft tissue healing technique. *J. Prosthet. Dent.* **2015**, *113*, 91–95. [CrossRef]
9. Rayyan, M.M.; Aboushelib, M.; Sayed, N.M.; Ibrahim, A.; Jimbo, R. Comparison of interim restorations fabricated by CAD/CAM with those fabricated manually. *J. Prosthet. Dent.* **2015**, *114*, 414–419. [CrossRef]
10. Taşın, S.; Ismatullaev, A.; Usumez, A. Comparison of surface roughness and color stainability of 3-dimensionally printed interim prosthodontic material with conventionally fabricated and CAD-CAM milled materials. *J. Prosthet. Dent.* **2021**. [CrossRef]
11. Díez-Quijano, C.; Azevedo, L.; Antonaya-Martín, J.L.; Del Río-Highsmith, J.; Gómez-Polo, M. Evaluation of the clinical behavior of 2 different materials for implant-supported interim fixed partial prostheses: A randomized clinical trial. *J. Prosthet. Dent.* **2020**, *124*, 351–356. [CrossRef] [PubMed]
12. Burns, D.R.; Beck, D.A.; Nelson, S.K. A review of selected dental literature on contemporary provisional fixed prosthodontic treatment: Report of the Committee on Research in Fixed Prosthodontics of the Academy of Fixed Prosthodontics. *J. Prosthet. Dent.* **2003**, *90*, 474–497. [CrossRef] [PubMed]
13. Güth, J.F.; Almeida ESilva, J.S.; Beuer, F.F.; Edelhoff, D. Enhancing the predictability of complex rehabilitation with a removable CAD/CAM-fabricated long-term provisional prosthesis: A clinical report. *J. Prosthet. Dent.* **2012**, *107*, 1–6. [CrossRef]
14. Polychronakis, N.; Lagouvardos, P.; Polyzois, G.; Sykaras, N.; Zoidis, P. Color changes of polyetheretherketone (PEEK) and polyoxymethelene (POM) denture resins on single and combined staining/cleansing action by CIELab and CIEDE2000 formulas. *J. Prosthodont. Res.* **2020**, *64*, 159–166. [CrossRef] [PubMed]
15. Meenakshi, A.; Gupta, R.; Bharti, V.; Sriramaprabu, G.; Prabhakar, R. An Evaluation of Retentive Ability and Deformation of Acetal Resin and Cobalt-Chromium Clasps. *J. Clin. Diagn. Res.* **2016**, *10*, ZC37–ZC41. [CrossRef] [PubMed]
16. Jiao, T.; Chang, T.; Caputo, A.A. Load transfer characteristics of unilateral distal extension removable partial dentures with polyacetal resin. *Aust. Dent. J.* **2009**, *54*, 31–37. [CrossRef]
17. Zok, F.W.; Miserez, A. Property maps for abrasion resistance of materials. *Acta Mater.* **2007**, *55*, 6365–6371. [CrossRef] [PubMed]
18. Arikan, A.; Ozkan, Y.K.; Arda, T.; Akalin, B. An in vitro investigation of water sorption and solubility of two acetal denture base materials. *Eur. J. Prosthodont. Restor. Dent.* **2005**, *13*, 119–122.
19. Ozkan, Y.; Arikan, A.; Akalin, B.; Arda, T. A study to assess the colour stability of acetal resins subjected to thermocycling. *Eur. J. Prosthodont. Restor. Dent.* **2005**, *13*, 10–14.
20. Hassel, A.J.; Grossmann, A.C.; Schmitter, M.; Balze, Z.; Buzello, A.M. Interexaminer reliability in clinical measurement of L*C*h* values of anterior teeth using a spectrophotometer. *Int. J. Prosthodont.* **2007**, *20*, 79–84.
21. CIE (Commission Internationale de l'Éclairage). *Annuaire, Roster, Register, Annexeau Bulletin CIE*; Bureau Central de la CIE: Paris, France, 1976.
22. CIE Commission International de Eclairage (CIE). *Colorimetry*, 3rd ed.; CIE Publication No. 15; Central Bureau of the CIE: Vienna, Austria, 2004.
23. Paravina, R.D.; Pérez, M.M.; Ghinea, R. Acceptability and perceptibility thresholds in dentistry: A comprehensive review of clinical and research applications. *J. Esthet. Restor. Dent.* **2019**, *31*, 103–112. [CrossRef] [PubMed]
24. CIE. *Technical Report: Improvement to Industrial Colour-Difference Evaluation*; CIE Publication 142; CIE Central Bureau: Vienna, Austria, 2001.
25. Pecho, O.E.; Ghinea, R.; Alessandretti, R.; Pérez, M.M.; Della Bona, A. Visual and instrumental shade matching using CIELAB and CIEDE2000 color difference formulas. *Dent. Mater.* **2016**, *32*, 82–92. [CrossRef] [PubMed]
26. Khashayar, G.; Bain, P.A.; Salari, S.; Dozic, A.; Kleverlaan, C.J.; Feilzer, A.J. Perceptibility and acceptability thresholds for colour differences in dentistry. *J. Dent.* **2014**, *42*, 637–644. [CrossRef]
27. Douglas, R.D.; Steinhauer, T.J.; Wee, A.G. Intraoral determination of the tolerance of dentists for perceptibility and acceptability of shade mismatch. *J. Prosthet. Dent.* **2007**, *97*, 200–208. [CrossRef]

28. Azer, S.S.; Hague, A.L.; Johnston, W.M. Effect of pH on tooth discoloration from food colorant in vitro. *J. Dent.* **2010**, *38* (Suppl. S2), e106–e109. [CrossRef] [PubMed]
29. Humphrey, S.P.; Williamson, R.T. A review of saliva: Normal composition, flow, and function. *J. Prosthet. Dent.* **2001**, *85*, 162–169. [CrossRef] [PubMed]
30. Kul, E.; Abdulrahim, R.; Bayındır, F.; Matori, K.A.; Gül, P. Evaluation of the color stability of temporary materials produced with CAD/CAM. *Dent. Med. Probl.* **2021**, *58*, 187–191. [CrossRef]
31. Lee, Y.K.; Powers, J.M. Influence of salivary organic substances on the discoloration of esthetic dental materials-a review. *J. Biomed. Mater. Res. B Appl. Biomater.* **2006**, *76*, 397–402. [CrossRef]
32. Kapos, T.; Evans, C. CAD/CAM technology for implant abutments, crowns, and superstructures. *Int. J. Oral Maxillofac. Implants* **2014**, *29*, 117–136. [CrossRef]
33. Bauer, R.; Zacher, J.; Strasser, T.; Rosentritt, M. In vitro performance and fracture resistance of interim conventional or CAD-CAM implant-supported screw- or cement-retained anterior fixed partial dentures. *J. Prosthet. Dent.* **2021**, *126*, 575–580. [CrossRef]
34. Kwan, J.C.; Kwan, N. Clinical Application of PEEK as a Provisional Fixed Dental Prosthesis Retained by Reciprocated Guide Surfaces of Healing Abutments During Dental Implant Treatment. *Int. J. Oral Maxillofac. Implants* **2021**, *36*, 581–586. [CrossRef] [PubMed]
35. Köroğlu, A.; Sahin, O.; Dede, D.Ö.; Yilmaz, B. Effect of different surface treatment methods on the surface roughness and color stability of interim prosthodontic materials. *J. Prosthet. Dent.* **2016**, *115*, 447–455. [CrossRef] [PubMed]
36. Wimmer, T.; Ender, A.; Roos, M.; Stawarczyk, B. Fracture load of milled polymeric fixed dental prostheses as a function of connector cross-sectional areas. *J. Prosthet. Dent.* **2013**, *110*, 288–295. [CrossRef]
37. Karaokutan, I.; Sayin, G.; Kara, O. In vitro study of fracture strength of provi- sional crown materials. *J. Adv. Prosthodont.* **2015**, *7*, 27–31. [CrossRef]
38. Çakmak, G.; Yilmaz, H.; Aydoğ, Ö.; Yilmaz, B. Flexural strength of CAD-CAM and conventional interim resin materials with a surface sealant. *J. Prosthet. Dent.* **2020**, *124*, 800.e1–800.e7. [CrossRef] [PubMed]
39. Sadighpour, L.; Geramipanah, F.; Falahchai, M.; Tadbiri, H. Marginal adaptation of three-unit interim restorations fabricated by the CAD-CA systems and the direct method before and after thermocycling. *J. Clin. Exp. Dent.* **2021**, *13*, e572–e579. [CrossRef]
40. Stawarczyk, B.; Sener, B.; Trottmann, A.; Roos, M.; Ozcan, M.; Hammerle, C.H.F. Discoloration of manually fabricated resins and industrially fabricated CAD/CAM blocks versus glass-ceramic: Effect of storage media, duration, and subsequent polishing. *Dent. Mater. J.* **2012**, *31*, 377–383. [CrossRef]
41. Guth, J.-F.; Zuch, T.; Zwinge, S.; Engels, J.; Stimmelmayr, M.; Edelhoff, D. Optical properties of manually and CAD/CAM-fabricated polymers. *Dent. Mater.* **2013**, *32*, 865–871. [CrossRef]
42. Dayan, C.; Guven, M.C.; Gencel, B.; Bural, C. A Comparison of the Color Stability of Conventional and CAD/CAM Polymethyl Methacrylate Denture Base Materials. *Acta Stomatol. Croat.* **2019**, *53*, 158–167. [CrossRef]
43. Tieh, M.T.; Waddell, J.N.; Choi, J.J.E. Optical Properties and Color Stability of Denture Teeth-A Systematic Review. *J. Prosthodont.* **2021**. [CrossRef]
44. Anselm Wiskott, H.W.; Perriard, J.; Scherrer, S.S.; Dieth, S.; Belser, U.C. In vivo wear of three types of veneering materials using implant-supported restorations: A method evaluation. *Eur. J. Oral Sci.* **2002**, *110*, 61–67. [CrossRef] [PubMed]
45. Gujjari, A.K.; Bhatnagar, V.M.; Basavaraju, R.M. Color stability and flexural strength of poly (methyl methacrylate) and bis-acrylic composite based provisional crown and bridge auto- polymerizing resins exposed to beverages and food dye: An in vitro study. *Indian J. Dent. Res.* **2013**, *24*, 172–177. [CrossRef] [PubMed]
46. Sham, A.S.; Chu, F.C.; Chai, J.; Chow, T.W. Color stability of provisional prosthodontic materials. *J. Prosthet. Dent.* **2004**, *91*, 447–452. [CrossRef] [PubMed]
47. Watanabe, H.; Kim, E.; Piskorski, N.L.; Sarsland, J.; Covey, D.A.; Johnson, W.W. Mechanical properties and color stability of provisional restoration resins. *Am. J. Dent.* **2013**, *26*, 265–270.
48. Kang, A.; Son, S.A.; Hur, B.; Kwon, Y.H.; Ro, J.H.; Park, J.K. The color stability of silorane- and methacrylate-based resin composites. *Dent. Mater. J.* **2012**, *31*, 879–884. [CrossRef]
49. Prasad, D.K.; Alva, H.; Shetty, M. Evaluation of colour stability of provisional restorative materials exposed to different mouth rinses at varying time intervals: An in vitro study. *J. Indian Prosthodont. Soc.* **2014**, *14*, 85–92. [CrossRef]
50. Versari, A.; Parpinello, G.P.; Mattioli, A.U. Characterisation of color components and polymeric pigments of commercial red wines by using selected UV-Vis spectrophotometric methods. *S. Afr. J. Enol. Vitic.* **2007**, *28*, 6–10.
51. Quek, S.H.Q.; Yap, A.U.J.; Rosa, V.; Tan, K.B.C.; Teoh, K.H. Effect of staining beverages on color and translucency of CAD/CAM composites. *J. Esthet. Restor. Dent.* **2018**, *30*, E9–E17. [CrossRef]
52. Suarez-Feito, J.M.; Sicilia, A.; Angulo, J.; Banerji, S.; Cuesta, I.; Millar, B. Clinical performance of provisional screw-retained metal-free acrylic restorations in an immediate loading implant protocol: A 242 consecutive patients' report. *Clin. Oral Implants Res.* **2010**, *21*, 1360–1369. [CrossRef]
53. Ohlmann, B.; Bermejo, J.L.; Rammelsberg, P.; Schmitter, M.; Zenthofer, A.; Stober, T. Comparison of incidence of complications and aesthetic performance for posterior metal-free polymer crowns and metal-ceramic crowns: Results from a randomized clinical trial. *J. Dent.* **2014**, *42*, 671–676. [CrossRef]
54. Huettig, F.; Prutscher, A.; Goldammer, C.; Kreutzer, C.A.; Weber, H. First clinical experiences with CAD/CAM-fabricated PMMA-based fixed dental prostheses as long-term temporaries. *Clin. Oral Investig.* **2016**, *20*, 161–168. [CrossRef] [PubMed]

55. Pecho, O.E.; Ghinea, R.; Perez, M.M.; Della Bona, A. Influence of Gender on Visual Shade Matching in Dentistry. *J. Esthet. Restor. Dent.* **2017**, *29*, E15–E23. [CrossRef] [PubMed]
56. Alkhatib, M.N.; Holt, R.D.; Bedi, R. Smoking and tooth discolouration: Findings from a national crosssectional study. *BMC Public Health* **2005**, *5*, 27. [CrossRef] [PubMed]
57. Cacciafesta, V.; Sfondrini, M.F.; Lena, A.; Vallittu, P.K.; Lassila, L.V. Flexural strengths of fiber-reinforced composites polymerized with conventional light-curing and additional postcuring. *Am. J. Orthod. Dentofac. Ortho-Pedics* **2007**, *132*, 524–527. [CrossRef]
58. Pieniak, D.; Walczak, A.; Walczak, M.; Przystupa, K.; Niewczas, A.M. Hardness and Wear Resistance of Dental Biomedical Nanomaterials in a Humid Environment with Non-Stationary Temperatures. *Materials* **2020**, *13*, 1255. [CrossRef]

Disclaimer/Publisher's Note: The statements, opinions and data contained in all publications are solely those of the individual author(s) and contributor(s) and not of MDPI and/or the editor(s). MDPI and/or the editor(s) disclaim responsibility for any injury to people or property resulting from any ideas, methods, instructions or products referred to in the content.

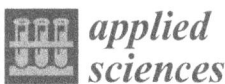

Article

Antifungal Efficacy of Sodium Perborate and Microwave Irradiation for Surface Disinfection of Polymethyl Methacrylate Polymer

Ziaullah Choudhry [1,*], Sofia Malik [2], Zulfiqar A. Mirani [3], Shujah A. Khan [4], Syed M. R. Kazmi [5], Waqas A. Farooqui [6], Muhammad A. Ahmed [7], Khulud A. AlAali [8], Abdullah Alshahrani [9], Mohammed Alrabiah [9], Ahmed H. Albaqawi [10] and Tariq Abduljabbar [9,*]

1. Prosthodontics Department, Dr Ishrat-ul-Ebad Khan Institute of Oral Health Sciences, Dow University of Health Sciences, Karachi 74200, Pakistan
2. Department of Science of Dental Material, Dr Ishrat-ul-Ebad Khan Institute of Oral Health Sciences, Dow University of Health Sciences, Karachi 74200, Pakistan; sofia.malik@duhs.edu.pk
3. Microbiology Section, Pakistan Council for Scientific and Industrial Research (PCSIR), Laboratories Complex Karachi, Karachi 75270, Pakistan; mirani_mrsa@yahoo.com
4. Prosthodontics Department, Liaquat College of Medicine and Dentistry, Darul Sehat Hospital, Karachi 75290, Pakistan; shujah.adil@gmail.com
5. Department of Surgery, Section of Dentistry, Aga Khan University, Karachi 74800, Pakistan; syed.murtaza@aku.edu
6. School of Public Health, Dow University of Health Sciences, Karachi 74200, Pakistan; waqas.ahmed@duhs.edu.pk
7. Department of Restorative Dental Sciences, College of Dentistry, King Faisal University, Al Ahsa 31982, Saudi Arabia; mshakeel@kfu.edu.sa
8. Department of Clinical Dental Sciences, College of Dentistry, Princess Nourah Bint Abdulrahman University, Riyadh 11564, Saudi Arabia; kaalaali@pnu.edu.sa
9. Prosthetic Dental Science Department, College of Dentistry, King Saud University, Riyadh 11451, Saudi Arabia; asalshahrani@ksu.edu.sa (A.A.); mohalrabiah@ksu.edu.sa (M.A.)
10. Department of Restorative Dental Science, College of Dentistry, University of Ha'il, Ha'il 55476, Saudi Arabia; a.albaqawi@uoh.edu.sa

* Correspondence: ziaullah.choudhry@duhs.edu.pk (Z.C.); tajabbar@ksu.edu.sa (T.A.); Fax: +966-14678639 (T.A.)

Abstract: Various disinfecting agents showing variable success in disinfecting polymethyl methacrylate (PMMA) are available. The aim of our study was to evaluate the antifungal efficacy of sodium perborate (denture cleaning tablet-DC), microwave irradiation, and their combination for eradicating candida albicans (*C. albicans*) from polymethyl methacrylate (PMMA) denture base polymer. One hundred and sixty-eight PMMA resin specimens (30 × 30 × 15 mm) were divided into four groups, including control (no disinfection), microwave disinfection in distilled water (MW-DW), sodium perborate with distilled water (DC-DW), and a combination of MW-DC-DW (n = 10). Biofilms of *C. albicans* were cultured on the PMMA resin denture base specimens for 96 h. The samples were exposed to three different antifungal regimes, i.e., MW, denture cleaning agent-sodium perborate (DC) and DW, and a combination of MW-DC-DW for 1 to 5 min. Scanning electron microscopy (SEM) was performed to evaluate colony formation. The colony-forming units (CFU) among the experimental groups were assessed using ANOVA, a Kruskal–Wallis test, and a Mann–Whitney test. The mean CFU values were compared with the control for each disinfecting regime at 96 h growth time. For MW-DC-DW, the CFU were significantly low at 2 and 3 min of exposure when compared with the control (DW) ($p < 0.05$). For the MW-DW treated group, the CFU were significantly low at 3 min of exposure when compared with the control (DW) ($p < 0.05$). It was also found that for DC-DW, the CFU were significantly low at 5 minutes when compared with the control specimens (DW) ($p < 0.05$). Microwave disinfection in combination with sodium perborate is a more effective disinfecting regime against *C. albicans* than that of microwave disinfection and sodium perborate alone.

Keywords: polymers; polymethyl methacrylate; dentures; candida; disinfection; oral health

Citation: Choudhry, Z.; Malik, S.; Mirani, Z.A.; Khan, S.A.; Kazmi, S.M.R.; Farooqui, W.A.; Ahmed, M.A.; AlAali, K.A.; Alshahrani, A.; Alrabiah, M.; et al. Antifungal Efficacy of Sodium Perborate and Microwave Irradiation for Surface Disinfection of Polymethyl Methacrylate Polymer. *Appl. Sci.* 2022, 12, 7004. https://doi.org/10.3390/app12147004

Academic Editors: Ricardo Castro Alves, José João Mendes and Ana Cristina Mano Azul

Received: 6 June 2022
Accepted: 4 July 2022
Published: 11 July 2022

Publisher's Note: MDPI stays neutral with regard to jurisdictional claims in published maps and institutional affiliations.

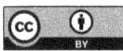

Copyright: © 2022 by the authors. Licensee MDPI, Basel, Switzerland. This article is an open access article distributed under the terms and conditions of the Creative Commons Attribution (CC BY) license (https://creativecommons.org/licenses/by/4.0/).

1. Introduction

Denture-related stomatitis (DRS) is an inflammatory reaction of the oral mucosa under different dental appliances [1]. Previous studies have revealed a 50% prevalence of DRS under removable dental prosthesis [2]. Among various etiological factors related to DRS, *fungi* are most often implicated in the pathogenesis of the disease [3]. Among *fungi*, Candida albicans (*C. albicans*) is considered the most common oral microbiota found in humans [4]. It presents all the properties of opportunistic pathogen, however, indicating that it can cause any pathologic infection when it finds the favorable environment. An infection caused by a *Candida* species can arise due to any local factors, such as poor hygiene, rough denture surface, and systemic conditions including diabetes mellitus, acquired immunodeficiency syndrome, and an immunocompromised state [5].

Moreover, the microorganisms present on a polymethyl methacrylate (PMMA) denture surface may transmit an infection from patients to the dental and laboratory staff [6]. A study by Powell et al. revealed that around 67% of the dentures sent to the dental laboratories from dental clinics have different types of opportunistic organisms on the surface [7]. Therefore, in order to reduce the incidence of DRS infections, denture disinfection is necessary. Various chemical agents are used for disinfection of PMMA dentures, including sodium perborate, sodium hypochlorite, glutaraldehyde and chlorine dioxide, 0.12% Chlorhexidine Gluconate, polymeric nanomaterials, and alkaline peroxide [8,9]. However, soaking dentures in chemical disinfectants may cause damage on the acrylic resin denture surface, alteration of material properties, and cytotoxicity [10,11]. Among several disinfectants used, chemical disinfecting agents in the form of denture cleaning tablets (containing sodium perborate) have gained widespread acceptance and are commonly used by denture patients [8]. Sodium-perborate decomposes into an alkaline peroxide solution, forming hydrogen peroxide, sodium metaborate, and oxygen in the presence of water [12]. The resulting peroxide releases oxygen bubbles, which help in mechanical and chemical cleaning [12,13]. In addition, the oxygen free radicals produced can cause effective antimicrobial activity through cell wall destruction [14]. However, sodium perborate was reported to show cytotoxic effects on human cells, including fibroblasts [15].

In order to overcome such disadvantages, alternatives for disinfecting PMMA denture bases have been researched. Among recent techniques, microwave oven sterilization has shown potential due to its antimicrobial efficacy and low cost [16]. It was also suggested that *fungi* and bacteria do not develop resistance against it. The literature has revealed that microwave sterilization for PMMA dentures is as potent as sodium hypochlorite alone [17,18]. While the mechanism of action for microwave irradiation is not yet clear, Companha et al. revealed in their study that microwave irradiation causes thermal alterations on bacterial and fungal cells' membrane permeability, thus causing cell death [19]. However, data related to its effectiveness as an antifungal denture disinfectant have not yet been determined and require further research.

According to the available indexed literature, microwave irradiation was used to disinfect PMMA dentures at higher watts, along with increased exposure times [20]. However, high temperature and exposure time negatively impacted the properties of the resin denture bases. Hence, the aim of our study was to evaluate the antifungal efficacy of sodium perborate (denture cleaning tablet-DC), microwave irradiation, and their combination for eradicating candida albicans (*C. albicans*) from a polymethyl methacrylate (PMMA) denture base polymer.

2. Materials and Methods

In our study, the sample preparation was performed at the Dr. Ishrat-ul-Ebad Khan Institute of Oral Health Sciences. (Department of Prosthodontics). The microbiological testing, along with disinfection interventions, were undertaken at the Pakistan Council of Scientific & Industrial Research Laboratories (PCSIR). The study protocol was reviewed by the ethics and review committee of the Dr. Ishrat-ul-Ebad Khan Institute of Oral Health Sciences and the Dow University of Health Sciences, with No. IRB-1101/DUHS/Approval/2020. The study was performed within the ethical guidelines of the declaration of Helsinki (2013). The study assessed the antifungal disinfection of PMMA denture resin using distilled water (DW), microwave irradiation (MW), and a denture cleaning agent (DC-sodium perborate), both individually and combined, at variable disinfecting durations (1 min, 2 min, and 3 min) on a candida culture incubated for 96 h.

2.1. Specimen Preparation

The sample size was obtained using Pass version 11 (NCSS Statistical software, Kaysville, UT, USA), employing one-way ANOVA with 99% confidence interval at 90% power, and with the means and standard deviation of viable cells in groups (DW = 7.47 ± 0.68, DC = 4.82 ± 0.73, DW + MW 1 min = 4.49 ± 0.45, DC + MW 1 min = 2.64 ± 0.59) from a previous study [21]. A sample size of ten per group was obtained using calculations (total 12 subgroups). A total of 128 specimens were fabricated (Table 1).

Table 1. Pairwise mean CFU comparison for *C. Albicans*.

Growth Time & Exposure Time vs. Control	Control CFU	MW-DC-DW	MW + DW	DC + DW
96 h	1400	MD (*p*-value)	MD (*p*-value)	MD (*p*-value)
1 min		−429 (0.008 **)	−197 (0.008 **)	−94 (0.008 **)
2 min		−447 (0.008 **)	−300 (0.008 **)	−98 (0.008 **)
3 min		−1388 (0.007 **)	−1344 (0.008 **)	−98 (0.007 **)
4 min		−1388 (0.008 **)	−1344 (0.008 **)	−200 (0.008 **)
5 min		−1388 (0.008 **)	−1344 (0.008 **)	−750 (0.008 **)

** Significant at 1% using the Mann–Whitney test; MW: microwave; DW: distilled water; DC: sodium perborate tablet. Values are represented as the mean difference (*p*-value).

In order to prepare the test specimens from PMMA acrylic resin, modelling wax (Yeti Dental, Berlin, Germany) was melted with help of a wax pot (Manfredi, Salerno, Italy) and poured into a three-part preformed metal mold with dimensions of 30 × 30 × 15 mm. Wax patterns were invested in a metallic denture flask filled with type III dental stone (Garrico Lab Stone, Rochester, NY, USA) to produce PMMA samples. De-waxing was performed using boiling water for 6 min. Heat-polymerized PMMA acrylic resin was mixed and packed at dough stage according to the manufacturer's recommendations at a powder-to-liquid ratio of 2.3 (grams of polymer powder) to 1 mL of liquid (monomer) (heat-cured acrylic provided by MR Dental, Plymouth, UK). A hydraulic press was used for packing the denture base resin, with a sheet of plastic separating the two halves. Heat-cured PMMA was polymerized in a thermostatically controlled water bath (Manfredi—Acrydig 12, Salerno, Italy) and processed at 74 °C for two hours, followed by 100 °C for one hour (Figure 1). The amount of residual monomer for heat-cured PMMA (2 h cycle) ranged from 16 to 40×10^{-3} v/v% [22]. However, the curing cycle protocol and storage conditions were standardized among all study specimens in order to standardize the residual monomer among samples.

All samples were cooled at room temperature before being deflasked and immersed in distilled water at room temperature for 48 h in order to eliminate residual monomer. A metal bur (Denfac acrylic trimming burs) was then used to trim excess resin, and the finishing was performed using abrasive paper in a hand-held micromotor. All the specimens were autoclaved at 121 °C for 15 min. For reliability, a single operator prepared all the samples. All specimens' dimensions were checked repeatedly. Intra-operator reliability was assessed at a kappa score of 0.85.

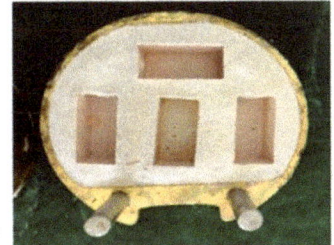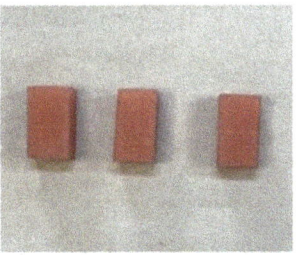

Figure 1. Fabrication of PMMA samples. (**A**) Dental stone mold. (**B**) Finished PMMA samples.

2.2. Study Groups

Based on the disinfection protocol, all the samples were randomly divided into the following groups.

Group MW-DW: The specimens were placed in a glass container filled with distilled water and disinfected with microwave (MW) radiation at 450 W. Depending on the MW radiation duration, the specimens were divided into MW-DW1 (1 min), MW-DW2 (2 min), and MW-DW3 (3 min). The protocol for MW disinfection was adopted from a previous study [23]. Different specimens in each subgroup were assessed at 96 h in a *C. Albicans* culture.

Group DC-DW: The specimens were dipped in a mixture of distilled water and denture cleaning tablet (DC) (Fittydent, Wien, Austria). Depending on the duration of immersion in the DC, the specimens were divided into DC-DW1 (1 min), DC-DW2 (2 min), and DC-DW3 (3 min). Different specimens in each subgroup were assessed at 96 h in a *C. Albicans* culture.

Group MW-DC-DW: In this group, the specimens were immersed in a glass beaker containing a mixture of distilled water and denture-cleaning tablet for five minutes. The glass beaker was placed in a microwave oven and irradiated at 650 W. Depending on the MW radiation's duration, the specimens were divided into MW-DC-DW1 (1 min), MW-DC-DW2 (2 min), and MW-DC-DW3 (3 min). The temperature of the solution was kept between 65 °C to 71 °C, with ±2 °C. The different specimens in each subgroup were assessed at 96 h in the culture.

Positive Control Group: In this group, specimens were dipped in a glass container filled with 200 mL of distilled water kept at room temperature. The container was placed in the microwave oven (Samsung 2450 MHz, 800 W) without irradiation.

Negative Control Group: The purpose of this group was to establish the sterilization of the specimens and the accuracy of the test. For *C. Albicans*, the sterilized specimens were placed in a container with sterilized water.

2.3. Biofilm Formation Assay

Tryptone Soya Broth (TSB) was used to enrich *C. albicans* (ATCC #90028) for 4 days. We then transferred 0.1 mL of this to 100 mL TSB that contained acrylic specimens (n = 163) and incubated it at 25 °C for 4 days. After 4 days' incubation, the growth was monitored, and acrylic specimens were collected from the flask, washed with sterile distilled water, placed in 100 mL PBS (pH-7.0), and vortexed [24] (Figure 2). This flask was exposed to three treatment regimes (DW+MW, DW+DC, & DC) at different exposure times, after which 1 mL of PBS was transferred to a sterile Petri plate, poured with Dichloran Rose-Bengal Chloramphenicol Agar (Merck, Germany) (Figure 3), and incubated at 25 °C for 48 h. The growth was monitored, and the CFU were counted.

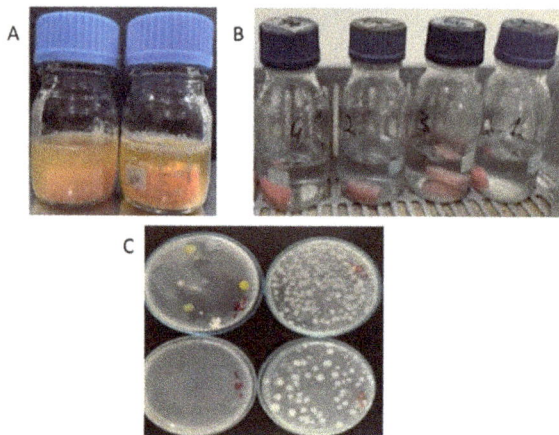

Figure 2. Procedure for biofilm formation assay. (**A**) TSB containing PMMA specimens. (**B**) Acquisition of PMMA specimens. (**C**) *Candida* incubation.

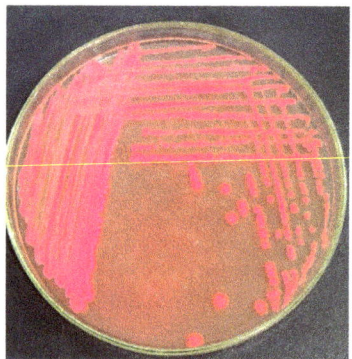

Figure 3. Pure culture of *C. albicans* on Dichloran Rose-Bengal Chloramphenicol Agar.

2.4. Quantification of Biofilm

All samples were incubated for 96 h for the biofilm assessment. The acrylic slides were collected between 24 h to 96 h, and the adhesion was monitored using a crystal violet binding assay as described earlier [25]. Briefly, the growth was fixed with acetic acid for 15 min, stained with 3% crystal violet (Ezzy Stain), washed with PBS at 7.0 pH, fixed gently by heating for 30 s, and finally washed with acetone. Each experiment was repeated four times to check the accuracy and precision of results. The colony-forming units (CFU) were evaluated by a single experienced microbiologist, and intra-operator reliability was observed (k = 0.84).

2.5. Scanning Electron Microscopy (SEM) Analysis

SEM was performed to analyze the production of the extracellular matrix material (ECM), as described earlier. All slides with biofilm were divided into 4 mm sections and then rinsed with distilled water, followed by staining with 0.02% Uranyl acetate for about 30 s. These 4 mm slide were coated with platinum in a coating machine (JEOL 3000 FC, Tokyo, Japan). All sections then displayed the existence of biofilm material under the examination of a scanning electron microscope (JEOL, Japan).

2.6. Statistical Analysis

The data were analyzed using IBM SPSS Statistics software version 21 (IBM Inc., Armonk, NY, USA). For disinfectant exposure time comparison, the Kruskal–Wallis test was applied for the *C. albicans* by treatment and growth time, as the CFU count was not normally distributed (Shapiro–Wilk test). For pairwise comparison of each exposure time with the control, the Mann–Whitney test was applied by treatment and growth time. A *p*-value of 0.05 or less was considered as statistically significant.

3. Results

The mean CFU comparison for *C. albicans*, with the controls for each disinfection technique at 96 h of growth, is presented in Table 1. We observed that specimens in DC-DW, MW-DW, and MW-DC-DW showed significant differences in the mean CFU of *C. Albicans* in comparison with the control without disinfection ($p < 0.05$). The MW-DC-DW disinfection regime showed near-complete disinfection (99.14%) of *C. Albicans*, compared with the controls ($p < 0.05$). The specimens treated with MW-DW showed 96% disinfection at 3 min, which was significantly lower than the controls ($p < 0.05$). The treatment with denture cleaning tablets with sodium perborate (DC-DW) showed only 53.57% of disinfection, compared with the control CFU after 5 min of treatment.

In the treatment with MW without using a denture cleaning tablet (MW-DW), the CFU count was reduced to 14% at 1 min of exposure and 21% at 2 min, whereas 3 min of microwave irradiation reduced 96% of the CFU count. In the disinfection treatment with DC (sodium perborate-cleaning tablet), the CFU count for *C. Albicans* was reduced to 6% at 1 min of exposure and to 7% at 2 and 3 min of exposure (Figure 4). However, DC use showed a maximum of 96% CFU reduction at 5 min of treatment. The combination of MW with DC showed the maximum disinfection, with the lowest CFU levels at 3 min among all three groups. MW alone showed significantly lower CFU levels (better disinfection) compared with MW-DC-DW combined; however, it exhibited higher disinfection than sodium perborate (disinfection tablet) alone (DC-DW) at 3 min of treatment. For all three disinfection regimes, the duration of disinfection showed significant influence on CFU levels ($p < 0.05$), with 3 min showing higher disinfection than the disinfection at 1 and 2 min ($p < 0.05$) (Figure 5).

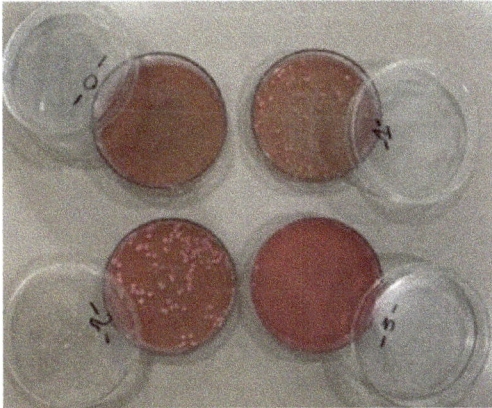

Figure 4. The effect of a denture cleaning tablet and MW 450 watt on the growth of *C. albicans*. Plate 0 was the untreated control, plate 1 was exposed for 1 min, plate 2 was exposed for 2 min, and plate 3 was exposed for 3 min.

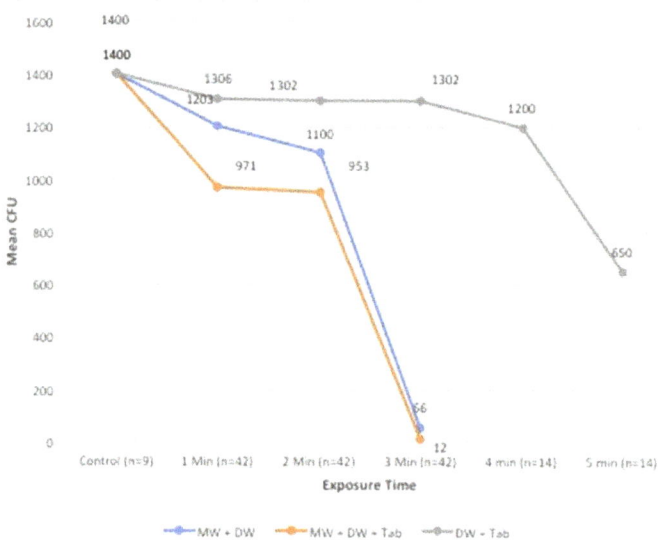

Figure 5. Colony-forming units of *C. Albicans* for different antifungal protocols at 96 h of growth.

A SEM analysis of the samples showed oval yeast-budding forms of *C. Albicans* cells, along with single-celled *C. Albicans*. Using SEM, the live cells of *C. Albicans* adhered to the PMMA polymer specimens were observed (Figure 6). After the disinfection procedure, the dead cells attached to PMMA surface were observed in the form of a cluster of irregular organelles.

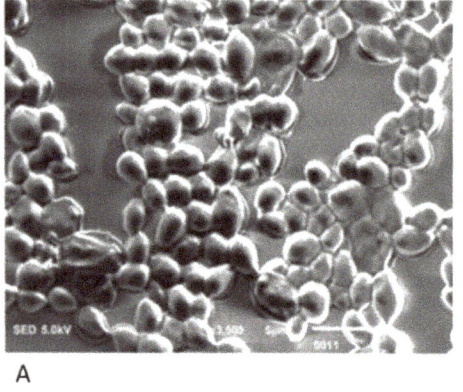
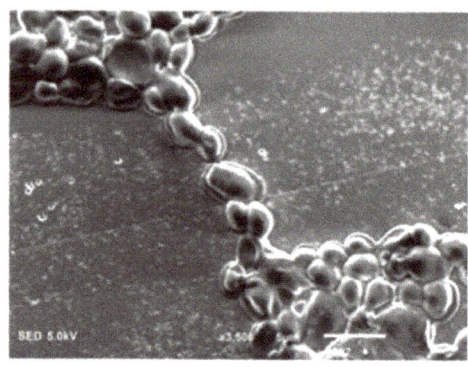

A B

Figure 6. *Cont.*

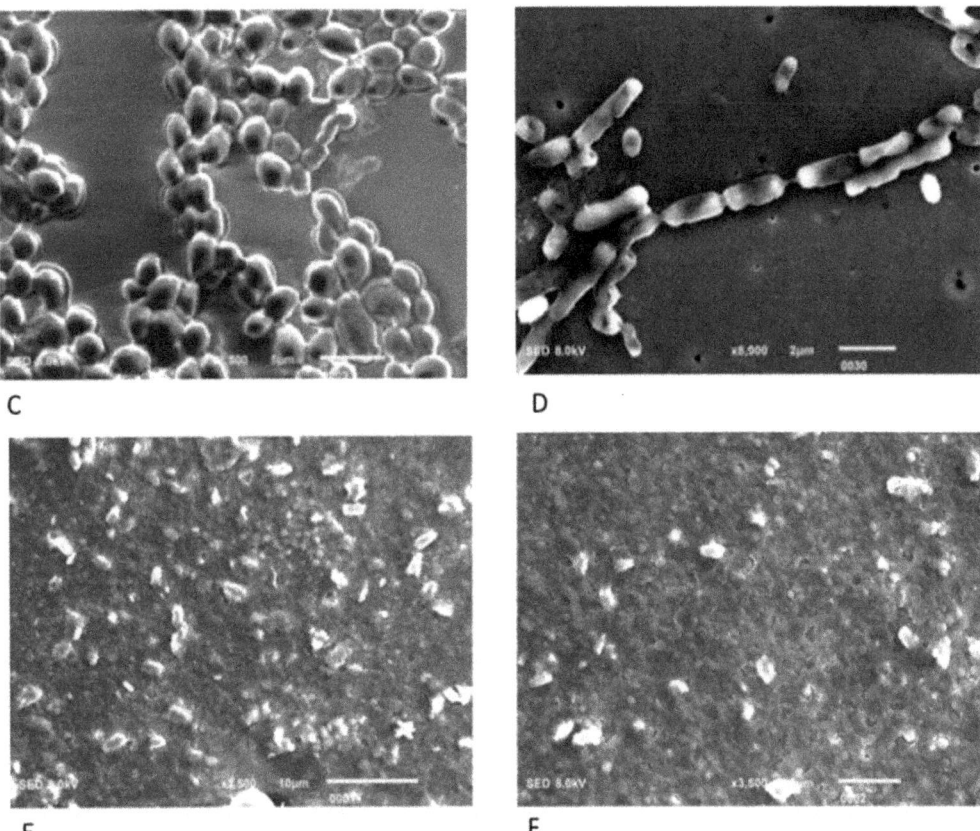

Figure 6. SEM micrographs presenting the attachment of *C. albicans* to PMMA samples. (**A**) Control sample with *C. albicans* growth. (**B**) MC-DC-DW sample at 1 min treatment. (**C**) MW-DW sample at 1 min treatment. (**D**) DC-DW sample at 5 min. (**E**) MW-DC-DW disinfection sample at 3 min. (**F**) MW-DW sample at 3 min.

4. Discussion

This study was performed to analyze the cumulative disinfection efficacy of a denture cleaning tablet (sodium perborate) and microwave irradiation on the eradication of *C. albicans* cultured on a PMMA denture base polymer. Our study was based on the hypothesis that there would be no significant difference in the disinfection efficacy of denture cleaning tablet, microwave irradiation, and their combination on the disinfection of *C. albicans* cultured on denture base. However, the postulated hypothesis was rejected as microwave irradiation combined with cleaning tablets (sodium perborate) (MW-DC-DW) showed better disinfection efficacy than that of microwave (MW) and cleaning tablets (DC) alone.

The outcomes of our study show that the CFU count of *C. albicans* was significantly reduced after 2 min of exposure to the MW-DW-DC group. However, 3 min of exposure to MW-DW-DC displayed a nearly zero CFU count of *C. albicans*. These results are in line with the findings of the study conducted by Sesma et al. [26]. Their study revealed that a combination of microwave and denture cleaning tablets demonstrated bactericidal as well as fungicidal effects against *C. albicans*. Moreover, they also identified that this combination possesses the ability to remove dead organisms from the PMMA denture bases. Denture cleaning tablets containing sodium perborate dissolve into peroxides, which results in the physical cleaning of the PMMA due to the bubbling and chemical destruction of the microbial cell walls [12–14]. Similar findings were also observed by Senna et al. [21]. They concluded that a denture cleaning tablet along with microwave irradiation caused the elimination of yeast cells from the PMMA resin base. Our study demonstrated almost 99% reduction in the CFU count of *C. albicans*. The slight difference observed in the previous studies may be due to the difference in the chemical composition of sodium perborate in the cleaning tablets and the different parameters of MW radiation [27,28].

Microwave disinfection is considered to be an effective and time-saving denture disinfection approach in clinical dentistry [29]. Microwaves disinfect by using thermal and non-thermal methods [30,31]. A thermal effect requires the presence of water or ionic molecules to produce a bactericidal influence at low energy levels [30], whereas high-energy, high-frequency microwaves cause cell wall and organelle destruction of microorganisms [31]. Our study found that microwave-disinfected samples displayed a significantly decreased CFU count of *C. albicans* at 3 min of exposure. Previous studies revealed that microwave disinfection initiates a change in the structure and permeability of the fungal cells, resulting in alterations in cell metabolism, causing cell death [32–34]. These results agree with the outcomes of the study conducted by Al-Saadi et al. [28]. In contrast, a study by Webb et al. showed a 1.3% survival rate of *C. albicans* when exposed to microwave irradiation at 350 W for 4 min [35]. In our study, MW irradiation disinfection was applied at higher power (450 Watts) for less time (3 min); therefore, a change in power and exposure time parameters may have ensured better disinfection. Moreover, in our study, the denture bases were immersed in distilled water prior to the exposure to MW irradiation. This technique may have provided the samples with a sterilized environment to prevent re-infection and a cleaner sample surface, compared with the dry sample's MW exposure. It was proposed that PMMA denture disinfection achieved by microwave irradiation is due to the presence of distilled water, which forms bubbles upon boiling, thus removing microorganisms from the sample surface [36,37]. A study by Najdovski et al. revealed that microwave irradiation at reduced power can be used for a high level of disinfection, but not for sterilization [22], which is in line with our findings.

In our study, fungal cell adhesion was analyzed by a crystal violet binding assay, and cell count was analyzed by an aerobic plate count assay. The plate count showed that the control acrylic slide carried 1400 cfu/mL of *C. albicans*. The results show that the subject isolate of *C. albicans* showed a high level of antimicrobial resistance against denture cleaning tablets (sodium perborate). This was attributed to biofilm formation, as *C. albicans* nullified the toxic effect of sodium perborate and survived even after 5 min of exposure. This agreed with the findings of the previous studies by Dills et al. and Drake et al. [32,38]. They both identified that alkaline peroxide denture cleansers are effective against the streptococcus species and do not show much activity against *C. albicans*. This also agrees with the study by Ferreira et al., who studied the effect of a denture cleaning tablet (Bonyplus) against *Candida* species and *S. mutans* and found that the denture cleansing solution did not show significant re-educating of *Candida* species [39]. In addition, the alkaline peroxide tablets were not effective against *S. mutans*.

Interestingly, samples were fabricated in our study by mixing powder and liquid. However, CAD-CAM dentures are also available, fabricated from prepolymerized PMMA resin blocks [40]. The prepolymerized resin dentures allow for fewer surface defects and irregularities, and the incidence of fungal infection among these dentures and their disinfection protocol may differ from conventional PMMA dentures. Therefore, studies assessing the disinfection of CAD-CAM PMMA dentures are warranted. Our study showed higher disinfection efficacy of MW with sodium perborate-disinfection tablets for the use of *Candida* in comparison with microwave (MW) and cleaning tablets (DC) alone. It is pertinent to mention that MW disinfection of PMMA denture bases can also result in distortion and discrepancy in their fit and adaptation on stone casts [17]. However, Pavan et al. showed that at high MW energy, distortion was observed for the PMMA denture, while at 500 W or below, the dimensional accuracy was comparable to the control [17]. As

MW disinfection in our study was performed at 450 W power, the PMMA resin specimens when exposed to our study's protocol for disinfection were dimensionally accurate and therefore could be clinically utilized. In addition, our study displayed some inherent limitations. Primarily, the study was based on in vitro design, assessing a single species of *Candida*, which may have limited the clinical implications. Moreover, only one type of denture disinfecting tablet was used; however, cleansing agents with hydrogen peroxide, sodium hypochlorite, and Chlorhexidine are also available. Therefore, further studies assessing the different candida species with contemporary denture cleansing agents are warranted to investigate the antimicrobial efficacy of microwave irradiation.

5. Conclusions

The microwave disinfection of PMMA for 3 min at 450 W in combination with a denture cleaning tablet (sodium perborate) is a more effective disinfecting regime against *C. albicans* than that of microwave and sodium perborate alone. Further studies assessing the efficacy of low-level MW irradiation on the disinfection of various bacterial species is recommended.

Author Contributions: Conceptualization, Z.C., S.A.K., S.M., S.M.R.K., W.A.F., M.A.A. and Z.A.M.; methodology, K.A.A., S.A.K., M.A.A., W.A.F., S.M.R.K., A.H.A. and A.A. software, K.A.A., W.A.F., S.M.R.K., A.A., A.H.A., M.A. and T.A.; validation, Z.C., A.A., W.A.F. and S.M.; formal analysis, S.A.K., Z.A.M., A.A., S.M.R.K., M.A. and K.A.A.; resources, A.H.A., T.A., M.A.A. and A.A.; data curation, S.A.K., Z.A.M., Z.C., M.A.A., S.M.R.K., W.A.F. and A.A.; writing—original draft preparation, K.A.A., T.A., M.A. and Z.C.; writing—review and editing, S.M.R.K., S.A.K., A.A., T.A., A.H.A. and K.A.A. All authors have read and agreed to the published version of the manuscript.

Funding: This research was funded by Princess Nourah bint Abdulrahman University researchers, supporting project number PNURSP2022R6, Princess Nourah bint Abdulrahman University, Riyadh, Saudi Arabia.

Institutional Review Board Statement: The study protocol was reviewed by the ethics and review committee of Dr. Ishrat-ul-Ebad Khan Institute of Oral Health Sciences and the Dow University of Health Sciences, with No. IRB-1101/DUHS/Approval/2020.

Informed Consent Statement: No human patients or human tissue was included in the study.

Data Availability Statement: The data are available on contact from the corresponding author.

Acknowledgments: The authors wish to thank the Princess Nourah bint Abdulrahman University researchers, supporting project number PNURSP2022R6, Princess Nourah bint Abdulrahman University, Riyadh, Saudi Arabia.

Conflicts of Interest: The author declares no conflict of interest.

References

1. Hayran, Y.; Sarikaya, I.; Aydin, A.; Tekin, Y.H. Determination of the effective anticandidal concentration of denture cleanser tablets on some denture base resins. *J. Appl. Oral Sci.* **2018**, *26*, e20170077. [CrossRef] [PubMed]
2. Gendreau, L.; Loewy, Z.G. Epidemiology and etiology of denture stomatitis. *J. Prosthodont.* **2011**, *20*, 251–260. [CrossRef] [PubMed]
3. Marsh, P.D.; Percival, R.S.; Challacombe, S.J. The influence of denture-wearing and age on the oral microflora. *J. Dent. Res.* **1992**, *71*, 1374–1381. [CrossRef] [PubMed]
4. Berger, J.C.; Driscoll, C.F.; Romberg, E.; Luo, Q.; Thompson, G. Surface roughness of denture base acrylic resins after processing and after polishing. *J. Prosthodont. Implant Esthet. Reconstr. Dent.* **2006**, *15*, 180–186. [CrossRef]
5. Busscher, H.J.; Weerkamp, A.H.; Van Der Mei, H.C.; Van Pelt, A.W.; De Jong, H.P.; Arends, J. Measurement of the surface free energy of bacterial cell surfaces and its relevance for adhesion. *Appl. Environ. Microbiol.* **1984**, *48*, 980–983. [CrossRef]
6. De Freitas Fernandes, F.S.; Pereira-Cenci, T.; Da Silva, W.J.; Ricomini Filho, A.P.; Straioto, F.G.; Cury, A.A. Efficacy of denture cleansers on Candida spp. biofilm formed on polyamide and polymethyl methacrylate resins. *J. Prosthet. Dent.* **2011**, *105*, 51–58. [CrossRef]
7. Powell, G.L.; Runnells, R.D.; Saxon, B.A.; Whisenant, B.K. The presence and identification of organisms transmitted to dental laboratories. *J. Prosthet. Dent.* **1990**, *64*, 235–237. [CrossRef]

8. Cakan, U.; Kara, O.; Kara, H.B. Effects of various denture cleansers on surface roughness of hard permanent reline resins. *Dent. Mater. J.* **2015**, *34*, 246–251. [CrossRef]
9. Yudaev, P.; Chuev, V.; Klyukin, B.; Kuskov, A.; Mezhuev, Y.; Chistyakov, E. Polymeric Dental Nanomaterials: Antimicrobial Action. *Polymers* **2022**, *14*, 864. [CrossRef]
10. Coenye, T.; De Prijck, K.; Nailis, H.; Nelis, H.J. Prevention of Candida albicans Biofilm Formation. *Open Mycol. J.* **2011**, *5*, 9–20. [CrossRef]
11. Yasui, M.; Ryu, M.; Sakurai, K.; Ishihara, K. Colonisation of the oral cavity by periodontopathic bacteria in complete denture wearers. *Gerodontology* **2012**, *29*, e494–e502. [CrossRef] [PubMed]
12. Yatabe, M.; Seki, H.; Shirasu, N.; Sone, M. Effect of the reducing agent on the oxygen-inhibited layer of the cross-linked reline material. *J. Oral Rehabil.* **2001**, *28*, 180–185. [CrossRef] [PubMed]
13. Budtz-Jørgensen, E. Materials and methods for cleaning dentures. *J. Prosthet. Dent.* **1979**, *42*, 619–623. [CrossRef]
14. Shakouie, S.; Milani, A.S.; Eskandarnejad, M.; Rahimi, S.; Froughreyhani, M.; Galedar, S.; Ranjbar, E. Antimicrobial activity of tetraacetylethylenediamine-sodium perborate versus sodium hypochlorite against Enterococcus faecalis. *J. Dent. Res. Dent. Clin. Dent. Prospect.* **2016**, *10*, 43–47. [CrossRef]
15. Fernandes, A.M.; Marques, M.M.; Camargo, S.E.A.; Cardoso, P.E.; Camargo, C.H.R.; Valera, M.C. Cytotoxicity of non-vital dental bleaching agents in human gingival fibroblasts. *Braz. Dent. Sci.* **2013**, *16*, 59–65. [CrossRef]
16. Arendorf, T.; Walker, D. Denture stomatitis: A review. *J. Oral Rehabil.* **1987**, *14*, 217–227. [CrossRef]
17. Pavan, S.; Arioli Filho, J.N.; Santos, P.H.d.; Mollo, F.d.A., Jr. Effect of microwave treatments on dimensional accuracy of maxillary acrylic resin denture base. *Braz. Dent. J.* **2005**, *16*, 119–123. [CrossRef]
18. Sanita, P.V.; Vergani, C.E.; Giampaolo, E.T.; Pavarina, A.C.; Machado, A.L. Growth of Candida species on complete dentures: Effect of microwave disinfection. *Mycoses* **2009**, *52*, 154–160. [CrossRef]
19. Campanha, N.H.; Pavarina, A.C.; Brunetti, I.L.; Vergani, C.E.; Machado, A.L.; Spolidorio, D.M.P. Candida albicans inactivation and cell membrane integrity damage by microwave irradiation. *Mycoses* **2007**, *50*, 140–147. [CrossRef]
20. Silva, M.M.; Vergani, C.E.; Giampaolo, E.T.; Neppelenbroek, K.H.; Spolidorio, D.M.; Machado, A.L. Effectiveness of microwave irradiation on the disinfection of complete dentures. *Int. J. Prosthodont.* **2006**, *19*, 272–278.
21. Senna, P.M.; Sotto-Maior, B.S.; da Silva, W.J.; Cury, A.A.D.B. Adding denture cleanser to microwave disinfection regimen to reduce the irradiation time and the exposure of dentures to high temperatures. *Gerodontology* **2013**, *30*, 26–31. [CrossRef] [PubMed]
22. Huda, I.; Nabi, A.T.; Turner, P.S.; Hegde, C. Study to determine and estimate residual monomer leached out in heat cure polymethylmethacrylate Resins of commonly used brands using different polymerization cycles: (An invitro study). *IP Ann. Od Prosthodont. Restor. Dentistry* **2019**, *5*, 28–36. [CrossRef]
23. Najdovski, L.; Dragaš, A.; Kotnik, V. The killing activity of microwaves on some non-sporogenic and sporogenic medically important bacterial strains. *J. Hosp. Infect.* **1991**, *19*, 239–247. [CrossRef]
24. Mirani, Z.; Urooj, S.; Khan, M.; Khan, A.; Shaikh, I.; Siddiqui, A. An effective weapon against biofilm consortia and small colony variants of MRSA. *Iran. J. Basic Med. Sci.* **2020**, *23*, 1494–1498. [PubMed]
25. Haney, E.; Trimble, M.; Cheng, J.; Vallé, Q.; Hancock, R. Critical assessment of methods to quantify biofilm growth and evaluate antibiofilm activity of host defence peptides. *Biomolecules* **2018**, *8*, 29. [CrossRef]
26. Sesma, N.; Rocha, A.L.; Laganá, D.C.; Costa, B.; Morimoto, S. Effectiveness of denture cleanser associated with microwave disinfection and brushing of complete dentures: In vivo study. *Braz. Dent. J.* **2013**, *24*, 357–361. [CrossRef]
27. Dantas, A.; Consani, R.L.X.; Sardi, J.; Mesquita, M.; Silva, M.; Sinhoreti, M. Biofilm formation in denture base acrylic resins and disinfection method using microwave. *J. Res. Pract. Dent.* **2014**, *2014*, 112424. [CrossRef]
28. Al-Saadi, M.H. Effectiveness of chemical and microwave disinfection on denture biofilm fungi and the influence of disinfection on denture base adaptation. *J. Indian Prosthodont. Soc.* **2014**, *14*, 24–30. [CrossRef]
29. Arita, M.; Nagayoshi, M.; Fukuizumi, T.; Okinaga, T.; Masumi, S.; Morikawa, M.; Kakinoki, Y.; Nishihara, T. Microbicidal efficacy of ozonated water against Candida albicans adhering to acrylic denture plates. *Oral Microbiol. Immunol.* **2005**, *20*, 206–210. [CrossRef]
30. Anaraki, M.R.; Mahboubi, S.; Pirzadeh, T.; Lotfipour, F.; Torkamanzad, N. Disinfection effect of microwave radiation on Bacillus subtilis as indicator organism on contaminated dental stone casts under dry and wet conditions. *GMS Hyg. Infect. Control* **2017**, *12*, 294.
31. Banik, S.; Bandyopadhyay, S.; Ganguly, S. Bioeffects of microwave—A brief review. *Bioresour. Technol.* **2003**, *87*, 155–159. [CrossRef]
32. Mese, A.; Mese, S. Effect of Microwave Energy on Fungal Growth of Resilient Denture Liner Material. *Biotechnol. Biotechnol. Equip.* **2007**, *21*, 91–93. [CrossRef]
33. Tarbet, W.J. Denture plaque: Quiet destroyer. *J. Prosthet. Dent.* **1982**, *48*, 647–652. [CrossRef]
34. Dills, S.; Olshan, A.; Goldner, S.; Brogdon, C. Comparison of the antimicrobial capability of an abrasive paste and chemical-soak denture cleaners. *J. Prosthet. Dent.* **1988**, *60*, 467–470. [CrossRef]
35. Webb, B.C.; Thomas, C.J.; Harty, D.W.; Willcox, M. Effectiveness of two methods of denture sterilization. *J. Oral Rehabil.* **1998**, *25*, 416–423. [CrossRef] [PubMed]
36. Polyzois, G.L.; Zissis, A.J.A.; Yannikakis, S. The effect of glutaraldehyde and microwave disinfection on some properties of acrylic denture resin. *Int. J. Prosthodont.* **1995**, *8*, 150–154. [PubMed]

37. Neppelenbroek, K.; Pavarina, A.C.; Spolidorio, D.M.P.; Vergani, C.E.; Mima, E.G.D.O.; Machado, A.L. Effectiveness of microwave sterilization on three hard chairside reline resins. *Int. J. Prosthodont.* **2003**, *16*, 264–270.
38. Drake, D.; Wells, J.; Ettinger, R. Efficacy of denture cleansing agents in an in vitro bacteria-yeast colonization model. *Int. J. Prosthodont.* **1992**, *5*, 300–307.
39. Ferreira, M.F.; Pereira-Cenci, T.; De Vasconcelos, L.M.R.; Rodrigues-Garcia, R.C.M.; Cury, A.A.D.B. Efficacy of denture cleansers on denture liners contaminated with Candida species. *Clin. Oral Investig.* **2009**, *13*, 237–242. [CrossRef]
40. Heikal, M.M.A.; Nabi, N.A.; Elkerdawy, M.W. A study comparing patient satisfaction and retention of CAD/CAM milled complete dentures and 3D printed CAD/CAM complete dentures versus conventional complete dentures: A randomized clinical trial. *Braz. Dent. Sci.* **2022**, *3*, 25. [CrossRef]

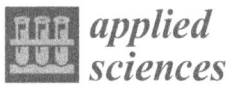

Article

Evaluation of the Retentive Forces from Removable Partial Denture Clasps Manufactured by the Digital Method

Vitor Anes [1,2,3,*], Cristina B. Neves [4,*], Valeria Bostan [5], Sérgio B. Gonçalves [3] and Luís Reis [3]

1. Instituto Superior de Engenharia de Lisboa, 1959-007 Lisboa, Portugal
2. Instituto Politécnico de Lisboa, 1549-020 Lisboa, Portugal
3. IDMEC, Instituto Superior Técnico, Universidade de Lisboa, 1049-001 Lisboa, Portugal; sergio.goncalves@tecnico.ulisboa.pt (S.B.G.); luis.g.reis@tecnico.ulisboa.pt (L.R.)
4. Biomedical and Oral Sciences Research Unit (UICOB), Faculdade de Medicina Dentária, Universidade de Lisboa, 1600-277 Lisboa, Portugal
5. Faculdade de Medicina Dentária, Universidade de Lisboa, 1600-277 Lisboa, Portugal; valeriabostan@campus.ul.pt
* Correspondence: vitor.anes@isel.pt (V.A.); mneves@edu.ulisboa.pt (C.B.N.)

Abstract: The purpose of this study was to evaluate the retentive forces over time of removable partial denture clasps fabricated by the digital method. Occlusal rest seats were fabricated on three premolar teeth fixed in acrylic blocks (9 × 20 × 40 mm). Digitization of the teeth was performed using a laboratory scanner (Zirkonzahn Scanner S600 GmbH, Gais, Italy). After the analysis and determination of the insertion axis, two types of clasps with mesial occlusal rests were designed per tooth: the back-action and the reverse back-action clasps, using the Partial Planner Zirkonzahn program. The file was sent for fabrication of six metal clasps from a cobalt-chromium SP2 alloy in the EOSINT M270 system by a direct laser sintering process. The Instron 5544 universal testing machine was used to perform 20,000 cycles of clasp insertion and removal in the corresponding tooth with a load cell of 100 N and a speed of 2.5 mm/s. The retentive force was recorded for each of the 1000 cycles, and the change in retention over time was calculated. Statistical analysis was performed using the nonparametric Mann–Whitney test and a significance level of 5%. At 16,000 cycles, a maximum change in retention of 3.74 N was recorded for the back-action clasps and a minimum of −24.28 N at 1000 cycles for the reverse back-action clasps. The reverse back-action clasps exhibited statistically significant lower change in retention than the reverse-action clasps at 4000 and 5000 cycles. No differences were observed in the remaining cycles. During the 20,000 cycles, the change in retention was low regardless of the type of clasp. For most cycles, there were no differences in the change in retention between the two types of clasps.

Keywords: removable partial denture metal framework; direct laser sintering; back-action clasp; reverse back-action clasp; retentive force; experiments; additive manufacturing; CAD-CAM

Citation: Anes, V.; Neves, C.B.; Bostan, V.; Gonçalves, S.B.; Reis, L. Evaluation of the Retentive Forces from Removable Partial Denture Clasps Manufactured by the Digital Method. *Appl. Sci.* **2023**, *13*, 8072. https://doi.org/10.3390/app13148072

Academic Editor: George Eliades

Received: 12 June 2023
Revised: 8 July 2023
Accepted: 8 July 2023
Published: 11 July 2023

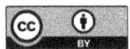

Copyright: © 2023 by the authors. Licensee MDPI, Basel, Switzerland. This article is an open access article distributed under the terms and conditions of the Creative Commons Attribution (CC BY) license (https://creativecommons.org/licenses/by/4.0/).

1. Introduction

Over the years and with scientific and technological progress, society has given more importance to oral health maintenance, promoting campaigns and prevention programs while developing dental materials and treatment options [1–3]. These efforts have led to a decrease in tooth loss during life and an increase in the number of cases of partial rather than complete edentulism [1–4].

In addition, mortality has decreased, and average life expectancy has increased, leading to an aging society [2,3,5]. For this reason, the need for treatment with fixed or removable prostheses is increasing every year [2]. In this sense, the rehabilitation of edentulous patients is crucial for their quality of life as it preserves masticatory function, phonetics and esthetics [1,6].

Fixed rehabilitation with implants has high success rates and has become increasingly popular in recent years. However, not all patients are good candidates for this type of treatment due to health, financial, anatomical, or psychological circumstances [7]. One alternative is the rehabilitation of edentulous areas with removable prostheses, which is still widely used in clinical practice [5,8]. Removable partial dentures (RPD) are prostheses that restore edentulous areas in partial edentulism, and can be performed rapidly with esthetic and functional benefits [5,9–11].

The development of this type of prosthesis remains a challenge. Proper planning and selection of RPD materials is key to reducing the incidence of complications.

When designing RPD, it is important that the framework has stability and a correct fit which is mostly provided by the major connector and clasps [12]. It should also provide support and retention, and not interfere with abutment teeth and other supporting structures when masticatory forces are applied [13,14]. The choice of the correct clasp geometry starts with the analysis of the Kennedy class and the insertion axis of the prosthesis, which determines the equator and the retentive zone of the tooth [12,13]. A clasp assembly consists of an occlusal rest, a reciprocal arm and a retentive arm [12]. All clasps must provide retention, stability, support, reciprocity and passivity and cover the largest possible area of the tooth [12,15,16]. The retentive arm provides primary retention of the prosthesis and must be able to deform as it passes the equator of the tooth and return to its original position without exerting damaging forces on the tooth [15,17,18].

In partial edentulous patients with bilateral (Class I Kennedy) or unilateral (Class II Kennedy) distal extension, retention, stability and support are very important [19]. The selected clasp must provide good retention, transfer forces parallel to the tooth axis, and minimize the application of damaging forces to the abutment tooth [12,19]. In these situations, it is common to use clasps with mesial occlusal rests, such as the reverse back-action clasp when buccal retention is on the distal side and the back-action clasp when there is mesial retention [16,19,20].

Of the various materials available for the manufacture of the metal framework, cobalt–chromium (Co–Cr) alloy has been the most commonly used material since 1929 [21]. This material is known for its low cost and adequate mechanical properties, such as lower density and higher modulus of elasticity than gold, as well as its high corrosion resistance, which is related to biocompatibility [4,17,18,21]. This metallic alloy contains about 53% to 67% Co, 25% to 32% Cr, 2% to 6% Mo, and a mixture of other elements [22,23].

The lost waxing casting or conventional method is most commonly used to produce metal frameworks [9,23]. The quality of the production largely depends on the experience of the laboratory technician and the quality of the impressions taken by the clinician, which is a time-consuming and expensive method [9,24]. Normally, this technique is prone to several errors that can result in 75% of frameworks not fitting properly on the supporting structures at the time of insertion into the patient's oral cavity [12,25,26]. Thus, over the years, the need to develop new techniques has increased, and scientific advances have made it possible to improve the process of RPD framework production, reducing the time and cost of fabrication, and improving the fit and functional efficiency of rehabilitations [1,3].

With the advent of digital technology, manufacturing methods have changed with the introduction of digital processes such as computer-aided design (CAD) and computer-aided manufacturing (CAM) [6,27]. With the development of these new methods, the results have become more predictable, reproducible, and accurate, which improves the longevity of the rehabilitations [4,28]. The use of CAD/CAM offers the advantages of digital planning and analysis, reduction in material waste and use of innovative materials, better communication between laboratory and clinician, reduction in the number of steps and errors, easy cast reproduction, and better quality control of the production [4,29–31].

The production of these structures can be performed by two digital methods: addition (AM—additive manufacturing) or subtraction (milling) [29]. The AM method makes use of sintering technology, such as: SLM—Selective Laser Melting, SLS—Selective Laser Sintering or DMLS—Direct Metal Laser Sintering [9,18]. This technology offers high productivity, improves the properties of materials by increasing density and homogeneity, and is a precise and cost-effective method [4,9]. Basically, additive manufacturing is based on the production of metal objects in 3D by sintering metal powders with a high-power laser [9,32]. In DMLS, a powder consisting of several metals is partially fused with a high-power Yb fiber laser [18,32]. This technique uses a powder with a mixture of metals whose melting temperatures are different to produce the solid metal structure [9,18]. The composition of Co–Cr powder is mainly Co and Cr, but also contains metals such as Mo, W, Si, Ce, F, Mn and C [33,34].

Since there is little information on the behavior of metal framework production by the digital method, it is important to evaluate the change over time of the retention forces of the RPD clasps.

In this sense, the aim of this study was to evaluate the retentive forces and the change in retention over time of RPD clasps produced by the digital method. Another objective was to compare the retentive force of clasps fabricated with different designs.

2. Materials and Methods

2.1. Production of Models

Three different intact premolar teeth were selected from a reservoir of the BIOMAT laboratory of the Faculty of Dental Medicine, University of Lisbon. Longitudinal undercuts were created around each tooth root to increase its adherence to the resin block. Then, it was scanned with the Zirkonzahn Scanner S600 equipment (Zirkonzahn GmbH, Gais, Italy) (Figure 1).

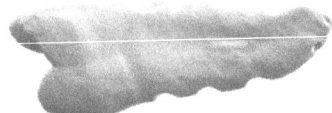

Figure 1. Digitized premolar with undercuts.

In the Autodesk Meshmixer program (2017, version 3.5.474), a 3D-printed resin block measuring 9 × 20 × 40 mm was designed for each tooth so that the long axis of the sinus (negative) of the root was perpendicular to the occlusal plane. The block was then printed using the NextDent 5100 3D printer (NextDent BV, Soesterberg, The Netherlands) (Figure 2), using NextDent Model 2.0 resin (Next Dent BV, Soesterberg, The Netherlands). Each tooth was embedded in one acrylic resin block and placed in a LC-3DPrint Box unit (NextDent, BV, Soesterberg, The Netherlands) for light curing for 30 min (Figure 3).

Mesial occlusal rest seats were performed on the selected teeth (Figure 4), according to the support principles: rounded triangular and concave shape, angle formed by the occlusal rest and the minor connector lower than 90°, minimum thickness of 1 mm and extension of one third in the mesiodistal and buccolingual lengths [12].

Finally, the model was scanned with a laboratory scanner (S600 Arti, Zirkonzahn GmbH, Italy) (Figure 5) and the final digital model was created, on which the clasps were later designed.

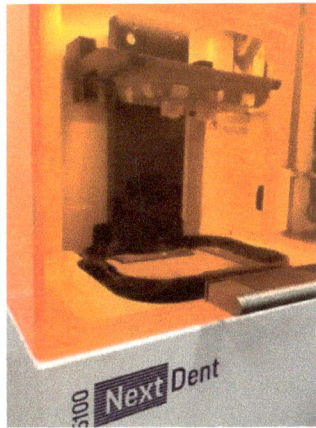

Figure 2. Next Dent 5100 3D printing machine, 3D Systems.

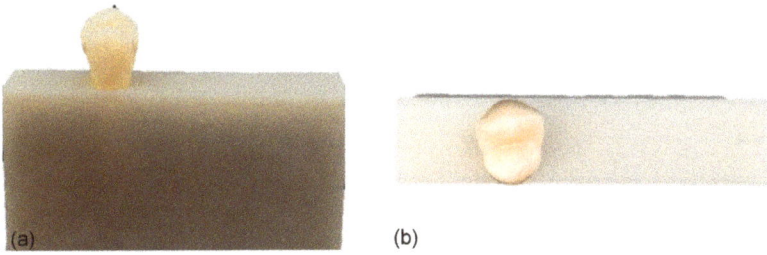

Figure 3. Acrylic block with embedded tooth 1: (**a**) Lingual view, (**b**) Occlusal view.

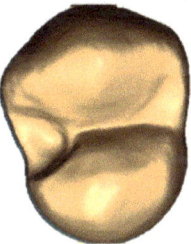

Figure 4. Occlusal view of mesial occlusal rest seat of tooth 1.

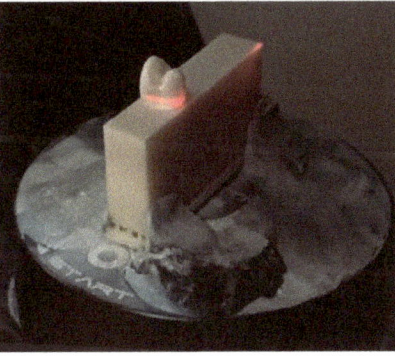

Figure 5. Digitization of the tooth with occlusal rest seat.

2.2. Production of Clasps

The digitized model was used with the clasp design using the Partial Planner program (Zirkonzahn, GmbH, Italy). Two types of clasps were designed with mesial occlusal rest, reciprocal arm in lingual tooth surface and retentive arm in the buccal tooth surface: back-action clasp (active tip of retentive arm in mesial direction) and reverse back-action (active tip of retentive arm in distal direction). In both cases, the longitudinal axis of the tooth was determined and used as the insertion axis for the clasp. The equator of the tooth was determined, and the retentions were removed. Then, in the case of the back-action clasp, a retention of 0.25 mm was sought on the mesial buccal surface, while in the case of the reverse back-action clasp, a retention of 0.25 mm was sought on the distal buccal surface.

After this step, the position of the retentive and reciprocal arms of the two clasps were determined. The reciprocal arm and the body of the retentive arm were located above the equator of the tooth, while the tip of the retentive arm was located below, in the previously selected zone. In addition, the mesial occlusal rest and the distal minor connector were added (Figures 6 and 7) [12]. A cylinder with a diameter of 5 mm and a height of 20 mm was attached to the distal end of the minor connector to serve as a support for the test machine (Figure 8). Finally, a digital design of each clasp in standard tessellation language (STL) file was created and sent to a commercial laboratory production center (Sineldent, Spain).

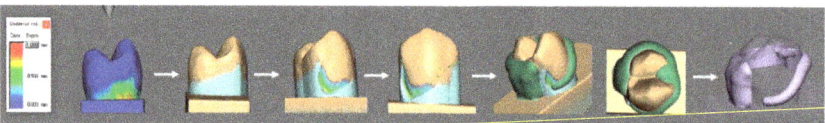

Figure 6. Diagram of the steps for making the back-action clasp.

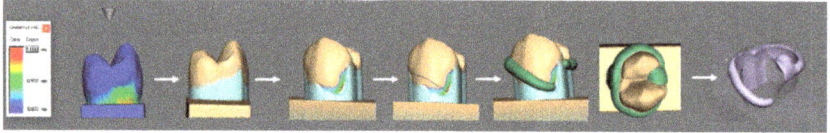

Figure 7. Diagram of the steps for making the reverse back-action clasp.

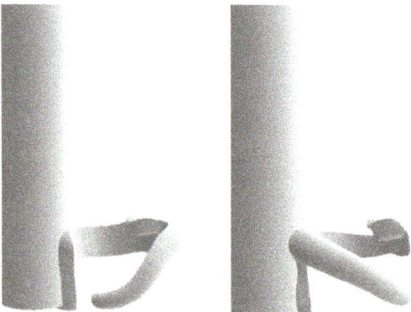

Figure 8. Clasps, final testing model.

A total of six Co–Cr clasps were fabricated, namely, two back-action clasps and two reversal back-action clasps for each of the three selected teeth.

The clasps were fabricated from SP2 Co–Cr alloy (EOS GmbH, Krailling, Germany) with 420 HV of hardness and 1350 MPa of tensile strength [35], using an EOSINT M270 system (EOS GmbH, Germany) with the direct metal laser sintering method and then heat treated for 45 min to remove the internal stresses of the metal. The clasps were then placed in an electrolytic bath (Polytherm compact, Dentaurum GmbH & Co. KG, Ispringen, Germany) for 3 min and finished with brushes, special polishing rubbers, and polishing paste by the same technician to diminish the high roughness of the metal surface. After this step, the fit of the clasps on the tooth was tested. A good fit was considered to be when the occlusal rest rested on the respective seat, in continuity with the tooth and when the clasp arms were in contact with the respective tooth surface (Figure 9).

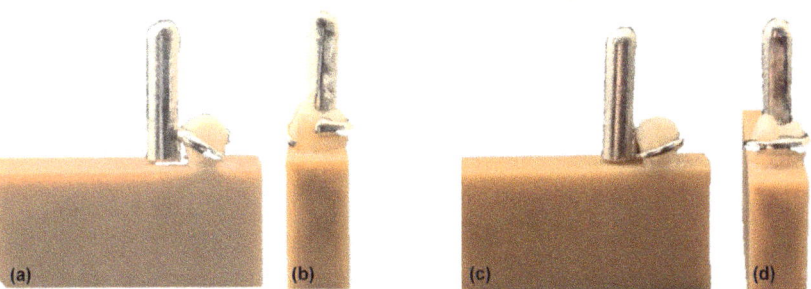

Figure 9. Back-action clasp, of tooth 2: (**a**) buccal view, (**b**) mesial view and reverse back-action clasp of tooth 2 (**c**) buccal view, (**d**) mesial view.

2.3. Test Conditions

For the evaluation of the retentive forces, repetitive cycles of insertion and removal of the clasps were performed using a universal mechanical testing machine Instron 5544 Tensile Tester (Instron, Norwood, MA, USA) equipped with a 100 N load cell. Mechanical claws were used to fix the resin block in which the tooth is fixed (BioPlus, Cat.: 2752-005, Charlotte, NC, USA) and a drill adapter with serial number 107,943 (Instron, Norwood, MA, USA) was used to fix the vertical cylinder to the clasp (Figures 10 and 11).

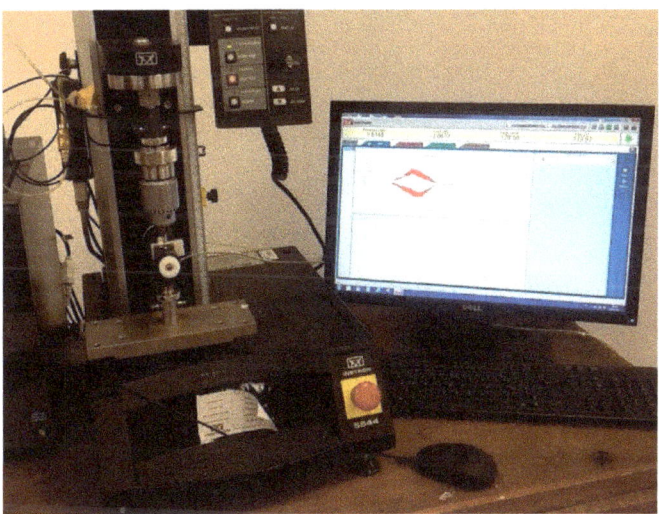

Figure 10. Instron 5544 tensile mechanical testing machine.

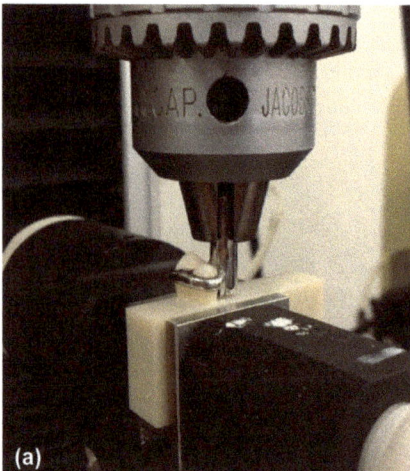
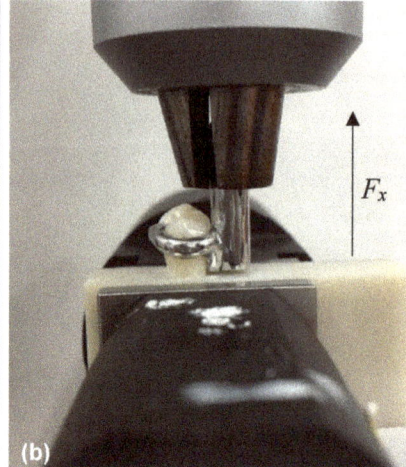

Figure 11. Mounting of the test models on the test device, reverse back-action clasp on tooth 1: (**a**) perspective view, (**b**) lingual view.

A total of 20,000 cycles of vertical movements, parallel to the longest axis of the tooth and to the axis of insertion of the clasps, were performed to simulate thirteen years of usage of the RPD, after assuming that the patient performs four cycles of insertion and removal of the RPD per day. This movement was performed at a constant rate of 2.5 mm/s. The force required to remove each clasp was recorded using the Bluehill version 3.0 program (Instron, Norwood, MA, USA).

The change in retention when the clasp is removed was calculated using Equation (1):

$$\Delta F = F_0 - F_x \qquad (1)$$

In the formula, ΔF corresponds to the change in retention, F_0 to the force required to remove the clasp at 0 cycles, and F_x to the force required to remove the clasp after x cycles. The retentive forces were recorded every 1000 cycles until 20,000 cycles were reached. The percentage change in retention was also calculated using Equation (2):

$$\frac{\Delta F}{F_0} \cdot 100\% \qquad (2)$$

For the teeth tested, the buccal and lingual surfaces were observed before and after the tests using an optical microscope (Nikon Optiphot, Tokyo, Japan) and a stereo zoom microscope (Optika Microscopes. SLX series, Ponteranica, Italy). On each tooth, points were marked on the buccal surface—mesial and distal—and on the lingual surface of the tooth for reference. A photographic evaluation of the wear of the tooth was made using the photographic record before and after the tests for each clasp.

2.4. Statistical Analysis

A descriptive analysis of the retentive forces of each clasp was performed every 1000 cycles and for each tooth. The median and interquartile range of change in retention and the percent change in retention by clasp type were calculated. Inferential statistical analysis of change in retention by clasp type was performed using the nonparametric Mann–Whitncy test. The significance level was set at 5% ($\alpha = 0.05$).

3. Results

Figure 12 shows the retentive forces of the two types of clasps for each of the three teeth used. The back-action clasp had an initial retentive force (cycle = 0) of 9.64 N, 10.87 N, and 11.24 N on tooth 1, 2, and 3, respectively, and a final retentive force (cycle = 20,000) of 8.88 N, 11.78 N, and 9.55 N, respectively. The reverse back-action clasp had an initial retentive force (cycle = 0) of 8.58 N, 12.97 N, and 11.76 N on tooth 1, 2, and 3, respectively, and a final retentive force (cycle = 20,000) of 12.10 N, 10.49 N, and 12.05 N, respectively.

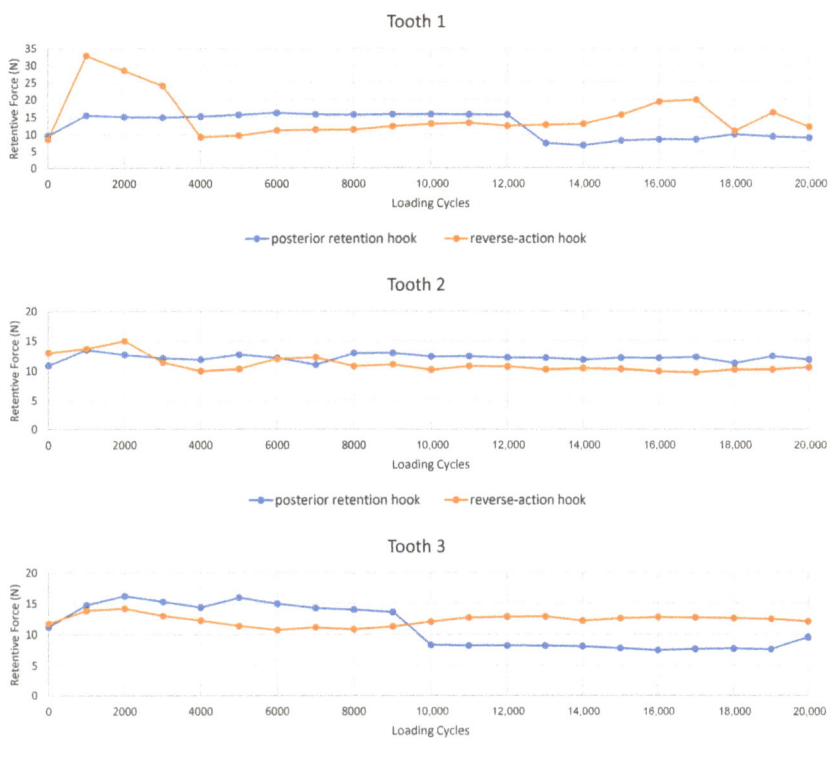

Figure 12. Diagram showing the retentive forces of the two clasps over the cycles on tooth 1, 2 and 3.

In tooth 1, the reverse back-action clasp initially showed higher values for retentive force than those of the back-action clasp. At 4000 cycles these values decreased, and at 13,000 cycles exceeded the values of the back-action clasp (Figure 12). In tooth 2, the reverse back-action clasp showed higher values of retentive force at the beginning of the test compared to the back-action clasp, but at 8000 cycles it had lower values. The back-action clasp initially had higher values of retentive forces than the reverse back-action clasp, but at 10,000 cycles it showed lower values (Figure 12).

Figures 13 and 14 show the percent change in retention over cycles by clasp type. For teeth 1 and 3, the back-action clasps experienced an abrupt loss of retention at 9000 and 13,000 cycles, respectively (Figure 13).

In the reverse back-action clasps, there were a few losses of retention over time in teeth 2 and 3 and an apparent loss of retention up to 4000, followed by a slight increase in retention in tooth 1 (Figure 14).

Descriptive analysis of the change in retention over the 20,000 cycles by clasp type is shown in Figure 15 and Table 1. The table shows the median, interquartile range, and maximum and minimum values of the variation in retention for each clasp type. There was a maximum force variation of 3.74 N (16,000 cycles for the reverse back-action clasp) and a minimum of −24.28 N (1000 cycles for the reverse back—action clasp). Negative values of change mean that the retentive force increases with the number of cycles and positive values of change mean that the retentive force decreases.

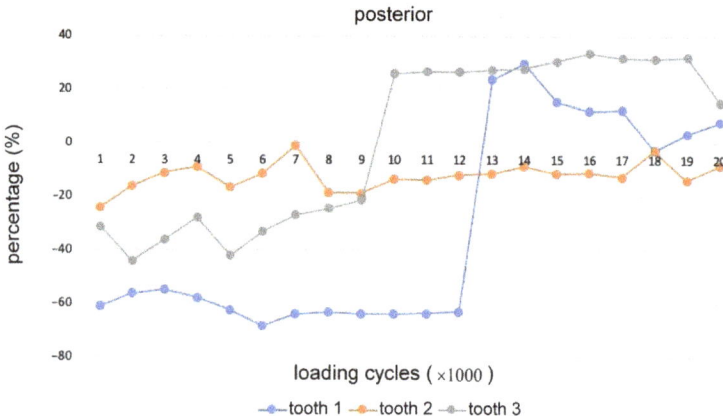

Figure 13. Percentage change in retention over loading cycles—back-action clasp on each tooth.

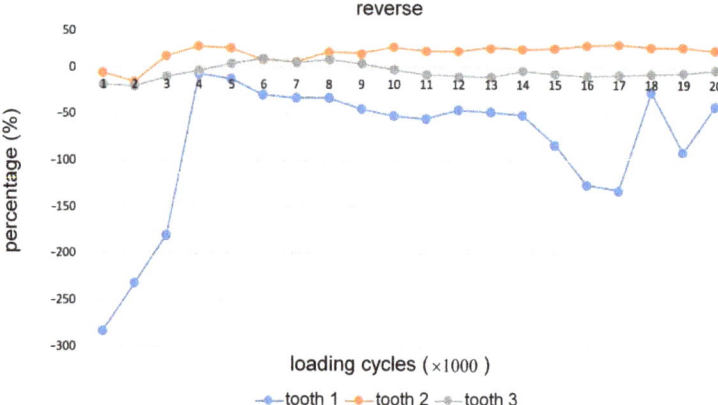

Figure 14. Percent change in retention over loading cycles—reverse back-action clasp on each tooth.

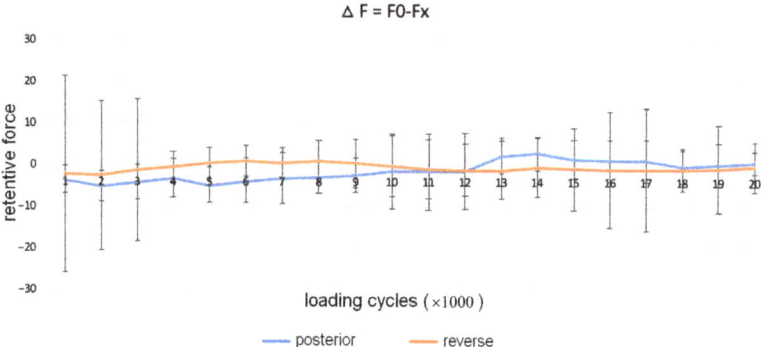

Figure 15. Change in retention of the two types of claps during insertion and removal.

Table 1. Median, interquartile range, maximum and minimum variation of retentive forces ($\Delta F = F_0 - F_x$) by clasp type, units in [N].

	Back-Action Clasp				Reverse Back-Action Clasp			
Cycles	Median	Amplitude Interquartile	Maximum	Mínimum	Median	Amplitude Interquartile	Maximum	Minimum
It 1000	−3.53	3.263	−2.64	−5.90	−2.12	23.587	−0.69	−24.28
2000	−4.98	3.655	−1.77	−5.43	−2.42	17.883	−1.97	−19.85
3000	−4.07	4.062	−1.22	−5.28	−1.21	17.044	1.62	−15.41
4000	−3.14	4.611	−0.97	−5.58	−0.46	3.627	3.03	−0.58
5000	−4.73	4.221	−1.80	−6.03	0.44	3.738	2.68	−1.05
6000	−3.72	5.36	−1.23	−6.59	1.03	3.623	1.09	−2.53
7000	−3.04	6.050	−0.10	−6.16	0.65	3.576	0.77	−2.79
8000	−2.75	4.079	−2.02	−6.10	0.93	5.045	2.24	−2.80
9000	−2.40	4.115	−2.05	−6.16	0.48	5.730	1.98	−3.74
10,000	−1.46	9.067	2.89	−6.16	−0.27	7.272	2.83	−4.43
11,000	−1.50	9.133	2.98	−6.14	−0.93	6.987	2.27	−4.71
12,000	−1.29	9.069	2.98	−6.08	−1.09	6.183	2.32	−3.86
13,000	2.27	4.284	3.04	−1.23	−1.11	6.923	2.82	−4.10
14,000	2.84	4.053	3.11	−0.93	−0.42	6.993	2.62	−4.36
15,000	1.49	4.658	3.42	−1.23	−0.79	9.792	2.75	−7.04
16,000	1.16	4.955	3.74	−1.21	−0.98	13.844	3.11	−10.73
17,000	1.18	4.939	3.56	−1.37	−0.92	14.591	3.31	−11.27
18,000	−0.27	3.850	3.52	−0.32	−0.82	5.109	2.85	−2.25
19,000	0.32	5.120	3.61	−1.50	−0.70	10.531	2.82	−7.70
20,000	0.76	2.602	1.68	−0.91	−0.29	6.006	2.48	−3.52

According to the inferential analysis, there was only a statistically significant difference between the change in retention of the two types of clasps at 4000 (Figure 16) and 5000 cycles (Figure 17). The reverse back-action clasp showed less change in retention at 4000 cycles ($p = 0.049$) and at 5000 cycles ($p = 0.049$) compared to the back-action clasp.

There were no statistically significant differences when comparing the change in retention in the remaining cycles between the two clasp groups ($p > 0.05$).

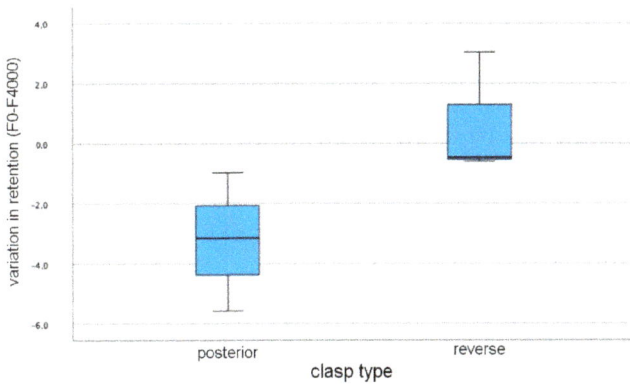

Figure 16. Boxplot diagrams of the change in retention of the two clasp types at 4000 cycles. Variation of retention in (N).

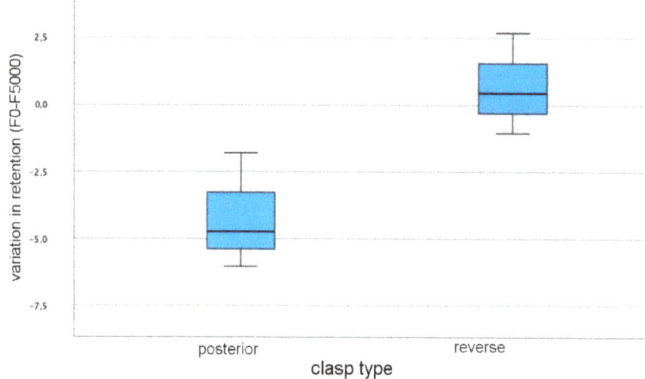

Figure 17. Boxplot diagrams of the change in retention of the two clasp types at 5000 cycles. Change in retention in (N).

4. Discussion

The objective of this study was to evaluate the retentive forces and their change over time of clasps with different designs that were digitally manufactured.

The prosthetic clasps are subject to daily movement during insertion and removal of the RPD by the patient. Several studies have examined the retentive force over multiple cycles of insertion and removal: 15,000 [8], 16,000 [15], 25,000 [34] and others [4,16,18,21,36,37]. In the present study, 20,000 cycles were performed, corresponding to a lifetime of 13 years, since changes in retention were observed only around this number of cycles.

The clasp retentive force is the force required to remove it from the tooth. It has been suggested that the retentive force for proper denture function is 5 N [12,21]. In the present study, it was shown that the initial retentive force of the back-action clasp was 10.58 N on average, and for the reverse back-action clasp was 11.10 N. This is consistent with the study of Tanaka, whose initial retentive force of Co–Cr clasps was 13 ± 4 N [38].

When evaluating the initial retentive forces versus the final retentive forces per tooth, the back-action clasp had lower initial and final retentive forces at tooth 1 compared to the reverse back-action clasp, but at tooth 2, the final retentive forces were higher for back-action forces. At tooth 3, the initial force of the back-action clasp was higher than that of the reverse back-action clasp, but the final force was lower. These discrepancies may be caused by differences in the tooth crown morphology. To address these discrepancies, the change in retention was calculated using Equation (1) to determine the variations in retention forces across cycles and to account for the initial retention force of each clasp. It is also important to highlight the fact that of the three teeth used, tooth 2 had a less retentive morphology and therefore had more constant values across cycles.

Both types of clasps have been shown to have some loss of retention over the loading cycles. However, the clasp with the back-action clasp was the one that showed the greatest change in retention at the end of the tests.

At the beginning of the experiments, both clasps showed a negative change in force, i.e., the retention values increased compared to the initial evaluation. This phenomenon was also found in other studies [4,8,36,39]. This can be justified because the tests were performed under cold conditions, and the insertion axis given by the testing machine was parallel to the longitudinal axis of the tooth, which is not the only axis that patients use when removing the removable framework [36]. The initial increase in retention forces can also be explained by the wear of the tooth and the inner surface of the clasp, which could have led to an increase in roughness at the beginning of the tests [8].

In Figures 13 and 14 the back-action clasp shows a tendency to decrease retention, with discrepancies between the values of the individual teeth. The reverse back-action clasp generally tends to maintain the values relatively constant. The fact that the reverse back-action clasp has a longer arm may mean that it is more flexible, which may result in more constant values, while the back-action clasp with its shorter retention arm loses more retention over time [15].

In a study by Helal et al. the comparison of the retentive forces of two types of clasps, namely the back-action clap and the conventional Akers clasp, showed a statistically significant difference in retentive forces at 4000 cycles [15]. This is consistent with the results of the present study, which showed that design affected the change in retention at 4000 cycles (p = 0.049) and 5000 cycles (p = 0.049). However, there was no effect on the change in retention in the remaining cycles, which contradicts the results of Kato et al., Tannous et al. and Torii et al. 2018, that showed a continuous decrease in retentive forces during the test [8,17,34].

In agreement with the studies of Hebel et al. and Helal et al., tooth wear was observed [15,39] in the area where the active tip of the retention arm of the clasp contacts the tooth surface (Figures 18 and 19). This analysis was only a qualitative analysis, unlike the previously mentioned studies that used mathematical calculations to quantify wear. In this sense, wear was observed in all teeth and in both types of clasps on both the buccal and lingual sides of the tooth. This suggests that the clasps, although made with a digital method, also cause enamel wear.

However, as in previous studies, tooth wear was found to be very low, in the order of 20 microns, and therefore it can be assumed that the decrease in retentive force is not due to tooth wear but due to changes in the clasp [38,40]. In addition, it can be assumed that the retentive arm of the clasp causes minimal wear on the tooth surface over the years and regardless of the design.

The present study has several limitations, such as the fact that the three teeth used are morphologically different, which resulted in different retentive forces for the same type of clasp. This limitation was reduced by using variation of change values for the retentive force, which removed the influence of the initial retentive force of each clasp. Another limitation was that the tests were performed in a dry environment, which may result in higher frictional resistance between surfaces [36], and the result could have been different if the tests had been performed in an artificial saliva environment.

With the present study, it was possible to perform a comparison of the retentive forces and the change in retention over 13 years of use simulation between two different designs of clasps manufactured by the digital method.

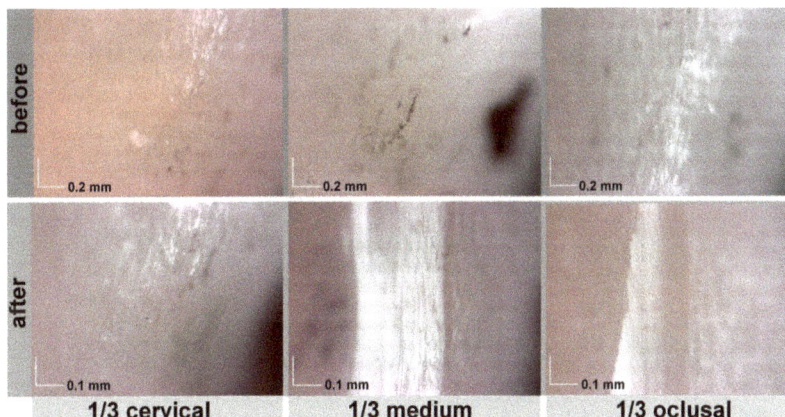

Figure 18. Buccal surface of tooth 3, before and after two trials with the back-action clasp, 5× magnification, scale of the upper images of 0.2 mm and the lower of 1.0 mm.

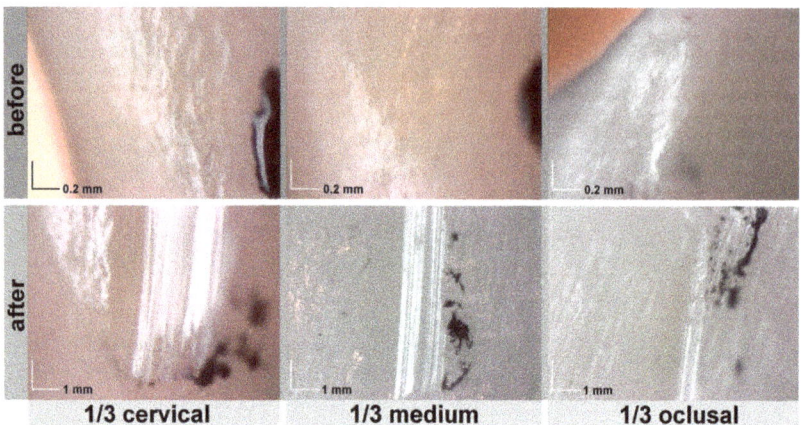

Figure 19. Distal and buccal surface of tooth 3, before and after two trials with the reverse back-action Clasp, 5× magnification, scale of the upper images is 0.2 mm and the lower is 1.0 mm.

The results show that, in general, there is no difference in retentive forces between the two types of clasps. However, there was no significant loss of retention force over time for either type of clasp, even when considering wear of the teeth, which, if relevant, would result in a loss of retentive force of the clasp.

In the future, it would be important to perform a comparison between the conventional and digital methods of RPD fabrication to determine if there are differences between these two clasp types, as there is little literature to compare them.

5. Conclusions

Based on the objectives of the present study and considering the limitations pointed out, it can be concluded that:

- Over 20,000 cycles, a reduced change in retention was verified in the clasps produced by the digital method, regardless of the type of clasp studied, which means that it will lose little retention over time.
- From this study, it can also be concluded that for most of the load cycles studied, no difference is observed between the changes in retention for the two types of clasps, leading to the conclusion that the design of the clasp does not have a great influence on the retentive force.

Author Contributions: Conceptualization, C.B.N., V.A. and V.B.; methodology, C.B.N.; software, S.B.G.; validation, V.A., C.B.N. and L.R.; formal analysis, C.B.N.; investigation, V.B.; resources, C.B.N. and L.R.; data curation, V.A.; writing—original draft preparation, V.B.; writing—review and editing, V.A.; visualization, V.B.; supervision, C.B.N.; project administration, C.B.N.; funding acquisition, C.B.N. All authors have read and agreed to the published version of the manuscript.

Funding: This research received no external funding.

Institutional Review Board Statement: Not applicable.

Informed Consent Statement: Not applicable.

Acknowledgments: This work was supported by FCT, through IDMEC, under LAETA, project UIDB/50022/2020.

Conflicts of Interest: The authors declare no conflict of interest.

References

1. Bajunaid, S.O.; Altwaim, B.; Alhassan, M.; Alammari, R. The Fit Accuracy of Removable Partial Denture Metal Frameworks Using Conventional and 3D Printed Techniques: An in Vitro Study. *J. Contemp. Dent. Pract.* **2019**, *20*, 476–481. [CrossRef] [PubMed]
2. Kim, J.J. Revisiting the Removable Partial Denture. *Dent. Clin.* **2019**, *63*, 263–278. [CrossRef]
3. Lima, J.M.C.; Anami, L.C.; Araujo, R.M.; Pavanelli, C.A. Removable Partial Dentures: Use of Rapid Prototyping. *J. Prosthodont.* **2014**, *23*, 588–591. [CrossRef] [PubMed]
4. Schweiger, J.; Güth, J.-F.; Erdelt, K.-J.; Edelhoff, D.; Schubert, O. Internal Porosities, Retentive Force, and Survival of Cobalt-Chromium Alloy Clasps Fabricated by Selective Laser-Sintering. *J. Prosthodont. Res.* **2020**, *64*, 210–216. [CrossRef] [PubMed]
5. Benso, B.; Kovalik, A.C.; Jorge, J.H.; Campanha, N.H. Failures in the Rehabilitation Treatment with Removable Partial Dentures. *Acta Odontol. Scand.* **2013**, *71*, 1351–1355. [CrossRef] [PubMed]
6. Almufleh, B.; Emami, E.; Alageel, O.; de Melo, F.; Seng, F.; Caron, E.; Abi Nader, S.; Al-Hashedi, A.; Albuquerque, R.; Feine, J. Patient Satisfaction with Laser-Sintered Removable Partial Dentures: A Crossover Pilot Clinical Trial. *J. Prosthet. Dent.* **2018**, *119*, 560–567. [CrossRef]
7. Lang, L.A.; Tulunoglu, I. A Critically Appraised Topic Review of Computer-Aided Design/Computer-Aided Machining of Removable Partial Denture Frameworks. *Dent. Clin.* **2014**, *58*, 247–255. [CrossRef] [PubMed]
8. Tannous, F.; Steiner, M.; Shahin, R.; Kern, M. Retentive Forces and Fatigue Resistance of Thermoplastic Resin Clasps. *Dent. Mater.* **2012**, *28*, 273–278. [CrossRef]
9. Alageel, O.; Abdallah, M.-N.; Alsheghri, A.; Song, J.; Caron, E.; Tamimi, F. Removable Partial Denture Alloys Processed by Laser-Sintering Technique. *J. Biomed. Mater. Res. Part B Appl. Biomater.* **2018**, *106*, 1174–1185. [CrossRef]
10. Campbell, S.D.; Cooper, L.; Craddock, H.; Hyde, T.P.; Nattress, B.; Pavitt, S.H.; Seymour, D.W. Removable Partial Dentures: The Clinical Need for Innovation. *J. Prosthet. Dent.* **2017**, *118*, 273–280. [CrossRef] [PubMed]
11. Hwang, H.H.-M.; Chou, C.-W.; Chen, Y.-J.; Yao, C.-C.J. An Overview of Digital Intraoral Scanners: Past, Present and Future-from an Orthodontic Perspective. *Taiwan. J. Orthod.* **2018**, *30*, 3.
12. Frank, R.P.; Brudvik, J.S.; Leroux, B.; Milgrom, P.; Hawkins, N. Relationship between the Standards of Removable Partial Denture Construction, Clinical Acceptability, and Patient Satisfaction. *J. Prosthet. Dent.* **2000**, *83*, 521–527. [CrossRef] [PubMed]
13. Bohnenkamp, D.M. Removable Partial Dentures: Clinical Concepts. *Dent. Clin.* **2014**, *58*, 69–89.
14. Arnold, C.; Hey, J.; Schweyen, R.; Setz, J.M. Accuracy of CAD-CAM-Fabricated Removable Partial Dentures. *J. Prosthet. Dent.* **2018**, *119*, 586–592. [CrossRef] [PubMed]
15. Helal, M.A.; Baraka, O.A.; Sanad, M.E.; Ludwig, K.; Kern, M. Effects of Long-Term Simulated RPD Clasp Attachment/Detachment on Retention Loss and Wear for Two Clasp Types and Three Abutment Material Surfaces. *J. Prosthodont. Implant Esthet. Reconstr. Dent.* **2012**, *21*, 370–377. [CrossRef] [PubMed]
16. Kato, Y.; Tasaka, A.; Kato, M.; Wadachi, J.; Takemoto, S.; Yamashita, S. Effects of Repetitive Insertion/Removal Cycles and Simulated Occlusal Loads on Retention of Denture Retainers. *Dent. Mater. J.* **2021**, *40*, 1277–1283. [CrossRef] [PubMed]
17. Tribst, J.P.M.; Dal Piva, A.M.d.O.; Borges, A.L.S.; Araújo, R.M.; da Silva, J.M.F.; Bottino, M.A.; Kleverlaan, C.J.; de Jager, N. Effect of Different Materials and Undercut on the Removal Force and Stress Distribution in Circumferential Clasps during Direct Retainer Action in Removable Partial Dentures. *Dent. Mater.* **2020**, *36*, 179–186. [CrossRef]
18. Kim, S.Y.; Shin, S.-Y.; Lee, J.H. Effect of Cyclic Bend Loading on a Cobalt-Chromium Clasp Fabricated by Direct Metal Laser Sintering. *J. Prosthet. Dent.* **2018**, *119*, 1027-e1. [CrossRef]
19. Hakkoum, M.A. New Clasp Assembly for Distal Extension Removable Partial Dentures: The Reverse RPA Clasp. *J. Prosthodont.* **2016**, *25*, 411–413. [CrossRef]
20. Eliason, C.M. RPA Clasp Design for Distal-Extension Removable Partial Dentures. *J. Prosthet. Dent.* **1983**, *49*, 25–27. [CrossRef] [PubMed]
21. Cheng, H.; Xu, M.; Zhang, H.; Wu, W.; Zheng, M.; Li, X. Cyclic Fatigue Properties of Cobalt-Chromium Alloy Clasps for Partial Removable Dental Prostheses. *J. Prosthet. Dent.* **2010**, *104*, 389–396. [CrossRef] [PubMed]
22. Puskar, T.; Jevremovic, D.; Williams, R.J.; Eggbeer, D.; Vukelic, D.; Budak, I. A Comparative Analysis of the Corrosive Effect of Artificial Saliva of Variable PH on DMLS and Cast Co-Cr-Mo Dental Alloy. *Materials* **2014**, *7*, 6486–6501. [CrossRef] [PubMed]
23. Dikova, T. *Properties of Co-Cr Dental Alloys Fabricated Using Additive Technologies*; [Internet]; Biomaterials in Regenerative Medicine; InTech: London, UK, 2018. [CrossRef]
24. Rist, K.; Cimic, S. Selective Laser Melting Technique in Fabrication of Partial Denture Metal Framework. *Res. J. Pharm. Biol. Chem. Sci.* **2016**, *7*, 2039–2043.
25. Conceição, P.; Portugal, J.; Franco, M.; Alves, N.M.; Marques, D.; Neves, C.B. Comparison between Digital Superimposition and Microcomputed Tomography Methods of Fit Assessment of Removable Partial Denture Frameworks. *J. Prosthet. Dent.* **2023**, 6. [CrossRef] [PubMed]
26. Anan, M.T.M.; Al-Saadi, M.H. Fit Accuracy of Metal Partial Removable Dental Prosthesis Frameworks Fabricated by Traditional or Light Curing Modeling Material Technique: An in Vitro Study. *Saudi Dent. J.* **2015**, *27*, 149–154. [CrossRef] [PubMed]
27. Pereira, A.L.C.; de Medeiros, A.K.B.; de Sousa Santos, K.; de Almeida, É.O.; Barbosa, G.A.S.; Carreiro, A. da F.P. Accuracy of CAD-CAM Systems for Removable Partial Denture Framework Fabrication: A Systematic Review. *J. Prosthet. Dent.* **2021**, *125*, 241–248. [CrossRef]

28. Alghazzawi, T.F. Advancements in CAD/CAM Technology: Options for Practical Implementation. *J. Prosthodont. Res.* **2016**, *60*, 72–84. [CrossRef]
29. Bilgin, M.S.; Baytaroğlu, E.N.; Erdem, A.; Dilber, E. A Review of Computer-Aided Design/Computer-Aided Manufacture Techniques for Removable Denture Fabrication. *Eur. J. Dent.* **2016**, *10*, 286–291. [CrossRef]
30. Abduo, J.; Lyons, K.; Bennamoun, M. Trends in Computer-Aided Manufacturing in Prosthodontics: A Review of the Available Streams. *Int. J. Dent.* **2014**, *2014*, 783948. [CrossRef] [PubMed]
31. Conceição, P.R.; Pinto, R.; Marques, D.; Portugal, J.; Neves, C.B.; Franco, M.; Alves, N. Fit Accuracy Assessment of RPD Metal Framework by Digital Superimposition. In *Advances and Current Trends in Biomechanics*; Belinha, J., Campos, J.C.R., Fonseca, E., Silva, M.H.F., Marques, M.A., Costa, M.F.G., Oliveira, S., Eds.; CRC Press: Boca Raton, FL, USA, 2022; pp. 331–334. [CrossRef]
32. Venkatesh, K.V.; Nandini, V.V. Direct Metal Laser Sintering: A Digitised Metal Casting Technology. *J. Indian Prosthodont. Soc.* **2013**, *13*, 389–392. [CrossRef]
33. Revilla-León, M.; Özcan, M. Additive Manufacturing Technologies Used for 3D Metal Printing in Dentistry. *Curr. Oral Health Rep.* **2017**, *4*, 201–208. [CrossRef]
34. Torii, M.; Nakata, T.; Takahashi, K.; Kawamura, N.; Shimpo, H.; Ohkubo, C. Fitness and Retentive Force of Cobalt-Chromium Alloy Clasps Fabricated with Repeated Laser Sintering and Milling. *J. Prosthodont. Res.* **2018**, *62*, 342–346. [CrossRef] [PubMed]
35. Conceição, P.R.; Franco, M.C.; Alves, N.; Portugal, J.; Neves, C.B. Fit Accuracy of Removable Partial Denture Metal Frameworks Produced by CAD-CAM–a Clinical Study. *Rev. Port. Estomatol. Med. Dentária Cir. Maxilofac.* **2021**, *62*, 194–200. [CrossRef]
36. Phillips, R.W.; Leonard, L.J. A Study of Enamel Abrasion as Related to Partial Denture Clasps. *J. Prosthet. Dent.* **1956**, *6*, 657–671. [CrossRef]
37. Rodrigues, R.C.S.; Ribeiro, R.F.; de Mattos, M.d.G.C.; Bezzon, O.L. Comparative Study of Circumferential Clasp Retention Force for Titanium and Cobalt-Chromium Removable Partial Dentures. *J. Prosthet. Dent.* **2002**, *88*, 290–296. [CrossRef]
38. Tanaka, A.; Miyake, N.; Hotta, H.; Takemoto, S.; Yoshinari, M.; Yamashita, S. Change in the Retentive Force of Akers Clasp for Zirconia Crown by Repetitive Insertion and Removal Test. *J. Prosthodont. Res.* **2019**, *63*, 447–452. [CrossRef]
39. Sato, Y.; Tsuga, K.; Abe, Y.; Asahara, S.; Akagawa, Y. Finite Element Analysis on Preferable I-Bar Clasp Shape. *J. Oral Rehabil.* **2001**, *28*, 413–417. [CrossRef]
40. Kim, H.R.; Jang, S.H.; Kim, Y.K.; Son, J.S.; Min, B.K.; Kim, K.H.; Kwon, T.Y. Microstructures and Mechanical Properties of Co-Cr Dental Alloys Fabricated by Three CAD/CAM-Based Processing Techniques. *Materials* **2016**, *9*, 596. [CrossRef]

Disclaimer/Publisher's Note: The statements, opinions and data contained in all publications are solely those of the individual author(s) and contributor(s) and not of MDPI and/or the editor(s). MDPI and/or the editor(s) disclaim responsibility for any injury to people or property resulting from any ideas, methods, instructions or products referred to in the content.

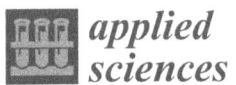

Review

The Use of Autogenous Teeth for Alveolar Ridge Preservation: A Literature Review

João Cenicante [1], João Botelho [1,2], Vanessa Machado [1,2], José João Mendes [1,2], Paulo Mascarenhas [3], Gil Alcoforado [1] and Alexandre Santos [1,*]

[1] Clinical Research Unit (CRU), Centro de Investigação Interdisciplinar, Egas Moniz (CiiEM),
Egas Moniz–Cooperativa de Ensino Superior, 2829-511 Almada, Portugal; joaopcenicante@gmail.com (J.C.); jbotelho@egasmoniz.edu.pt (J.B.); vmachado@egasmoniz.edu.pt (V.M.); jmendes@egasmoniz.edu.pt (J.J.M.); galcoforado@egasmoniz.edu.pt (G.A.)
[2] Evidence-Based Hub, Clinical Research Unit (CRU), Centro de Investigação Interdisciplinar, Egas Moniz (CiiEM), Egas Moniz–Cooperativa de Ensino Superior, 2829-511 Almada, Portugal
[3] Oral and Biomedical Sciences Research Unit, Faculty of Dental Medicine, University of Lisbon, 1649-004 Lisbon, Portugal; pmascarenhas@iro.pt
* Correspondence: alex_santos_30@hotmail.com; Tel.: +351-212-946-800

Abstract: Alveolar ridge resorption is a natural consequence of teeth extraction, with unpleasant aesthetic and functional consequences that might compromise a future oral rehabilitation. To minimize the biological consequences of alveolar ridge resorption, several surgical procedures have been designed, the so-called alveolar ridge preservation (ARP) techniques. One important characteristic is the concomitant use of biomaterial in ARP. In the past decade, autogenous teeth as a bone graft material in post-extraction sockets have been proposed with very interesting outcomes, yet with different protocols of preparation. Here we summarize the available evidence on autogenous teeth as a biomaterial in ARP, its different protocols and future directions.

Keywords: extracted teeth; bone regeneration; bone graft; autogenous graft; autogenous tooth bone graft; human dentin; demineralized dentin

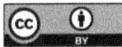

1. Introduction

A tooth is indicated for extraction when it is no longer possible to restore or maintain in acceptable conditions considering its health, function and/or aesthetics [1]. The extraction of a tooth triggers a series of events that further result in the decrease of height and width of the alveolar process, particularly on the buccal side and horizontally [2–7]. After extraction, this resorptive event occurs during the first three months of healing until one year, with potential aesthetic and functional consequences for prosthetic rehabilitation [2,8].

Due to the fallouts of alveolar ridge resorption after tooth extraction, a socket-filling procedure is frequently required when dental implants are planned to rehabilitate function, aesthetics and comfort [9]. To this end, alveolar ridge preservation (ARP) in post-extraction sockets is a well described surgical technique able to prevent bone resorption partially but not completely [10,11].

Several graft materials have been advocated in ARP including bone substitutes, such as allografts, xenografts, alloplasts and autografts (i.e., autogenous bone) [4]. Bone graft materials must have three main properties: osteoconduction (the ability to provide scaffold for bone regeneration), osteoinduction (the capacity to recruit primitive, undifferentiated and pluripotent cells that are developed into having a bone-forming capacity) and osteogenesis (presence of cells that promote bone regeneration) [12,13]. Autogenous bone is widely accepted as the gold standard bone graft material as it contemplates all three characteristics [9]. Nonetheless, autogenous bone has limited intra-oral availability, causes high donor site morbidity and presents elevated resorption rates [9,12].

A recently proposed material was autogenous teeth, commonly seen as dental waste after dental extractions [14]. Chemically, dentin is very similar to bone, with an osteoconductive and osteoinductive matrix, and therefore is a viable candidate for bone grafting [15,16]. Autogenous teeth have fair intra-oral availability and may be obtained through standard procedures with low morbidity [17]. Nonetheless, it is important to bear in mind that the amount of dentin graft is dependent on the condition of the discarded teeth [12].

Ever since, several protocols have been proposed for ARP using autogenous teeth as a graft material and, so far, three different methods of dentin processing have been developed: demineralized dentin matrix (DDM), partially demineralized dentin matrix (PDDM) and undemineralized dentin (UDD) (Figure 1) [12,14]. However, these different methods present clinical pros and cons that deserve attention. For this reason, this review summarizes the available evidence on autogenous teeth as graft material, its different types and its applicability in ARP.

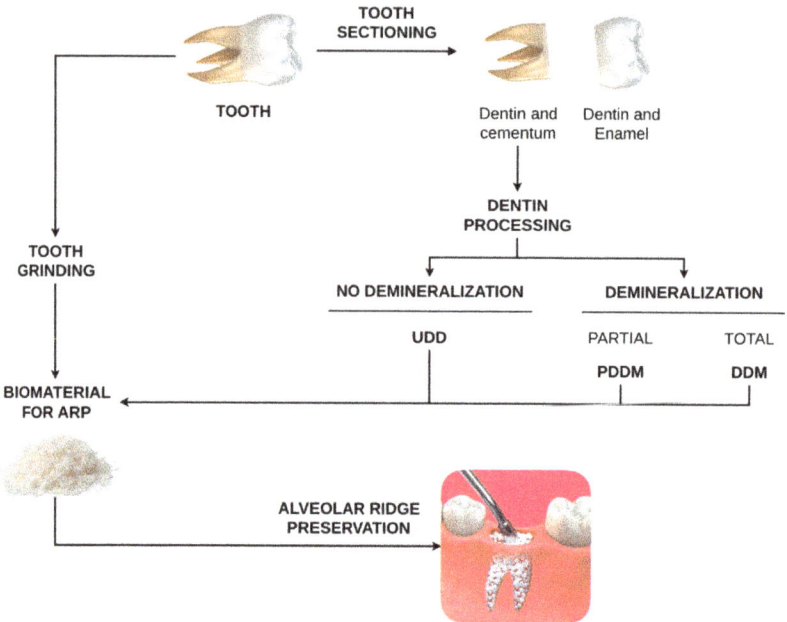

Figure 1. Schematic diagram explaining different dentin processing approaches. UDD—undemineralized dentin matrix; PDDM—partially demineralized dentin matrix; DDM—demineralized dentin matrix).

2. Alveolar Ridge Preservation in Extraction Sockets

2.1. Biological Effect of a Tooth Extraction

Tooth extraction sets off a series of biological events, with a local inflammatory response and an irreversible structural transformation of the periodontium [3]. In terms of hard tissues, as previously stated, it can be expected a bone resorption, mainly in the first three months, causing both vertical and horizontal changes in the alveolar process [5,10].

These anatomical changes are more buccally and horizontally pronounced [3–7], with an average horizontal reduction of 3.79–3.87 mm and an average vertical reduction on the buccal side of 0.64–1.24 mm [5,7].

Concerning the soft tissues, the socket defect will determine the healing process through secondary intention resulting in cell proliferation, whereas the gingival form mostly depends on the external shape of the alveolar bone [5].

In order to diminish the biological effect of a tooth extraction, an appropriate treatment plan and technique are central [3]. As for the surgical technique, a flapless approach is considered a simple, atraumatic and conservative method, being the usual choice to reduce post-surgery healing period, discomfort and inflammation [4]. This surgical approach is characterized by the nondetachment of the periosteum, preserving the blood supply to the buccal bone, which, as mentioned before, suffers a more pronounced resorption [18].

2.2. Alveolar Ridge Preservation: Concept and Bone Graft Materials Used

The biological effect subsequent to a tooth extraction might have a devastating impact on the rehabilitation treatment, affecting both hard and soft tissues [3]. While bone availability might decrease, which is a key factor in the implant placement, the aesthetic result may also be compromised, by damaging the soft tissue [8,19].

Under the rationale of ARP, filling a socket with grafting materials might reduce alveolar ridge resorption comparing to natural healing via blood clot [19]. Overall, ARP comprises three essential goals: (1) the maintenance of the existing soft and hard tissue envelope; (2) the preservation of a stable alveolar ridge in order to maximize the functional and aesthetic outcome; and (3) the simplification of the treatment procedures following the alveolar ridge regeneration [20].

When considering ridge resorption in this procedure, one must not only analyze the socket graft material and the surgical protocol but also the systemic and local characteristics that can play a role in this clinical procedure [1]. Among the factors that might affect ARP are number of adjacent teeth to be extracted, socket morphology (single versus multirooted teeth), integrity of the socket walls, periodontal biotype (assessing its thickness), smoking status, systemic factors (e.g., bone metabolic disorders, uncontrolled diabetes) and patient compliance [1,3,8].

Regarding the numerous biomaterials used for socket grafting, many approaches have been described in the literature [2,6,21]. Examples of these approaches are: using only bone grafting alone, including autografts (e.g., autogenous bone), allografts (including cortical mineralized freeze-dried bone and cortical demineralized freeze-dried bone) xenografts (derived from bovine bone), alloplasts (including medical-grade calcium sulfate, hydroxyapatite and beta-tricalcium phosphate (β-TCP)) [2,6,21].

Finally, it has been also described the application of a membrane alone (resorbable or non-resorbable), or combined with a grafting material [2,6,21].

Several systematic reviews have addressed ARP effectiveness. While some of these reviews points out to a rather scarce evidence with no significant conclusions [2,19,20], more recent systematic reviews showed more promising results [1,3,4,6,8,10,11,21–23]. Comprehensively, there is general consensus that ARP does not avoid completely the inevitable dimensional loss that exists [1,3,4].

While xenogenic or allogenic materials have been associated with better results when compared with alloplastic grafts [1,3,4], others highlight the positive influence of the use of barrier membranes, resorbable and non-resorbable [8,10,21] or the combined use of a bone graft with a resorbable membrane [6]. Nonetheless, other studies advocate that although the benefit of this procedure exists, the evidence available is insufficient to state which method is best in reducing the dimensional changes addressed before [8,11,23].

The reason behind this limited evidence can be explained by the high heterogeneity present in the existing systematic reviews [1–4,6,8,10,11,19–23]. This heterogeneity is dependent on the broad definition of alveolar ridge regeneration, where many aspects enter the equation. Some examples are: type of graft material used, with or without resorbable or non-resorbable membrane, use of growth factors, with or without raising a flap when extracting the tooth, achieving primary or secondary intention closure, with damaged or intact sockets, multi rooted teeth or single rooted teeth, mandible or maxilla, among other patient related factors mentioned before [3,10,19,21,22].

Another technique that has also been described with promising results is the socket-shield [24]. The hypothesis behind this technique is that by retaining a section of the buccal side of the root during implant placement the extensive bone loss that occurs on the buccal side of the bone will be reduced [24–26]. Regarding this technique, some modifications have appeared since it was first presented, showing promising results [25]. However, more high level evidence studies are required to better assess this approach [25,26].

3. Autogenous Teeth as a Bone Graft Material

3.1. Biological Plausibility

In order to understand the use of human teeth as a bone graft material, we must bear in mind the chemical composition of human teeth and alveolar bone. The ratio inorganic/organic/water of the various components of the teeth goes as follows: enamel (95%/0.6%/4%), dentin (70–75%/20%/10%) and cementum (45–55%/50–55%) [12,16]. When comparing with the alveolar bone ratio, (65%/35%/0%), the similarity between bone and especially dentin becomes clear [16].

Considering this potential, researches started looking for the different hard tissues present in teeth. Yeomans and Urist pioneer study on the potential bone-inducing properties of dentin opened up new boundaries on graft materials [27]. Yeomans and Urist firstly reported the bone induction capacity of autogenous demineralized dentin matrix [27]. In the same year, Bang and Urist also referred the similarity between dentin collagenous matrix and bone matrix in terms of osteoinductive capacity [28]. Only in 2009, the Korean Tooth Bank, in Seoul, Korea, developed an autogenous tooth bone graft material, which lead to a significant increase of studies in this field regarding the clinical performance of this material [29].

Given the role and highly percentage of dentin in autogenous tooth [30], several studies have focused on different methods of treating dentin matrix towards the optimization of the procedure clinical effectiveness [14].

In the inorganic component of dentin, X-ray diffraction analysis showed that, unlike enamel hydroxyapatite, dentin hydroxyapatite (which consists of 70% of the dentin in its weight volume) is structured with low-crystalline calcium phosphate, which in turn, allows the osteoclasts to easily decompose this mineral, promoting an effective bone remodeling [15,30]. This property is not only similar to bone tissue, also mainly composed by low-crystalline calcium phosphate, but also essential in alveolar ridge regeneration, ensuring osteoconductive capacity [12,16,29]. Besides hydroxyapatite, there are other three biological calcium phosphates such as: tricalcium phosphate, octacalcium phosphate and amorphous calcium phosphate [31]. All these forms interact with each other, playing a positive role in bone remodeling [15].

In the organic component of the dentin matrix, a dense network of type 1 collagen fibrils represents 90% of its content [12]. The other 10% is formed by the so-called non-collagenous proteins such as: osteocalcin, osteonectin, sialoprotein and phosphoprotein, which are known to be involved in bone calcification [15]. Additionally, growth factors are also present, including bone morphogenetic proteins (BMP), LIM mineralization protein 1, transforming growth factor-β among others [12,14]. Bessho et al. compared the dentin-matrix derived BMP with the bone-matrix derived BMP, concluding that although they are not identical, both induce bone formation [32]. Similarly, Boden et al. demonstrated that LIM mineralization protein 1 is a positive regulator of the osteoblast differentiation [33]. These growth factors, alongside other non-collagenous proteins have a proven osteoinductive capacity [12,15,16,29,32–35].

One important aspect that can be beneficial in terms of implant placement is the healing period. In the literature, this period usually varies from 4 to 6 months [36,37], although in some cases, dental implants may be placed 2 to 3 months after alveolar ridge preservation [38]. Several authors compared the use of autogenous tooth graft versus a xenograft [17,39,40]. While some studies assess the performance of the implants immediately placed after graft [17,40], one study compared the two grafts after a healing period of 6 months [39]. Regarding this matter, thanks to the reduced resorption rate of the autogenous tooth graft (4 to 6 months) an earlier placement of the implant can be done, reducing the healing period [38,41].

3.2. Dentin Processing

As aforementioned, autogenous teeth can be used as bone graft material with osteoconductive and osteoinductive potential [9,12]. However, several concerns have been addressed regarding the need for any dentin processing prior to bone grafting for the purpose of clinical optimization. Some examples are the extraction of non-collagenous proteins [42], elimination of the organic matrix [14] and finally, one of the most commonly used, dentin preparation by demineralization [12].

The hypothesis of demineralization is that through this procedure, the organic substances (type 1 collagen fibrils, non-collagenous proteins and growth factors) will be more exposed, decreasing the graft crystallinity and increasing its porosity and surface area [16,35,43]. This process releases growth factors and non-collagenous proteins, which in turn, results in an enhanced osteoinductive activity [14].

Although protocols vary from study to study, a general protocol includes tooth extraction, removal of soft tissue, carious lesions and filling materials of any nature [17,44–46], sectioning into blocks or particles and finally choosing the degree of demineralization [47]. Among the demineralization agent are ethylenediaminetetraacetic acid (EDTA), phosphoric acid, chloridric acid, nitric acid, hydrogen oxide, ethyl ether and ethyl alcohol [14]. Hence, dentin materials were categorized into 3 categories: demineralized dentin matrix (DDM), partially demineralized dentin matrix (PDDM) and undemineralized dentin (UDD) [12].

While some investigators have reported success when using DDM (or PDDM) [17,37,39,40,44,48–50] others prefer using in its undemineralized form [38,51–57].

Mineralized dentin particles offer a mechanical stability, creating a solid site for implant placement [38,52]. With the use of a mineralized graft, although the osteoinductive properties of dentin may be delayed, the low crystallinity of dentin hydroxyapatite allows the progressive bone remodeling [15,30].

Due to a lack of uniformity and standardization in the literature, it is difficult to determine with certainty which form of graft is advantageous for which clinical indication. Regarding ARP procedures, several authors have reported success when using DDM, PDDM and UDD, indicating that each form can be a viable option [38,40,41]. Nonetheless, some authors suggest an approach patient-based. DDM and PDDM can be indicated when the socket walls have already been resorbed or destroyed due to pathological causes [58]. The exposure of growth factors and non-collagenous proteins, as previously stated, will allow an earlier regeneration [14,38]. The UDM on the other hand, thanks to the mechanical stability inherent to the graft, may allow an earlier placement of dental implants [38].

As previously stated, the amount of biomaterial that the clinician can gather is dependent on the extension of carious lesions and filling materials [17,44–46], nonetheless, one possible approach that can overcome this limitation is the extraction of impacted third molars, when it is required a larger amount of biomaterial [51,59].

In order to obtain a demineralized graft, the Korea Tooth Bank, established in Seoul, was one of the first to be available for clinicians [60]. However, due to this time-consuming option, several devices appeared on the market for this purpose.

The VacuaSonic® (Cosmobiomedicare, Seoul, Korea) produces a demineralized graft. This system comes with a powder reagent (DecalSi® DM Powder reagent) and a block reagent (DecalSi® DM Block reagent), giving the clinician a choice, on which form of graft he prefers. According to the manufacturer, the process takes 30 min for powder graft and 2 h for block graft [50].

Another system that can be used is the Smart Dentin Grinder™ (Kometa Bio ltd., Holon, Israel) which is a device that grinds the tooth to particles of 250–1200 μm, according to the manufacturer. Alongside this grinder, comes a disposable griding chamber (single-use) as well as a dentin cleanser (0.5 M NaOH and 30% ethanol (V/V)) which is applied for 5 min and a phosphate buffer saline (PBS) solution with calcium and magnesium with an application time of 1 min, repeating this last step. This device can be used in order to produce a mineralized or partially demineralized graft, which in this last case, a 10% solution of EDTA during 2 min is added [38].

Finally, another system commonly used to produce a demineralized graft is the Tooth Transformer device (TT Tooth Transformer srl. Milan, Italy). This device comes with a tooth grinder and a series of disposable accessories that contacts with the resulting autologous material and liquid responsible for the demineralization. According to Minetti, this process takes approximately 25 min [61]. Regarding prices, while the VacuaSonic® (Cosmobiomedicare, Seoul, Korea) costs around 12365 €, the Smart Dentin Grinder™ (Kometa Bio ltd., Holon, Israel) costs around 1277 € and finally the Tooth Transformer (TT Tooth Transformer srl. Milan, Italy) device has a price of around 2000 €.

Due to the potential of the autogenous tooth as a bone substitute, several clinical applications have appeared in the literature besides ARP procedures [9,12,35].

One study performed lateral alveolar ridge augmentation comparing the use of autogenous tooth roots versus the use of autogenous bone blocks [62]. In this particular study, after 26 weeks of healing, the implants were placed with no significant difference between groups ($p > 0.05$) in terms of primary implant stability quotient [62].

The use of autogenous tooth graft was also associated with the treatment of grade II and III furcation defects by one study, which compared the clinical and radiologic performance of this graft material with the use of freeze-dried bone allograft [63]. The results of this study point out the potential benefit that autogenous tooth can have as a bone graft material, demonstrating a significant reduction in vertical bone depth, horizontal bone depth as well as radiographically bony defect [63].

Another possible application for autogenous tooth is in sinus floor elevation procedures [64,65]. One particular study compared the use of autogenous tooth versus the bovine-derived xenograft Bio-Oss (Geistlich Pharma AG, Wolhusen, Switzerland) [64]. With a follow up period of 4 months, there was no significant difference between the two groups after a clinical, radiologic and histomorphometry assessment [64]. In another study, Kim et al. performed a micromorphometry and histological evaluation 9 months after sinus bone graft using autogenous tooth [65]. This evaluation concluded that autogenous tooth showed excellent bone healing, proving to be a viable option for this kind of procedure [65].

4. Demineralized Dentin Matrix (DDM)

4.1. Preclinical Studies

Two preclinical studies have confirmed the potential of human DDM placed in extraction sockets as well as the influence that this biomaterial has on proteins and growth factors such as BMP-2, BMP-4 and vascular endothelial growth factor (VEGF) [45,46]. In both studies, there was a common protocol: after the removal of caries lesions, pulp tissues and periodontal ligament, the agent responsible for the demineralization was a 10% EDTA solution with a pH varying from 7.2 to 7.3 [45,46]. After cutting with a cryostat, one study stored the material in a sterile phosphate buffered saline (PBS) with penicillin and streptomycin for decontamination [46].

4.1.1. Histologic and Histomorphometric Outcomes

A histologic and morphometric analysis showed that human DDM integrated newly formed bone after 14 days showing histological features of mature bone, proving its osteoconductivity [45,46].

4.1.2. Immunohistochemistry Outcomes

One interesting aspect regarding these studies results from the immunohistochemistry evaluation. Oliveira et al. found that with the degradation of the human DDM, the number of BMP-2 and BMP-4 immunostained cells increased at day 10, suggesting that this event is key in stimulating cellular differentiation and consequently bone formation [46]. A similar result can be seen in Reis-Filho et al.'s study after a period of 14 and 21 days, where with the human DDM resorption, the expression of VEGF increased, indicating angiogenesis, which in turn accelerates the healing process [45]. Both these results support the evidence of the osteoinductive capacity of the DDM [45,46].

4.2. Clinical Studies

Furthermore, several clinical studies have been published endorsing the use of DDM in ARP despite diverging in terms of the protocol used for dentin processing [17,37,39,40,44,48–50,66,67].

The removal of carious lesions, fillings and soft tissues seems shoes an apparent unanimity [17,37,39,44,66], however, while most authors use dentin, enamel and cementum, some eliminate these last two [40], or simply use the root portion of the tooth [37]. Some investigators defend the use of dentin alone due to its osteoconductive and osteoinductive properties being similar to alveolar bone [35,43] and in this way enamel shall be removed because it has high-crystalline calcium phosphate and therefore might complicate the absorption process [15,30]. On the other hand, it is described in some protocols the use of the whole tooth as a bone graft material, combining the chemical properties of dentin with the mechanical advantage that enamel brings, allowing an earlier placement of dental implants [38,52,57].

In the majority of these studies, the demineralization agent was not specified [17,39,44,48–50,66], but rather the explanation that the autogenous graft went through a dehydration, defatting, demineralized and lyophilized course [39,66]. Nonetheless, studies often report the use of 70% ethyl alcohol, 0.6 N chloridric acid and 2% nitric acid [37,40,67]. The size of the graft particles varies from 200 to 1000 μm [37,39,40,66].

These studies evaluated the efficacy of this biomaterial in the clinical, radiologic, histologic and morphometric scenario.

4.2.1. Clinical Outcomes

Overall, grafted sites healed without any clinical manifestation of infection, wound dehiscence, or implant failure, in the cases where dental implants were placed [17,44,50]. In these studies, the primary stabilization ranged from 71.8 to 74 implant stability quotient (ISQ) [37,39,49].

Several intervention studies performed an interesting evaluation comparing the clinical, radiologic and histologic efficacy between DDM and a standard xenograft (Bio-Oss (Geistlich Pharma AG, Wolhusen, Switzerland) with excellent and proven efficacy [17,39,40]. Both groups, showed comparable healing process, implant stability and bone formation ration, proving that this biomaterial can be a viable alternative to the xenograft, with the advantage of being autogenous [17,39,40]. Furthermore, from the patient's perspective, autogenous teeth were associated with low levels of pain and swelling [17].

4.2.2. Radiologic Outcomes

Regarding radiologic outcomes, the studies presented favorable results. The mean density of the graft decreased with time, with the architecture of the DDM becoming increasingly more similar to that of the surrounding bone, suggesting a satisfactory bone healing [40,50,67].

4.2.3. Histologic and Histomorphometric Outcomes

Histologic and histomorphometric analysis showed a good tissue integration with a direct union between the new bone and the graft material, evidencing osteoconductive and osteoinductive properties [39,66]. It was reported a dense lamellar bone formation [48–50] associated with connective tissue reach in angiogenesis [37], fulfilling the goal of minimizing the alveolar bone loss in extraction sockets [44]. The follow-up period on which these results were found varied from 3.5 to 6 months [39,44,48,66].

The most important limitations when comparing these studies are the variety of protocols and adjuvant materials used, for instance absorbable [44,50] or non-absorbable membranes [67], or the use of platelet-rich fibrin (PRF) [40].

5. Partially Demineralized Dentin Matrix (PDDM)

Regarding PDDM, only two interventional studies have studied its clinical potential for ARP, one pilot on PDDM associated with platelet-rich plasma [36], and another randomized trial concerning PDDM alone [41].

In terms of protocol for dentin processing, both studies present slight changes. In both studies, the soft tissues, caries and calculus were removed with the teeth being crushed with the auxiliary of different grinders, who generated graft particles varying between 300 and 800 μm [36,41]. The main difference in terms of protocol is the agent used for partial demineralization. On the one side, Minamizato et al. used a 2% HNO_3 solution (pH 1.0) for 10 min, followed by an extensive 10 min rinse with 0.1 M Tris-HCl (pH 7.4) [36]. On the other side, Joshi et al. used lactic acid (1N) for a 15–20 min period and later a sterile normal saline solution [41]. The reason behind the choice of an organic acid was, according to Joshi et al., the contact between the residues with human tissues [41].

5.1. Clinical Outcomes

Clinically speaking, the postoperative follow-up occurred uneventfully [36,41]. In the Minamizato trial, dental implants were placed at 4–6 months postoperative with primary stability and insertion torque varying from 25 to 40 N cm [36]. At the time of the second surgery, the implant stability quotient (ISQ) was over 60 in all cases, suggesting a positive osteointegration [36]. One factor that could help the healing process is the demineralization the occurred, enhancing the antimicrobial activity of some dentin components [36]. In the Joshi Trial, although no implants were placed, after a period of 4 months, the authors reported that the sockets grafted with PDDM showed visually less width shrinkage when compared with the sites grafted with β-TCP and non-grafted sites [41].

5.2. Radiologic Outcomes

Radiographic assessment was made by X-ray panoramic and cone beam computed tomography (CBCT). This analysis showed that the radiopacity of the PDDM decreased gradually with the lamina dura around the graft becoming progressively indistinguishable [36]. Comparing the dimensional changes of the alveolar ridge between PDDM and β-TCP, the width and height loss was lower in the PDDM group, with these values being statistically significant [41]. In terms of ridge height, while in the PDDM group there was a reduction of 0.28 ± 0.13 mm, in the β-TCP group there was a reduction of 1.72 ± 0.56 mm and in the control group it was reported a reduction of 2.60 ± 0.88 mm ($p < 0.05$) [41]. In terms of width, a similar result was achieved, with the control group showing an increased reduction (2.29 ± 0.40 mm), followed by the β-TCP group (1.45 ± 0.40 mm) and finally the PDDM group (0.15 ± 0.08 mm) ($p < 0.05$) [41].

5.3. Histologic Outcomes

Finally, histologic analysis showed a positive integration of the PDDM at 4 to 6 months postoperative. Histologic specimens of the PDDM group showed newly formed bone in both studies [36,41], with a higher percentage of osteoid formation, when comparing to the β-TCP group [41].

These two studies point out the use of PDDM as a viable option in alveolar ridge regeneration, displaying good clinical, radiologic and histologic outcomes.

6. Undemineralized Dentin Matrix (UDD)

In terms of UDD, a solid number of preclinical and clinical studies have been performed evaluating its efficacy [38,51–57,68].

6.1. Preclinical Studies

The protocol used for the preparation of this biomaterial was very similar in all of the preclinical studies. The crown portion of the tooth was removed, as well as pulp tissues and periodontal ligament still attached [52,53,68]. This was made by using curettes, ultrasonic devices, hand instruments and specific burs [52,53,68]. In all studies, the preparation was rinsed with a saline solution along with a basic alcohol cleanser [52,53,68]. Finally, either using the Smart Dentin Grinder™ (Kometa Bio ltd., Holon, Israel) [52,53] or a specific grinder [68], the teeth were grinded into particles with diameters over 300 μm and less than 1200 μm [52,53], or between 350 and 500 μm [68].

Histologic and Histomorphometric Outcomes

After assessing the viability of UDD under radiologic, histologic and histomorphometry analysis, some preclinical studies reached opposite conclusions. In 2015, one study, after histologic and histomorphometry analysis, reported that the use of UDD, after 8 weeks did not offered any improvement in bone regeneration, showing in terms of ratio of bone to total area of each probe 170 ± 16 μm^3 for the control group (no bone graft material used) and 71 ± 14 μm^3 for the UDD group, with a significant difference ($p < 0.05$) [68].

The opposite was concluded in two other preclinical studies [52,53]. When compared to a healing without any bone graft material, after a 90 days observation period, the added benefit of the UDD was proven [52,53]. In one study, the percentage of newly bone formation was $91.32 \pm 0.8\%$ in the UDD group and $65.89 \pm 0.6\%$ in the control group ($p < 0.05$) [52]. In the other study, the percentage of immature bone was $14.2 \pm 0.66\%$ in the UDD group and $35.17 \pm 0.74\%$ in the control group ($p < 0.05$) [53].

6.2. Clinical Studies

Equivalently to the studies mentioned before, these clinical studies applied a similar protocol when preparing UDD. Generally speaking, after the teeth extraction, removal of crowns, fillings of any nature, pulp tissues and periodontal ligament, the biomaterial was grinded in order to generate particles with a diameter varying from 300 to 1200 μm [38,51,54–57,59]. In most of the studies, a basic alcohol cleanser consisting of 0.5 M of NaOH and 30%/20% alcohol as well as a sterile phosphate buffered saline were applied to the samples gathered [38,55,56]. This step is important in order to remove organic debris and also possible bacteria and toxins found in dentine [38,55,56].

When assessing the efficacy of the UDD in these studies, one aspect that is worthy of mention is that in some studies a combination of UDD was used either with platelet-rich fibrin [54] or with leukocyte-platelet-rich fibrin and fibrinogen [57], which can be seen as a drawback when analyzing this biomaterial due to lack of standardization as well as understanding the real influence of the UDD.

6.2.1. Clinical Outcomes

Clinically, the healing process was satisfactory, with no major post-operative complications, with less inflammation and rejection response, one potential limitation of other types of bone grafts [38,57].

One particular split-mouth randomized double-blind study deviated from the usual analysis of this subject. This study used UDD from lower third molar extractions and evaluated clinical outcomes such as: pocket depth, recession, clinical attachment level regarding the lower second molar, as well as patient-related outcomes: pain, healing and swelling [51]. After a 3-month observation period, in terms of pocket depth (control group: 3.43 ± 0.79, UDD group: 2.86 ± 0.9), gingival recession (control group: -2.29 ± 1.25, UDD group: -2.86 ± 0.9) and clinical attachment level (control group: 1.14 ± 1.57, UDD group: 0 ± 0), the differences found were not statistically significant ($p > 0.05$) [51]. Finally, regarding patient-related outcomes (pain, healing and swelling), similar results were found, with no statistically significant differences found between groups ($p > 0.05$) [51]. A similar result was found in a split-mouth clinical trial where the use of the lower third molar as a bone substitute resulted in a significant reduction of the pocket depth, mainly in the first 3 months [59]. After a 6-month-period, the bone density found in the test group was greater, with statistically significant difference ($p < 0.001$) [59].

6.2.2. Radiologic Outcomes

Radiologically, CBCT images showed that alveolar ridge dimensions were preserved in most cases [54,55,57]. In the study by Andrade et al. the vertical and horizontal dimensions of the sockets grafted were preserved, and in some cases increased [57]. One particular study by Pohl et al. performed a retrospective radiographic cone-beam computed tomography in order to better assess the efficacy of this graft in terms of volume stability [54]. Comparing the preoperative and the postoperative (4 months after ARP procedure) dimensions, the reduction in the buccal bone plate thickness at 1 mm, 3 mm and 5 mm bellow the buccal crest was, respectively: -0.87 ± 0.84 mm; -0.60 ± 0.70 mm and -0.41 ± 0.55 mm [54]. Following the same level measurements, the mean ridge width changes were, respectively: 1.38 ± 1.24 mm, 0.82 ± 1.13 mm, and 0.43 ± 0.89 mm [54]. Finally, the authors concluded that the average mid-buccal bone height gain was 1.1% and the mid-lingual height gain was 5.6% [54]. Another study that evaluated through CBCT analysis the alveolar ridge dimensions before and 4 months after the ARP procedure reported a loss of 0.76 mm in the vertical dimension and a loss of 1.1 mm in the horizontal dimension [69].

6.2.3. Histologic and Histomorphometry Outcomes

Regarding histologic and histomorphometry analyses, UDD generated moderate osteoblastic activity, presenting some dentin fragments as well as connective tissue, suggesting a gradual increase in the graft resorption and consequently bone formation [54,56,57]. Additionally, Andrade et al. reported a consecutive increase of the bone percentage (26.3% at 4 months and 66.5% at 6 months), and a decrease on dentin (10.4% at 4 months and 0.9% at 6 months) and connective tissue (63.3% at 4 months and 32.6% at 6 months) in the socket, substantiating a gradual bone formation along with graft resorption [57].

7. Conclusions

Autogenous teeth as a biomaterial for ARP present osteoconductive and osteoinductive properties, which suggests that they can be an equally effective bone substitute. In some cases, autogenous teeth have superior clinical performance when compared with other grafts. According to this literature review, autogenous teeth, in every form of processing, present potential within the clinical, radiologic and histologic outcomes.

Nonetheless, further research, with standardized protocols in terms of patient selection, dentin processing, surgery procedure and comparison with other grafts are essential in order to reach a definitive conclusion about this graft efficacy. Particularly, there is a scarcity of studies comparing the different dentin processing protocols with each other, though the difference between each method may only rely on the advantages and fallouts of the method itself (demineralization vs. non-demineralization) and not in the clinical potential per se.

Author Contributions: Conceptualization, J.C., J.B., and A.S.; validation, A.S.; writing—original draft preparation, J.C., J.B., V.M., and A.S.; writing—review and editing, J.C., J.B., V.M., J.J.M., P.M., G.A. and A.S. All authors have read and agreed to the published version of the manuscript.

Funding: This research received no external funding.

Institutional Review Board Statement: Not applicable.

Informed Consent Statement: Not applicable.

Conflicts of Interest: The authors declare no conflict of interest.

References

1. Avila-Ortiz, G.; Elangovan, S.; Kramer, K.W.O.; Blanchette, D.; Dawson, D.V. Effect of alveolar ridge preservation after tooth extraction: A systematic review and meta-analysis. *J. Dent. Res.* **2014**, *93*, 950–958. [CrossRef]
2. Ten Heggeler, J.M.A.G.; Slot, D.E.; Van Der Weijden, G.A. Effect of socket preservation therapies following tooth extraction in non-molar regions in humans: A systematic review. *Clin. Oral Implants Res.* **2011**, *22*, 779–788. [CrossRef]

3. Avila-Ortiz, G.; Chambrone, L.; Vignoletti, F. Effect of alveolar ridge preservation interventions following tooth extraction: A systematic review and meta-analysis. *J. Clin. Periodontol.* **2019**, *46*, 195–223. [CrossRef]
4. Jambhekar, S.; Kernen, F.; Bidra, A.S. Clinical and histologic outcomes of socket grafting after flapless tooth extraction: A systematic review of randomized controlled clinical trials. *J. Prosthet. Dent.* **2015**, *113*, 371–382. [CrossRef]
5. Tan, W.L.; Wong, T.L.T.; Wong, M.C.M.; Lang, N.P. A systematic review of post-extractional alveolar hard and soft tissue dimensional changes in humans. *Clin. Oral Implants Res.* **2012**, *23*, 1–21. [CrossRef]
6. Troiano, G.; Zhurakivska, K.; Lo Muzio, L.; Laino, L.; Cicciù, M.; Lo Russo, L. Combination of Bone Graft and Resorbable Membrane for Alveolar Ridge Preservation: A Systematic Review, Meta-analysis and Trial Sequential Analysis. *J. Periodontol.* **2017**, *89*, 46–57. [CrossRef]
7. Van Der Weijden, F.; Dell'Acqua, F.; Slot, D.E. Alveolar bone dimensional changes of post-extraction sockets in humans: A systematic review. *J. Clin. Periodontol.* **2009**, *36*, 1048–1058. [CrossRef] [PubMed]
8. Vignoletti, F.; Matesanz, P.; Rodrigo, D.; Figuero, E.; Martin, C.; Sanz, M. Surgical protocols for ridge preservation after tooth extraction: A systematic review. *Clin. Oral Implants Res.* **2012**, *23*, 22–38. [CrossRef] [PubMed]
9. Ramanauskaite, A.; Sahin, D.; Sader, R.; Becker, J.; Schwarz, F. Efficacy of autogenous teeth for the reconstruction of alveolar ridge deficiencies: A systematic review. *Clin. Oral Investig.* **2019**, *23*, 4263–4287. [CrossRef] [PubMed]
10. Bassir, S.; Alhareky, M.; Wangsrimongkol, B.; Jia, Y.; Karimbux, N. Systematic Review and Meta-Analysis of Hard Tissue Outcomes of Alveolar Ridge Preservation. *Int. J. Oral Maxillofac. Implants* **2018**, *33*, 979–994. [CrossRef] [PubMed]
11. Stumbras, A.; Kuliesius, P.; Januzis, G.; Juodzbalys, G. Alveolar Ridge Preservation after Tooth Extraction Using Different Bone Graft Materials and Autologous Platelet Concentrates: A Systematic Review. *J. Oral Maxillofac. Res.* **2019**, *10*, 1–15. [CrossRef]
12. Gual-Vaqués, P.; Polis-Yanes, C.; Estrugo-Devesa, A.; Ayuso-Montero, R.; Marí-Roig, A.; López-López, J. Autogenous teeth used for bone grafting: A systematic review. *Med. Oral Patol. Oral Cir. Bucal* **2018**, *23*, e112–e119. [CrossRef] [PubMed]
13. Albrektsson, T.; Johansson, C. Osteoinduction, osteoconduction and osseointegration. *Eur. Spine J.* **2001**, *10*, S96–S101. [CrossRef] [PubMed]
14. Tabatabaei, F.S.; Tatari, S.; Samadi, R.; Moharamzadeh, K. Different methods of dentin processing for application in bone tissue engineering: A systematic review. *J. Biomed. Mat. Res. Part A* **2016**, *104*, 2616–2627. [CrossRef] [PubMed]
15. Kim, Y.-K. Bone graft material using teeth. *J. Korean Assoc. Oral Maxillofac. Surg.* **2012**, *38*, 134–138. [CrossRef]
16. Kim, Y.-K.; Lee, J.; Um, I.-W.; Kim, K.-W.; Murata, M.; Akazawa, T.; Mitsugi, M. Tooth-derived bone graft material. *J. Korean Assoc. Oral Maxillofac. Surg.* **2013**, *39*, 103. [CrossRef] [PubMed]
17. Wu, D.; Zhou, L.; Lin, J.; Chen, J.; Huang, W.; Chen, Y. Immediate implant placement in anterior teeth with grafting material of autogenous tooth bone vs xenogenic bone. *BMC Oral Health* **2019**, *19*, 1–11. [CrossRef] [PubMed]
18. Barone, A.; Borgia, V.; Covani, U.; Ricci, M.; Piattelli, A.; Iezzi, G. Flap versus flapless procedure for ridge preservation in alveolar extraction sockets: A histological evaluation in a randomized clinical trial. *Clin. Oral Implants Res.* **2015**, *26*, 806–813. [CrossRef]
19. Barallat, L.; Ruíz-Magaz, V.; Levi, P.A.; Mareque-Bueno, S.; Galindo-Moreno, P.; Nart, J. Histomorphometric results in ridge preservation cases comparing various graft materials in extraction sockets with nongrafted sockets in humans: A systematic review. *Implant Dent.* **2014**, *23*, 539–554. [CrossRef]
20. De Risi, V.; Clementini, M.; Vittorini, G.; Mannocci, A.; De Sanctis, M. Alveolar ridge preservation techniques: A systematic review and meta-analysis of histological and histomorphometrical data. *Clin. Oral Implants Res.* **2015**, *26*, 50–68. [CrossRef]
21. Vittorini Orgeas, G.; Clementini, M.; De Risi, V.; De Sanctis, M. Surgical Techniques for Alveolar Socket Preservation: A Systematic Review. *Int. J. Oral Maxillofac. Implants* **2013**, *28*, 1049–1061. [CrossRef]
22. Horváth, A.; Mardas, N.; Mezzomo, L.A.; Needleman, I.G.; Donos, N. Alveolar ridge preservation. A systematic review. *Clin. Oral Investig.* **2013**, *17*, 341–363. [CrossRef]
23. Chan, H.-L.; Lin, G.-H.; Fu, J.-H.; Wang, H.-L. Alterations in Bone Quality After Socket Preservation with Grafting Materials: A Systematic Review. *Int. J. Oral Maxillofac. Implants* **2013**, *28*, 710–720. [CrossRef] [PubMed]
24. Hürzeler, M.B.; Zuhr, O.; Schupbach, P.; Rebele, S.F.; Emmanouilidis, N.; Fickl, S. The socket-shield technique: A proof-of-principle report. *J. Clin. Periodontol.* **2010**, *37*, 855–862. [CrossRef] [PubMed]
25. Mourya, A.; Mishra, S.K.; Gaddale, R.; Chowdhary, R. Socket-shield technique for implant placement to stabilize the facial gingival and osseous architecture: A systematic review. *J. Investig. Clin. Dent.* **2019**, *10*, e12449. [CrossRef]
26. Gharpure, A.S.; Bhatavadekar, N.B. Current evidence on the socket-shield technique: A systematic review. *J. Oral Implantol.* **2017**, *43*, 395–403. [CrossRef]
27. Yeomans, J.D.; Urist, M.R. Bone Induction by Decalcified Dentine Implanted into Oral, Osseous and Muscle Tissues. *Arch. Oral Biol.* **1967**, *12*, 999–1008. [CrossRef]
28. Bang, G.; Urist, M.R. Bone Induction in Excavation Chambers in Matrix of Decalcified Dentin. *Arch. Surg* **1967**, *94*, 781–789. [CrossRef]
29. Kim, Y.-K.; Lee, J.K.; Kim, K.-W.; Um, I.-W.; Murata, M. *Healing Mechanism and Clinical Application of Autogenous Tooth Bone Graft Material*; Pignatello, R., Ed.; IntechOpen: London, UK, 2013; Volume 395, ISBN 978-953-51-1051-4.
30. Kim, Y.-K.; Kim, S.G.; Oh, J.S.; Jin, S.C.; Son, J.S.; Kim, S.Y.; Lim, S.Y. Analysis of the inorganic component of autogenous tooth bone graft material. *J. Nanosci. Nanotechnol.* **2011**, *11*, 7442–7445. [CrossRef] [PubMed]
31. Kim, Y.K.; Kim, S.G.; Bae, J.H.; Um, I.W.; Oh, J.S.; Jeong, K.I. Guided bone regeneration using autogenous tooth bone graft in implant therapy: Case series. *Implant Dent.* **2014**, *23*, 138–143. [CrossRef]

32. Bessho, K.; Tanaka, N.; Matsumoto, J.; Tagawa, T.; Murata, M. Human Dentin-matrix-derived Bone Morphogenetic Protein. *J. Dent. Res.* **1991**, *70*, 171–175. [CrossRef]
33. Boden, S.D.; Liu, Y.; Hair, G.A.; Helms, J.A.; Hu, D.; Racine, M.; Nanes, M.S.; Titus, L. LMP-1, A LIM-Domain Protein, Mediates BMP-6 Effects on Bone Formation. *Endocrinology* **1998**, *139*, 5125–5134. [CrossRef]
34. Um, I.W. Demineralized Dentin Matrix (DDM) As a Carrier for Recombinant Human Bone Morphogenetic Proteins (rhBMP-2). In *Advances in Experimental Medicine and Biology*; Springer: Berlin, Germany, 2018; Volume 1077, pp. 487–499. ISBN 9789811309472.
35. Um, I.-W.; Young-Kyun Kim, Y.-K.; Mitsugi, M. Demineralized dentin matrix scaffolds for alveolar bone engineering. *J. Indian Prosthodont. Soc.* **2017**, *17*, 120–127. [CrossRef]
36. Minamizato, T.; Koga, T.; Takashi, I.; Nakatani, Y.; Umebayashi, M.; Sumita, Y.; Ikeda, T.; Asahina, I. Clinical application of autogenous partially demineralized dentin matrix prepared immediately after extraction for alveolar bone regeneration in implant dentistry: A pilot study. *Int. J. Oral Maxillofac. Surg.* **2017**, *47*, 125–132. [CrossRef]
37. Kim, S.Y.; Kim, Y.K.; Park, Y.H.; Park, J.C.; Ku, J.K.; Um, I.W.; Kim, J.Y. Evaluation of the healing potential of demineralized dentin matrix fixed with recombinant human bone morphogenetic protein-2 in bone grafts. *Materials* **2017**, *10*, 49. [CrossRef] [PubMed]
38. Binderman, I.; Hallel, G.; Nardy, C.; Yaffe, A.; Sapoznikov, L. A Novel Procedure to Process Extracted Teeth for Immediate Grafting of Autogenous Dentin. *JBR J. Interdiscip. Med. Dent. Sci.* **2014**, *2*, 2–6. [CrossRef]
39. Pang, K.-M.; Um, I.-W.; Kim, Y.-K.; Woo, J.-M.; Kim, S.-M.; Lee, J.-H. Autogenous demineralized dentin matrix from extracted tooth for the augmentation of alveolar bone defect: A prospective randomized clinical trial in comparison with anorganic bovine bone. *Clin. Oral Implants Res.* **2016**, *28*, 809–815. [CrossRef]
40. Li, P.; Zhu, H.C.; Huang, D.H. Autogenous DDM versus Bio-Oss granules in GBR for immediate implantation in periodontal postextraction sites: A prospective clinical study. *Clin. Implant Dent. Relat. Res.* **2018**, *20*, 923–928. [CrossRef]
41. Joshi, C.P.; Dani, N.H.; Khedkar, S.U. Alveolar ridge preservation using autogenous tooth graft versus beta-tricalcium phosphate alloplast: A randomized, controlled, prospective, clinical pilot study. *J. Indian Soc. Periodontol.* **2016**, *20*, 429–434. [CrossRef] [PubMed]
42. Huang, B.; Sun, Y.; MacIejewska, I.; Qin, D.; Peng, T.; McIntyre, B.; Wygant, J.; Butler, W.T.; Qin, C. Distribution of SIBLING proteins in the organic and inorganic phases of rat dentin and bone. *Eur. J. Oral Sci.* **2008**, *116*, 104–112. [CrossRef]
43. Park, M.; Mah, Y.J.; Kim, D.H.; Kim, E.S.; Park, E.J. Demineralized deciduous tooth as a source of bone graft material: Its biological and physicochemical characteristics. *Oral Surg. Oral Med. Oral Pathol. Oral Radiol.* **2015**, *120*, 307–314. [CrossRef]
44. Minetti, E.; Giacometti, E.; Gambardella, U.; Contessi, M.; Ballini, A.; Marenzi, G.; Celko, M.; Mastrangelo, F. Alveolar socket preservation with different autologous graft materials: Preliminary results of a multicenter pilot study in human. *Materials* **2020**, *13*, 1153. [CrossRef] [PubMed]
45. Reis-Filho, C.R.; Silva, E.R.; Martins, A.B.; Pessoa, F.F.; Gomes, P.V.N.; De Araújo, M.S.C.; Miziara, M.N.; Alves, J.B. Demineralised human dentine matrix stimulates the expression of VEGF and accelerates the bone repair in tooth sockets of rats. *Arch. Oral Biol.* **2012**, *57*, 469–476. [CrossRef]
46. De Oliveira, G.S.; Miziara, M.N.; Silva, E.R.D.; Ferreira, E.L.; Biulchi, A.P.F.; Alves, J.B. Enhanced bone formation during healing process of tooth sockets filled with demineralized human dentine matrix. *Aust. Dent. J.* **2013**, *58*, 326–332. [CrossRef]
47. Gharpure, A.S.; Bhatavadekar, N.B. Clinical efficacy of tooth-bone graft: A systematic review and risk of bias analysis of randomized control trials and observational studies. *Implant Dent.* **2017**, *26*, 119–134. [CrossRef] [PubMed]
48. Chung, J.-H.; Lee, J.-H. Study of bone healing pattern in extraction socket after application of demineralized dentin matrix material. *J. Korean Assoc. Oral Maxillofac. Surg.* **2011**, *37*, 365–374. [CrossRef]
49. Park, S.-M.; Um, I.-W.; Kim, Y.-K.; Kim, K.-W. Clinical application of auto-tooth bone graft material. *J. Korean Assoc. Oral Maxillofac. Surg.* **2012**, *38*, 1–8. [CrossRef]
50. Kim, E.-S. Autogenous fresh demineralized tooth graft prepared at chairside for dental implant. *Maxillofac. Plast. Reconstr. Surg.* **2015**, *37*, 4–9. [CrossRef]
51. Nadershah, M.; Zahid, T.M. Use of Autogenous Dentin Graft in Mandibular Third Molar Extraction Sockets: A Split-Mouth Randomized Double-Blind Study. *Int. J. Pharm. Res. Allied Sci.* **2019**, *8*, 73–79.
52. Calvo-Guirado, J.L.; Cegarra Del Pino, P.; Sapoznikov, L.; Delgado Ruiz, R.A.; Fernández-Domínguez, M.; Gehrke, S.A. A new procedure for processing extracted teeth for immediate grafting in post-extraction sockets. An experimental study in American Fox Hound dogs. *Ann. Anat.* **2018**, *217*, 14–23. [CrossRef]
53. Calvo-Guirado, J.L.; Maté-Sánchez De Val, J.E.; Ramos-Oltra, M.L.; Martínez, C.P.A.; Ramírez-Fernández, M.P.; Maiquez-Gosálvez, M.; Gehrke, S.A.; Fernández-Domínguez, M.; Romanos, G.E.; Delgado-Ruiz, R.A. The use of tooth particles as a biomaterial in post-extraction sockets. Experimental study in dogs. *Dent. J.* **2018**, *6*, 12. [CrossRef]
54. Pohl, S.; Binderman, I.; Tomac, J. Maintenance of alveolar ridge dimensions utilizing an extracted tooth dentin particulate autograft and platelet-rich fibrin: A retrospective radiographic cone-beam computed tomography study. *Materials* **2020**, *13*, 1083. [CrossRef]
55. Dwivedi, A.; Kour, M. A neoteric procedure for alveolar ridge preservation using autogenous fresh mineralized tooth graft prepared at chair side. *J. Oral Biol. Craniofac. Res.* **2020**, *10*, 535–541. [CrossRef]
56. Del Canto-Díaz, A.; De Elío-Oliveros, J.; Del Canto-Díaz, M.; Alobera-Gracia, M.A.; Del Canto-Pingarrón, M.; Martínez-González, J.M. Use of autologous tooth-derived graft material in the post-extraction dental socket. Pilot study. *Med. Oral Patol. Oral Cir. Bucal* **2019**, *24*, e53–e60. [CrossRef] [PubMed]

57. Andrade, C.; Camino, J.; Nally, M.; Quirynen, M.; Martínez, B.; Pinto, N. Combining autologous particulate dentin, L-PRF, and fibrinogen to create a matrix for predictable ridge preservation: A pilot clinical study. *Clin. Oral Investig.* **2019**, *24*, 1151–1160. [CrossRef] [PubMed]
58. Kim, Y.; Pang, K.; Yun, P.; Leem, D.; Um, I. Long-term follow-up of autogenous tooth bone graft blocks with dental implants. *Clin. Case Rep.* **2016**, *5*, 108–118. [CrossRef]
59. Sánchez-Labrador, L.; Martín-Ares, M.; Ortega-Aranegui, R.; López-Quiles, J.; Martínez-González, J.M. Autogenous dentin graft in bone defects after lower third molar extraction: A split-mouth clinical trial. *Materials* **2020**, *13*, 3090. [CrossRef] [PubMed]
60. Kim, Y.; System, B.; Kim, Y.; Um, I.; Murata, M. Clinical Report Tooth Bank System for Bone Regeneration-Safety Report. *J. Hard Tissue Biol.* **2014**, *23*, 371–376. [CrossRef]
61. Minetti, E.; Berardini, M.; Trisi, P. A New Tooth Processing Apparatus Allowing to Obtain Dentin Grafts for Bone Augmentation: The Tooth Transformer. *Open Dent. J.* **2019**, *13*, 6–14. [CrossRef]
62. Schwarz, F.; Hazar, D.; Becker, K.; Parvini, P.; Sader, R.; Becker, J. Short-term outcomes of staged lateral alveolar ridge augmentation using autogenous tooth roots. A prospective controlled clinical study. *J. Clin. Periodontol.* **2019**, *46*, 969–976. [CrossRef]
63. Reddy, G.V.; Abhinav, A.; Malgikar, S.; Bhagyashree, C.; Babu, P.R.; Reddy, G.J.; Sagar, S.V. Clinical and Radiographic Evaluation of Autogenous Dentin Graft and Demineralized Freeze-Dried Bone Allograft with Chorion Membrane in the Treatment of Grade II and III Furcation Defects: A Randomized Controlled Trial. *Indian J. Dent. Sci.* **2019**, *11*, 10–13. [CrossRef]
64. Jun, S.H.; Ahn, J.S.; Lee, J.I.; Ahn, K.J.; Yun, P.Y.; Kim, Y.K. A prospective study on the effectiveness of newly developed autogenous tooth bone graft material for sinus bone graft procedure. *J. Adv. Prosthodont.* **2014**, *6*, 528–538. [CrossRef]
65. Kim, Y.-K.; Jun, S.-H.; Um, I.-W.; Kim, S. Evaluation of the Healing Process of Autogenous Tooth Bone Graft Material Nine Months after Sinus Bone Graft: Micromorphometric and Histological Evaluation. *J. Korean Assoc. Maxillofac. Plast. Reconstr. Surg.* **2013**, *35*, 310–315. [CrossRef]
66. Kim, Y.K.; Kim, S.G.; Byeon, J.H.; Lee, H.J.; Um, I.U.; Lim, S.C.; Kim, S.Y. Development of a novel bone grafting material using autogenous teeth. *Oral Surg. Oral Med. Oral Pathol. Oral Radiol. Endodontol.* **2010**, *109*, 496–503. [CrossRef]
67. Gomes, M.F.; De Abreu, P.P.; Cantarelli Morosolli, A.R.; Araújo, M.M.; Vilela Goulart, M.D.G. Densitometric analysis of the autogenous demineralized dentin matrix on the dental socket wound healing process in humans. *Braz. Oral Res.* **2006**, *20*, 324–330. [CrossRef] [PubMed]
68. Kadkhodazadeh, M.; Ghasemianpour, M.; Soltanian, N.; Sultanian, G.R.; Ahmadpour, S.; Amid, R. Effects of fresh mineralized dentin and cementum on socket healing: A preliminary study in dogs. *J. Korean Assoc. Oral Maxillofac. Surg.* **2015**, *41*, 119–123. [CrossRef] [PubMed]
69. Valdec, S.; Pasic, P.; Soltermann, A.; Thoma, D.; Stadlinger, B.; Rücker, M. Alveolar ridge preservation with autologous particulated dentin—A case series. *Int. J. Implant Dent.* **2017**, *3*, 1–9. [CrossRef] [PubMed]

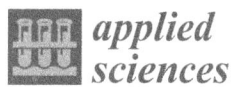

Article

Effect of Non-Thermal Atmospheric Pressure Plasma on Differentiation Potential of Human Deciduous Dental Pulp Fibroblast-like Cells

Masae Okuno, Sho Aoki, Saki Kawai, Rie Imataki, Yoko Abe, Kyoko Harada * and Kenji Arita

Department of Pediatric Dentistry, Osaka Dental University, 8-1 Kuzuha, Hanazono-cho, Hirakata, Osaka 573-1121, Japan; okuno-m@cc.osaka-dent.ac.jp (M.O.); sho-a@cc.osaka-dent.ac.jp (S.A.); sakky.925@gmail.com (S.K.); imataki-r@cc.osaka-dent.ac.jp (R.I.); abe-y@cc.osaka-dent.ac.jp (Y.A.); dent_ak@yahoo.co.jp (K.A.)
* Correspondence: kyoko-w@cc.osaka-dent.ac.jp; Tel.: +81-72-864-3085 or +81-72-864-3185

Abstract: Human mesenchymal stem cells can differentiate into various cell types and are useful for applications in regenerative medicine. Previous studies indicated that dental pulp exfoliated from deciduous teeth is a valuable alternative for dental tissue engineering because it contains stem cells with a relatively high proliferation rate. For clinical application, it is necessary to rapidly obtain a sufficient number of cells in vitro and maintain their undifferentiated state; however, the abundance of stem cells in the dental pulp tissue is limited. Non-thermal atmospheric pressure plasma (NTAPP) has been applied in regenerative medicine because it activates cell proliferation. Here, we examined the effects of NTAPP to activate the proliferation of human deciduous dental pulp fibroblast-like cells (hDDPFs) in vitro. Compared with untreated cells, NTAPP increased cell proliferation by 1.3-fold, significantly upregulated well-known pluripotent genes for stemness (e.g., *Oct4*, *Sox2*, and *Nanog*), and activated the expression of stem cell-specific surface markers (e.g., CD105). Overall, NTAPP activated the proliferation of various mesodermal-derived human adult stem cells while maintaining their pluripotency and stemness. In conclusion, NTAPP is a potential tool to expand the population of various adult stem cells in vitro for medical applications.

Keywords: non-thermal atmospheric pressure plasma (NTAPP); human deciduous dental pulp fibroblast-like cells; regenerative medicine

Citation: Okuno, M.; Aoki, S.; Kawai, S.; Imataki, R.; Abe, Y.; Harada, K.; Arita, K. Effect of Non-Thermal Atmospheric Pressure Plasma on Differentiation Potential of Human Deciduous Dental Pulp Fibroblast-like Cells. *Appl. Sci.* 2021, 11, 10119. https://doi.org/10.3390/app112110119

Academic Editors: Ricardo Castro Alves, José João Mendes and Ana Cristina Mano Azul

Received: 1 October 2021
Accepted: 26 October 2021
Published: 28 October 2021

Publisher's Note: MDPI stays neutral with regard to jurisdictional claims in published maps and institutional affiliations.

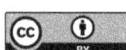

Copyright: © 2021 by the authors. Licensee MDPI, Basel, Switzerland. This article is an open access article distributed under the terms and conditions of the Creative Commons Attribution (CC BY) license (https://creativecommons.org/licenses/by/4.0/).

1. Introduction

Stem cells isolated from multiple tissues are used in regenerative medicine as they can differentiate into various tissues, including odontoblastic, chondrocytic, adipocytic, and osteoblastic cell lineages [1–4]. Previous in vivo studies demonstrated the differentiation of stem cells isolated from human dental pulp tissue into odontoblast-like cells lining the existing dentin surface [5] and the formation of a continuous layer of dentin-like tissue on the existing canal dentinal walls and mineral trioxide aggregate cement surfaces [6]. In addition, when stromal stem cells obtained from human dental pulp or bone fragments in vitro were transplanted into immunocompromised rats it resulted in the generation of a tissue structure with an integral blood supply similar to that of the human adult bone [7]. Stem cells from exfoliated human deciduous pulp show a higher proliferation rate than that of adult bone marrow stromal stem cells [8]. Similarly, fibroblast-like cells from exfoliated human deciduous dental pulp have a higher proliferation rate than that of those from permanent teeth [9]. Therefore, stem cells from exfoliated human deciduous pulp might be helpful in tissue regeneration, although those in the dental pulp tissue are present in minimal quantities. Some studies have reported that stem cells comprise 0.8% and 0.4% of human and mouse dental pulp, respectively [10,11]. Thus, it is necessary to proliferate cells and maintain the undifferentiated state of human dental pulp cells for clinical applications.

Various stimuli, such as drugs and incubation under hypoxia, have been used to activate pulp undifferentiation potential [12]; however, their use is currently limited because of safety and cost issues. Therefore, a safer and simpler alternative method is needed.

Recently, "plasma medicine", which involves the application of non-thermal atmospheric pressure plasma (NTAPP) for medical treatment, is a novel tool being applied in regenerative medicine. Plasma medicine aims at irradiating inorganic materials for surface modification or sterilization, whereas NTAPP combines irradiation at low temperatures and under atmospheric pressure, allowing the direct treatment of biological tissues for wound healing [13], selective apoptosis of cancer cells [14], and proliferation of pluripotent stem cells [15]. In the field of medical science, NTAPP has been studied worldwide for clinical applications. Although the information on the effects of direct plasma irradiation on the dental pulp and periapical soft tissues is limited, NTAPP is a simple, safe, and inexpensive tool that could be used in clinical dentistry.

In this study, we aimed to evaluate the effectiveness of NTAPP in activating the proliferation of undifferentiated human deciduous dental pulp fibroblast-like cells (hDDPFs). To this end, we examined the rate of cell multiplication in vitro, the expression of genes related to cell proliferation, and changes in mesenchymal stem cell (MSC) markers.

2. Materials and Methods

2.1. Cell Culture

Non-carious deciduous teeth (canine or molar) obtained from three healthy orthodontic patients at the pediatric dentistry in Osaka Dental University Hospital were kept in sterile 0.01 M phosphate-buffered saline (PBS; Wako Co., Ltd., Tokyo, Japan) and cut horizontally under sanitary conditions. The dental pulp tissue was gently removed, minced, and cultured in 35-mm tissue culture dishes, containing Dulbecco's modified Eagle medium (DMEM) supplemented with 10% fetal bovine serum (FBS; Wako, Tokyo, Japan), 100 U mL^{-1} penicillin (Life Technologies, Carlsbad, CA, USA), 100 μg mL^{-1} streptomycin (Life Technologies), and 4 mM L-glutamine (Life Technologies) at 37 °C in a humidified atmosphere of 5% CO_2. The culture medium was replaced with fresh medium every 3 days. hDDPFs isolated from the dental pulp tissues at passages 2–9 and expressed the markers CD105, CD44, and CD146 (data not shown) were used in this study. All experiments were approved by the Ethical Committee of Osaka Dental University (No. 111039). Informed consent was obtained from all study participants, and the study was conducted according to the principles of the Declaration of Helsinki.

2.2. NTAPP Stimulation Device

We used an argon-based NTAPP device in which the multi-gas plasma jet source has a columnar body similar to a pen and is connected to an AC power supply of 16 kHz and 9 kV and a gas cylinder (Plasma Concept Tokyo, Tokyo, Japan; Figure 1).

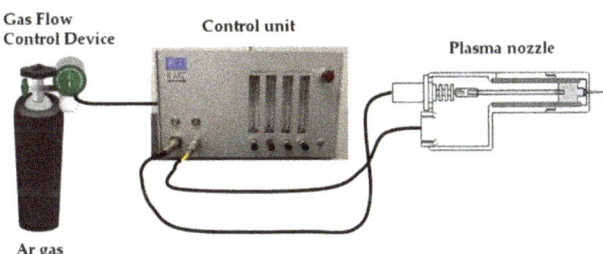

Figure 1. Argon-based non-thermal atmospheric pressure plasma (NTAPP) stimulation device used in this study. The multi-gas plasma jet source has a columnar body like a pen connected to an AC power supply of 16 kHz and 9 kV and a gas cylinder.

2.3. Cell Proliferation Assay

2.3.1. Investigation of NTAPP Irradiation Conditions

To investigate the effects of NTAPP, we first examined the cell proliferative potential after NTAPP irradiation. To expose cells to NTAPP, 1×10^4 cells seeded in 24-well culture plates were incubated for 96 h. The cells were exposed to the indicated doses of NTAPP (2.7 standard L/min, 20 V) for 10, 20, 30, and 40 s every hour, and the number of times was 1, 2, 3, and 4. The distance between the NTAPP stimulation device and cells was fixed to 2 cm, and 0.5 mL of medium was used. Then, the cells were further incubated for 72 h. After that, cell proliferation was evaluated using a Cell Titer96 Aqueous One Solution Cell Proliferation Assay kit (Promega, Madison, WI, USA), according to the manufacturer's instructions. Briefly, hDDPFs were cultured in 24-well plates at 1×10^4 cells per well for 96 h at 37 °C under a humidified atmosphere of 5% CO_2 and then treated with or without the indicated dose of NTAPP (2.7 standard L/min^{-1}, 20 V). The NTAPP-treated cells and non-treated cells (control) were further incubated for 72 h. Next, 3-(4,5-dimethylthiazol-2yl)-5-(3-carboxymethoxyphenyl)-2-(4-sulfophenyl)-2H-tetrazolium (MTS) and phenazine methosulfate were added to the cultures. Absorbances at 490 nm and 690 nm were measured using a Spectra Max5 microplate reader (Molecular Devices, Downingtown, PA, USA).

2.3.2. Effects of NTAPP on Culture Medium

Some studies have reported that NTAPP irradiation alters the culture medium and affects the cells [16,17]. Then, we wondered whether the cell proliferation induced by NTAPP was the direct effect of NTAPP, or the indirect outcome of the medium modified by NTAPP, or both.

To answer this question, we experimented with four groups. (Table 1) Groups 1 and 2 were not irradiated, whereas groups 3 and 4 were irradiated 3 times with NTAPP for 20 s. Immediately after irradiation, the cell culture media of groups 2 and 3 were exchanged. The cell proliferation was evaluated using the Cell Titer96 Aqueous One Solution Cell Proliferation Assay kit and the results were compared with the results of the earlier cell proliferation assay.

Table 1. Irradiation conditions for cells and culture medium.

Group	Cell	Medium
1	NTAPP(-)	NTAPP(-)
2	NTAPP(-)	NTAPP(+)
3	NTAPP(+)	NTAPP(-)
4	NTAPP(+)	NTAPP(+)

2.4. Reverse-Transcription Polymerase Chain Reaction (RT-PCR)

We examined the expression of *Oct4*, *Sox2*, and *Nanog* to determine whether hDDPFs irradiated with NTAPP 3 times for 20 s each time could maintain proliferative capacity and pluripotency. We also studied the expression of *Sox9*, a marker of pluripotency in undifferentiated neural crest cells, and that of *ALP*, a marker of pluripotency in undifferentiated osteoblasts. Complementary DNA (cDNA) was isolated from NTAPP-treated cells and non-treated cells after 72 h of incubation using a Cells-to-CT 1-Step TaqMan kit (Thermo-Fisher Scientific, Waltham, MA, USA), according to the manufacturer's instructions. RT-PCR was performed using a Step One Plus system (Thermo-Fisher Scientific) in a total volume of 20 µL, consisting of 5 µL Master Mix, 13 µL RNase-free water, 0.5 µL *Oct3/4* (Hs01654807_s1), *Sox2* (Hs01053049_s1), *Nanog* (Hs02387400_g1), *Sox9* (Hs00165814_m1), or *ALP* (Hs01029144_m1) primers, 0.5 µL glyceraldehyde-3-phosphate dehydrogenase (*GAPDH*; Hs02758991_g1) primers and 1 µL cDNA. In the TaqMan Gene Expression Assay (Life Technologies), the thermal conditions were as follows: 50 °C for 5 min, followed by

40 cycles at 95 °C for 20 s, 95 °C for 3 s, and 60 °C for 30 s. Gene expression in multiplex reactions was quantified using the comparative Ct method with normalization of the amount of the target (FAM) to endogenous GAPDH (VIC) expression. The relative expression levels were normalized to GAPDH expression.

2.5. Flow Cytometry

To detect stem cell-specific surface markers, NTAPP-treated cells and non-treated cells were detached with Accutase (Innovative Cell Technologies, San Diego, CA, USA), washed with FACS buffer (PBS, 1% FBS, 0.1% NaN_3 sodium azide), and centrifuged for 5 min at 1000 rpm and 4 °C. Cells were incubated with an optimal dilution of fluorescein-conjugated monoclonal antibodies (anti-CD44-allophycocyanin [APC], anti-CD105-fluorescein isothiocyanate [FITC], and anti-CD146-phycoerythrin [PE]; Biolegend, San Diego, CA, USA) for 1 h on ice. In total, 10,000 stained cells per assay were evaluated using BD FACSVerse (BD Biosciences, San Jose, CA, USA) and analyzed using FlowJo (BD Biosciences). To evaluate the fluorescence intensity, we measured the value of ΔMFI (the change of median fluorescence intensity). We compared the ΔMFIs of CD44, CD105, and CD146 in hDDPF treated with NTAPP.

2.6. Statistical Analysis

Data were expressed as means ± standard error of the mean (SE). Comparison among groups was performed with one-way ANOVA, followed by the Student-Newman–Keuls test. For comparisons between two groups with normally distributed data, two-tailed unpaired Student's t tests were used to determine statistical significance. Significance was set at a p-value of <0.05 (KaleidaGraph 4.00; SynergySoftware, Reading, PA, USA).

3. Results

3.1. Cell Proliferation Assay

3.1.1. Investigation of NTAPP Irradiation Conditions

We observed cell proliferation in hDDPFs treated 1–4 times with NATPP for 20 s compared with that in the non-treated group. When hDDPFs were irradiated with NTAPP 4 times, we observed cell detachment and irreversible disturbance of the proliferative capacity (Figure 2). Optimum NTAPP protocol (3 times with NTAPP for 20 s) was followed for all the following experiments.

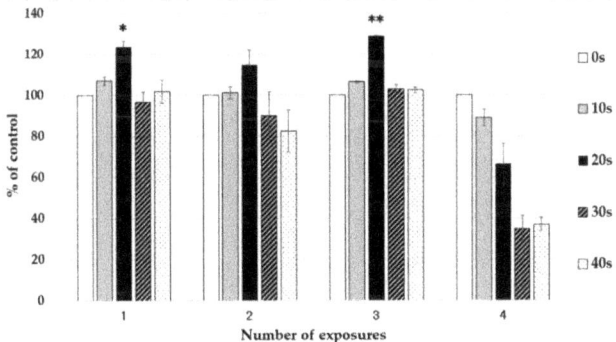

Figure 2. Direct effects of non-thermal atmospheric pressure plasma (NTAPP) on the proliferation of human deciduous dental pulp fibroblast-like cells (hDDPFs). These hDDPF (1×10^4 cells per well) were incubated for 96 h at 37 °C and 5% CO_2 in 24-well plates and then treated 1, 2, 3, or 4 times with NTAPP for 10, 20, 30, or 40 s per h. NTAPP-treated cells were incubated for 72 h at 37 °C and 5% CO_2. Cell proliferation was measured using the MTS assay. Data are presented as means ± SE (n = 4). Markers * and ** indicate significant differences at $p < 0.05$ and $p < 0.01$, respectively.

3.1.2. Effects on the Culture Medium

As shown in Figure 3, compared with the control (Group 1), in which neither cells nor culture medium were irradiated, a significant increase in the proliferative capacity of cells in Group 4 was confirmed, in which both cells and culture medium were irradiated.

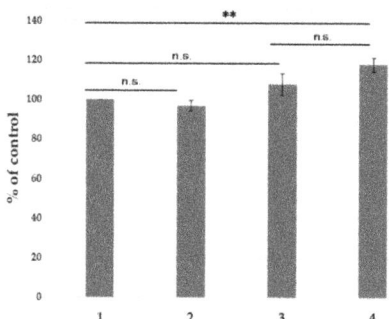

Figure 3. Effects of NTAPP on the culture medium. Group 4 (in which both cells and culture medium were NTAPP-irradiated) showed a significant increase in the proliferative capacity compared with the control (group 1) (in which neither cells nor culture medium was irradiated). Data are presented as means ± SE ($n = 4$). ** indicates significant differences at $p < 0.01$.

3.2. RT-PCR

The results showed NTAPP upregulated *Oct3/4*, *Sox2* and *Nanog* in hDDPFs (Figure 4).

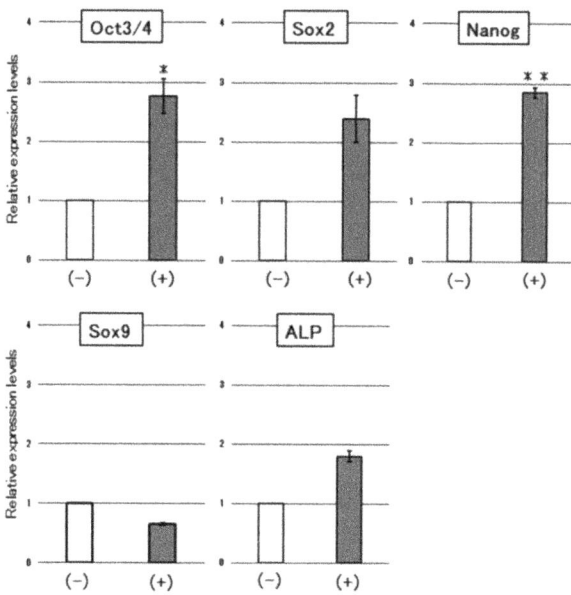

Figure 4. Effect of non-thermal atmospheric pressure plasma (NTAPP) on the expression of pluripotency markers (*Oct3/4*, *Sox2*, *Nanog*, *Sox9*, and *ALP*) in human deciduous dental pulp fibroblast-like cells (hDDPFs). (−) indicates the control group (non-NTAPP treated cells), and (+) indicates NTAPP-treated cells. Values were normalized using GAPDH as the internal control. Data are presented as means ± SE ($n = 5$). Data from five different experiments are shown. * and ** indicate significant differences at $p < 0.05$ and $p < 0.01$, respectively.

3.3. Flow Cytometry

The increased protein expression of stemness markers in NTAPP-treated hDDPFs was further confirmed using flow cytometry. We found that the ΔMFI of CD105 was significantly increased post-incubation for 72 h compared with that of non-treated cells, whereas no change was observed in CD44 and CD146 (Figure 5).

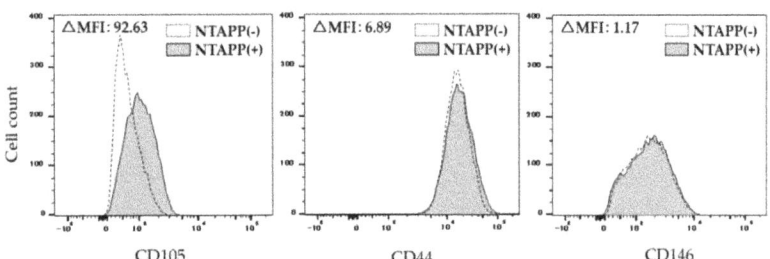

Figure 5. Effect of non-thermal atmospheric pressure plasma (NTAPP) on the expression of stem cell-specific markers (CD44, CD105, and CD146) in human deciduous dental pulp fibroblast-like cells (hDDPFs). ΔMFI (%), change in median fluorescence intensity.

4. Discussion

NTAPP is a partially ionized gas containing electrically charged particles and radicals at atmospheric pressure [18]. Previous studies reported that NTAPP exhibits various physiological effects beneficial for applications in regenerative medicine. It activates the proliferation of various mesoderm-derived adult stem cells, including human adipose tissue-derived stem cells, bone marrow-derived (BM)-MSCs, and hematopoietic stem cells, in vitro without affecting their stem-like properties [15,19].

In the present study, we investigated the effectiveness of NTAPP in activating the proliferation of cells from the deciduous dental pulp for potential use in regenerative dentistry. Our results showed that the cell proliferative capacity of cells treated 3 times with NTAPP for 20 s each time was approximately 1.2-fold higher than that of non-treated cells. In this study, the increased rate of cell proliferation was detected by MTS which is an indirect indicator. To confirm that proliferation (and not only metabolic activity) was increased by the NTAPP treatment, work should be carried out to directly compare cell numbers between the control group and the group treated with the optimum NTAPP protocol in future study. The optimal NTAPP conditions vary depending on plasma generator devices, the gas type used for plasma generation, and cell type. For instance, it has been reported that the proliferative potential of MSCs and hematopoietic stem cells is increased when treated with helium-based NTAPP 10 times for 50 s each time, in contrast to that of human synovial cells when treated with argon-based NTAPP for 60 s [19,20]. Here, the proliferative potential of hDDPFs decreased when treated >3 times with NTAPP for >20 s each time. Thus, the appropriate treatment conditions for each cell line need to be established before any clinical application.

In plasma medicine, NTAPP acts directly on cells and indirectly through the plasma-treated medium. For instance, NTAPP-activated media have anti-cancer effects on various human cancer cells [16], and He-based low-temperature atmospheric plasma jet-activated media have anti-bacterial properties [17,21]. Here, we found that cells cultured in NTAPP-treated medium had a higher proliferative capacity than those cultured in non-treated medium. Therefore, NTAPP enhanced cell proliferation both directly and indirectly by modifying the culture medium. Many oral periapical tissues contain large amounts of water. For instance, the dental pulp is a soft gelatinous tissue and water comprises 75–80% of its volume [22]. Therefore, it is essential to consider the effects of NTAPP on the cells and the surrounding fluid. Our findings showed the effectiveness of NTAPP in modifying the cell culture media, possibly expanding the applications of NTAPP using dental pulp.

Previous studies reported that *Oct4*, *Sox2*, and *Nanog* play essential roles in maintaining stem cell pluripotency and promoting cell proliferation in various adult stem cells [23–26]. To determine whether NTAPP treatment (3 times, 20 s each) could promote the proliferation of hDDPFs without affecting pluripotency, we examined the expression of *Oct4*, *Sox2*, and *Nanog*. We also studied the expression of *Sox9*, a marker of pluripotency of undifferentiated neural crest cells, and *ALP*, a marker of pluripotency of undifferentiated osteoblasts since hDDPFs are known to differentiate into chondrocytes and osteoblasts [27–29]. Our results showed that mRNA expression of *Oct3/4*, *Sox2* and *Nanog* was upregulated in NTAPP-treated cells.

A study on multipotent myoblasts has reported that the expression of *Sox9* increases after 3 to 5 days of incubation with material trioxide aggregate (MTA), which promotes hard tissue formation [30]. Therefore, in our experiments, confirming the expression of Sox9 in NTAPP-irradiated cells cultured for a longer period was necessary.

It has been reported that the MSC markers CD44, CD73, and CD90, as well as the stem cell markers CD105 and CD146, are expressed in dental pulp cells. Of these, CD105 is highly expressed in deciduous teeth [31]. In the present study, we studied CD44, CD105, and CD146 and found that they are all expressed in non-treated cells; however, only the expression of CD105 was increased after NTAPP treatment. It is known that MSCs from various human tissues and organs are adherent to plastic, have a fibroblastoid morphology, and are positive for CD73, CD90, and CD105 [32,33], but they vary in potency and self-renewal potential. Therefore, NTAPP treatment (3 times, 20 s each) is an effective tool that activates cell proliferation while maintaining and increasing MSC and stem cell markers in hDDPFs.

The multi-gas plasma jet source can generate atmospheric plasma of various gas species, including argon, oxygen, helium, nitrogen, air, and carbon dioxide, at low gas temperatures (<57 °C) [34]. Nevertheless, a study has reported that the effect of plasma depends on the type of gas, and different gases change the active species produced, thus changing the effectiveness and speed of the treatment. [35] For example, NTAPP using nitrogen and carbon dioxide is effective for hemostasis [36].

Helium and argon have been used in many plasma studies, but we preferred the latter because of the lower temperature, according to the manufacturer's instructions. We found that NTAPP based on argon gas was effective for promoting proliferation in hDDPFs; however, further research is necessary to examine other gas species and elucidate the complex biological effects of NTAPP on human stem cells.

5. Conclusions

Our study showed that argon-generated NTAPP activates the proliferative potential of hDDPFs both directly and indirectly through the culture medium. Furthermore, we revealed the possibility of enhancing the undifferentiated and proliferative cell potential, suggesting that NTAPP could be an effective tool in regenerative dentistry.

Author Contributions: K.H. and K.A. conceived and designed the experiments. M.O., S.A. and S.K. performed the experiments. R.I. and Y.A. analyzed the data, and M.O. and K.H. wrote the paper. All authors have read and agreed to the published version of the manuscript.

Funding: This work was supported by grants from Osaka Dental University Research Funds (21-12).

Institutional Review Board Statement: The study was conducted according to the Declaration of Helsinki, and approved by the Institutional Ethics Committee of Osaka Dental University (No.111039 date of approval: 29 July 2019).

Informed Consent Statement: Informed consent was obtained from all subjects involved in the study.

Data Availability Statement: Not applicable.

Acknowledgments: We are grateful to Hiroshi Inoue and Seiji Goda for their advice and assistance.

Conflicts of Interest: The authors declare no conflict of interest.

References

1. Prockop, D.J. Marrow stromal cells as stem cells for nonhematopoietic tissues. *Science* **1997**, *276*, 71–74. [CrossRef] [PubMed]
2. Yamashita, K.; Dennis, J.E.; Lennon, D.P.; Morimoto, H.; Kitamura, S.; Caplan, A.I. Dental pulp cells with multi-potential for differentiation to odontoblast and chondroblast. *J. Hard Tissue Biol.* **2003**, *12*, 49–55. [CrossRef]
3. Baghaban, E.M.; Vahabi, S.; Shariati, M.; Nazarian, H. In vitro growth and characterization of stem cells from human dental pulp of deciduous versus permanent teeth. *J. Dent. Res.* **2010**, *7*, 185–195.
4. Gronthos, S.; Mankani, M.; Brahim, J.; Robey, P.G.; Shi, S. Postnatal human dental pulp stem cells (DPSCs) in vitro and in vivo. *Proc. Natl. Acad. Sci. USA* **2000**, *97*, 13625–13630. [CrossRef]
5. Cordeiro, M.M.; Dong, Z.; Kaneko, T.; Zhang, Z.; Miyazawa, M.; Shi, S.; Smith, A.J.; Nör, J.E. Dental pulp tissue engineering with stem cells from exfoliated deciduous teeth. *J. Endod.* **2008**, *34*, 962–969. [CrossRef] [PubMed]
6. Huang, G.T.; Yamaza, T.; Shea, L.D.; Djouad, F.; Kuhn, N.Z.; Tuan, R.S.; Shi, S. Stem/progenitor cell–mediated de novo regeneration of dental pulp with newly deposited continuous layer of dentin in an in vivo model. *Tissue Eng. Part A* **2010**, *16*, 605–615. [CrossRef]
7. d'Aquino, R.; Graziano, A.; Sampaolesi, M.; Laino, G.; Pirozzi, G.; De Rosa, A.; Papaccio, G. Human postnatal dental pulp cells co-differentiate into osteoblasts and endotheliocytes: A pivotal synergy leading to adult bone tissue formation. *Cell Death Dis.* **2007**, *14*, 1162–1171. [CrossRef] [PubMed]
8. Miura, M.; Gronthos, S.; Zhao, M.; Lu, B.; Fisher, L.W.; Robey, P.G.; Shi, S. SHED: Stem cells from human exfoliated deciduous teeth. *Proc. Natl. Acad. Sci. USA* **2003**, *100*, 5807–5812. [CrossRef] [PubMed]
9. Nakamura, S.; Yamada, Y.; Katagiri, W.; Sugito, T.; Ito, K.; Ueda, M. Stem cell proliferation pathways comparison between human exfoliated deciduous teeth and dental pulp stem cells by gene expression profile from promising dental pulp. *J. Endod.* **2009**, *35*, 1536–1542. [CrossRef]
10. Honda, M.J.; Nakashima, F.; Satomura, K.; Shinohara, Y.; Tsuchiya, S.; Watanabe, N.; Ueda, M. Side population cells expressing $ABCG_2$ in human adult dental pulp tissue. *Int. Endod. J.* **2007**, *40*, 949–958. [CrossRef] [PubMed]
11. Kenmotsu, M.; Matsuzaka, K.; Kokubu, E.; Azuma, T.; Inoue, T. Analysis of side population cells derived from dental pulp tissue. *Int. Endod. J.* **2010**, *43*, 1132–1142. [CrossRef] [PubMed]
12. Kawai, S.; Harada, K.; Nagata, S.; Ohura, K.; Arita, K. Effect of 6-bromoindirubin-3′-oxime on human deciduous tooth dental pulp cells. *Jpn. Pharmacol. Ther.* **2012**, *31*, 87–95.
13. Shi, X.M.; Xu, G.M.; Zhang, G.J.; Liu, J.R.; Wu, Y.M.; Gao, L.G.; Yang, Y.; Chang, Z.S.; Yao, C.W. Low-temperature plasma promotes fibroblast proliferation in wound healing by ROS-activated NF-κB signaling pathway. *Curr. Med. Sci.* **2018**, *38*, 107–114. [CrossRef] [PubMed]
14. Chang, J.W.; Kang, S.U.; Shin, Y.S.; Kim, K.I.; Seo, S.J.; Yang, S.S.; Lee, J.S.; Moon, E.; Baek, S.J.; Lee, K.; et al. Non-thermal atmospheric pressure plasma induces apoptosis in oral cavity squamous cell carcinoma: Involvement of DNA-damage-triggering sub-G (1) arrest via the ATM/p53 pathway. *Arch. Biochem. Biophys.* **2014**, *545*, 133–140. [CrossRef] [PubMed]
15. Park, J.; Lee, H.; Lee, H.J.; Kim, G.C.; Kim, D.Y.; Han, S.; Song, K. Non-thermal atmospheric pressure plasma efficiently promotes the proliferation of adipose tissue-derived stem cells by activating NO-response pathways. *Sci. Rep.* **2016**, *6*, 39298. [CrossRef] [PubMed]
16. Kajiyama, H.; Utsumi, F.; Nakamura, K.; Tanaka, H.; Toyokuni, S.; Hori, M.; Kikkawa, F. Future perspective of strategic non-thermal plasma therapy for cancer treatment. *J. Clin. Biochem. Nutr.* **2017**, *60*, 33–38. [CrossRef] [PubMed]
17. Ikawa, S.; Kitano, K.; Hamaguchi, S. Effects of pH on bacterial inactivation in aqueous solutions due to low-temperature atmospheric pressure plasma application. *Plasma Process. Polym.* **2010**, *7*, 33–42. [CrossRef]
18. Hoffmann, C.; Berganza, C.; Zhang, J. Cold atmospheric plasma: Methods of production and application in dentistry and oncology. *Med. Gas Res.* **2013**, *3*, 21. [CrossRef]
19. Park, J.; Lee, H.; Lee, H.J.; Kim, G.C.; Kim, S.S.; Han, S.; Song, K. Non-thermal atmospheric pressure plasma is an excellent tool to activate proliferation in various mesoderm-derived human adult stem cells. *Free Radic. Biol. Med.* **2019**, *134*, 374–384. [CrossRef]
20. Hamaguchi, S. Interaction of plasmas with biological objectsin plasma medicine. *Plasma Fusion Res.* **2011**, *87*, 696–703.
21. Tasaki, T.; Ohshima, T.; Usui, E.; Ikawa, S.; Kitano, K.; Maeda, N.; Momoi, Y. Plasma-treated water eliminates Streptococcus mutans in infected dentin model. *Dent. Mater. J.* **2017**, *36*, 422–428. [CrossRef] [PubMed]
22. Yanagida, T.; Yamamoto, S.; Akisaka, T.; Sawada, T. *Tooth Development Tissue Lesion*, 1st ed.; Ishiyaku Publishers, Inc.: Tokyo, Japan, 1995; p. 92.
23. Shi, G.; Jin, Y. Role of Oct4 in maintaining and regaining stem cell pluripotency. *Stem Cell Res. Ther.* **2010**, *1*, 39. [CrossRef]
24. Tsai, C.C.; Hung, S.C. Functional roles of pluripotency transcription factors in mesenchymal stem cells. *Cell Cycle* **2012**, *11*, 3711–3712. [CrossRef] [PubMed]
25. Han, S.M.; Han, S.H.; Coh, Y.R.; Jang, G.; Ra, J.C.; Kang, S.K.; Lee, H.W.; Youn, H.Y. Enhanced proliferation and differentiation of Oct4-And Sox2-overexpressing human adipose tissue mesenchymal stem cells. *Exp. Mol. Med.* **2014**, *46*, e101. [CrossRef] [PubMed]
26. Sun, Z.; Han, Q.; Zhu, Y.S.; Li, Z.Y.; Chen, B.; Liao, L.M.; Bian, C.J.; Li, J.; Shao, C.S.; Zhao, R.C. NANOG has a role in mesenchymal stem cells' immunomodulatory effect. *Stem Cells Dev.* **2011**, *20*, 1521–1528. [CrossRef] [PubMed]

27. Fujita, N.; Takayasu, M.; Daito, M. In vitro chondrogenic differentiation potential of dental pulp stem cells. *Pediatric Dent. J.* **2008**, *46*, 548–554.
28. Mortada, I.; Mortada, R. Dental pulp stem cells and osteogenesis: An update. *Cytotechnology* **2018**, *70*, 1479–1486. [CrossRef]
29. Sato, R.; Namura, Y.; Tanabe, N.; Sakai, M.; Utsu, A.; Tomita, K.; Suzuki, N.; Motoyoshi, M. Atmospheric pressure plasma treatment with nitrogen induces osteoblast differentiation and reduces iNOS and COX-2 expressions. *J. Hard Tissue Biol.* **2021**, *30*, 131–136. [CrossRef]
30. Makoto, H. Biological effect of calcium ion released from mineral trioxide aggregate. *J. Jpn. Endod. Assoc.* **2019**, *40*, 1–6. [CrossRef]
31. Sato, M.; Ishida, C.; Iwasa, S.; Takei, H.; Honda, M.; Tetsuo Shirakawa, T. Characterization of cultured human mesenchymal stem cells from deciduous and permanent teeth. *Pediatr. Dent. J. Jpn.* **2014**, *52*, 417–424.
32. Beeravolu, N.; Khan, I.; McKee, C.; Dinda, S.; Thibodeau, B.; Wilson, G.; Perez-Cruet, M.; Bahado-Singh, R.; Chaudhry, G.R. Isolation and comparative analysis of potential stem/progenitor cells from different regions of human umbilical cord. *Stem Cell Res.* **2016**, *16*, 696–711. [CrossRef]
33. Beeravolu, N.; McKee, C.; Alamri, A.; Mikhael, S.; Brown, C.; Perez-Cruet, M.; Chaudhry, G.R. Isolation and characterization of mesenchymal stromal cells from human umbilical cord and fetal placenta. *J. Vis. Exp.* **2017**, *122*, e55224. [CrossRef] [PubMed]
34. Takamatsu, T.; Hirai, H.; Sasaki, R.; Miyahara, H.; Okino, A. Surface hydrophilization of polyimide films using atmospheric damage-free multigas plasma jet source. *IEEE Trans. Plasma Sci.* **2013**, *41*, 119–125. [CrossRef]
35. Takamatsu, T.; Uehara, K.; Sasaki, Y.; Miyahara, H.; Matsumura, Y.; Iwasawa, A.; Ito, N.; Azuma, T.; Kohno, M.; Okino, A. Investigation of reactive species using various gas plasmas. *RSC Adv.* **2014**, *4*, 39901–39905. [CrossRef]
36. Nomura, Y.; Takamatsu, T.; Kawano, H.; Miyahara, H.; Okino, A.; Yoshida, M.; Azuma, T. Investigation of blood coagulation effect of nonthermal multigas plasma jet in vitro and in vivo. *J. Surg. Res.* **2017**, *219*, 302–309. [CrossRef] [PubMed]

MDPI
St. Alban-Anlage 66
4052 Basel
Switzerland
www.mdpi.com

Applied Sciences Editorial Office
E-mail: applsci@mdpi.com
www.mdpi.com/journal/applsci

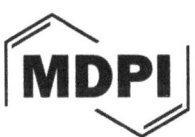

Disclaimer/Publisher's Note: The statements, opinions and data contained in all publications are solely those of the individual author(s) and contributor(s) and not of MDPI and/or the editor(s). MDPI and/or the editor(s) disclaim responsibility for any injury to people or property resulting from any ideas, methods, instructions or products referred to in the content.

www.ingramcontent.com/pod-product-compliance
Lightning Source LLC
LaVergne TN
LVHW070446100526
838202LV00014B/1679